DEDICATION

To Beth, Tina, and Pete, with love.

Anne-Marie Kiehne

To Bob.

Sue G. Thacker

STUDY GUIDE TO ACCOMPANY

Maternal-Child NURSING

SECOND EDITION

STUDY GUIDE TO ACCOMPANY

Maternal-Child NURSING

SECOND EDITION

Emily Slone McKinney, MSN, RN, C
Susan Rowen James, RN, PhD (c)
Sharon Smith Murray, MSN, RN, C
Jean Weiler Ashwill, MSN, RN

Prepared by

ANNE-MARIE KIEHNE, PhD, RN
College of Health Professions
Temple University
Philadelphia, Pennsylvania

SUE G. THACKER, RN, C, PhD
Professor of Nursing
Wytheville Community College
Wytheville, Virginia

ELSEVIER
SAUNDERS

ELSEVIER
SAUNDERS

11830 Westline Industrial Drive
St. Louis, Missouri 63146

STUDY GUIDE TO ACCOMPANY MATERNAL-CHILD NURSING, 2/E ISBN 1-4160-0255-3

Notice

Nursing is an ever-changing field. Standard safety precautions must be followed, but as new research and clinical experience broaden our knowledge, changes in treatment and drug therapy may become necessary or appropriate. Readers are advised to check the most current product information provided by the manufacturer of each drug to be administered to verify the recommended dose, the method and duration of administration, and contraindications. It is the responsibility of the licensed prescriber, relying on experience and knowledge of the patient, to determine dosages and the best treatment for each individual patient. Neither the publisher nor the editor assumes any liability for any injury and/or damage to persons or property arising from this publication.

Previous edition copyrighted 2000

International Standard Book Number 1-4160-0255-3

Executive Editors: Michael Ledbetter/Loren Wilson
Senior Developmental Editors: Lisa P. Newton/Nancy O'Brien
Publishing Services Manager: Catherine Jackson
Senior Project Manager: Celeste Clingan
Designer: Julia Dummitt

Printed in United States of America

Last digit is the print number: 9 8 7 6 5 4 3 2

Preface

The objective of this Study Guide to accompany Maternal-Child Nursing, second edition, is to facilitate your understanding of the vast amount of material presented in the textbook.

Organization

Each chapter in this Study Guide is meant to be used as a studying tool for its corresponding textbook chapter. Chapters are presented in the same numerical order as in the textbook. At the end of this manual, you will find answers to the learning exercises and Review Questions for all Study Guide chapters.

Features

Each chapter includes features that are designed to help you better comprehend and organize the textbook material.

Learning exercises are organized primarily to follow the order of content in the textbook and are also grouped by types of exercises. To emphasize the significant content of each chapter, we have presented questions in a variety of formats—matching, fill in the blank, short answer, true or false, and crossword puzzles. Bold topical headings corresponding to those in the textbook serve as transitions from one subject to the next. The answers for all these exercises are provided at the back of the Study Guide.

Critical Thinking Exercises and **Suggested Learning Activities** are opportunities for you to apply your knowledge to real-life situations, either clinical or personal.

Case Studies and **Student Learning Applications** are designed for you to apply your knowledge to hypothetical situations that mirror real-life events in pediatric nursing. In many cases, there may be no single correct answer, and we hope that by sharing your answers with other students, you will broaden your perspective of the clinical situation.

Review Questions are provided in multiple-choice format to give you an opportunity to review key content quickly. The answers to these questions are also provided at the back of the manual.

It is our intention that the learning activities presented in this Study Guide will help you to apply the content of the textbook directly to the practice of maternal-child nursing.

Anne-Marie Kiehne, PhD, RN

Contents

1

Foundations of Maternity and Pediatric Nursing

HELPFUL HINT

A fundamentals-of-nursing textbook can provide additional information on many of the topics covered in the chapter as they relate to the nursing profession.

MATCHING KEY TERMS

Match the terms with the correct definition.

1. ______ advocacy
2. ______ morbidity
3. ______ malpractice
4. ______ neonatal mortality
5. ______ intrapartum
6. ______ ethics
7. ______ lactation
8. ______ negligence

a. Infant deaths that occur in the first 28 days of life
b. Speaking or arguing in support of a policy or person's rights
c. Negligence by a professional person
d. Time of labor and childbirth
e. Ratio of sick to well persons in a defined population
f. Secretion of milk from the breasts
g. Rules or principles that govern conduct
h. Failure to act in the way a reasonable, prudent person of a similar background would act in a similar circumstance

HISTORICAL PERSPECTIVES

Maternity Nursing

1. Identify the three basic principles of family-centered maternity care.
   a. ______________
   b. ______________
   c. ______________
2. Describe each of these settings for childbirth.
   a. Traditional hospital setting

   b. Labor, delivery, and recovery (LDR) rooms

   c. Labor, delivery, recovery, and postpartum (LDRP) rooms

d. Birth centers

e. Home births

Pediatric Nursing

Answer as either true (T) or false (F).

1. ______ Throughout history, children have been valued and protected by society.
2. ______ During the 19th century, the most serious child health problems were directly related to poverty and overcrowding.
3. ______ The first public health program for mothers and children was initiated by Lillian Wald.
4. ______ Hospital policies have changed in response to an awareness of children's emotional and psychological needs.

CURRENT TRENDS IN MATERNITY AND PEDIATRIC CARE

1. How has cost containment affected maternity and pediatric care?

Answer as either true (T) or false (F).

2. ______ WIC provides supplemental food supplies to bottle-fed children but not for breastfeeding mothers.
3. ______ Premature births have increased in the past two decades.
4. ______ African-American women have lower maternal mortality rates than do white women.
5. ______ Infant mortality rates have continued to drop since 1950 due to better neonatal care.
6. ______ Accidents are the leading cause of death in children aged 1 to 19 years.
7. ______ There is no link between children living in poverty and poorer health outcomes.

ETHICAL PERSPECTIVES ON MATERNAL AND CHILD NURSING

1. Four of the most important ethical principles are ______________,
______________, ______________, and ______________.

LEGAL ISSUES

1. What are the four elements of negligence/malpractice?

   a. ____________

   b. ____________

   c. ____________

   d. ____________

2. Identify the four requirements for informed consent.

   a. ____________

   b. ____________

   c. ____________

   d. ____________

SUGGESTED LEARNING ACTIVITY

1. Gather additional information about one of the health care assistance programs (WIC, Medicaid's EPSDT program, Public Law 99-457, or the Healthy Start program) presented in this chapter.
2. Research agencies available in your town that offer assistance, such as health care, food, clothing, or emotional support, to pregnant women who are unable to pay for such assistance.

CRITICAL THINKING EXERCISE

1. Share with other students any legal situations you have encountered or read about that have involved nurses and maternity or pediatric clients.
2. Discuss the following situation with fellow students: Sally, who is 23 years old, is 24 weeks pregnant with her first child. She admits to her nurse-midwife that she continues to use several illegal drugs on a weekly basis. What are the nurse-midwife's legal and ethical responsibilities to the mother and to the fetus?

REVIEW QUESTIONS

Choose the correct answer.

1. Lillian Wald is recognized for which contribution to nursing?
   a. Discouraged the practice of tightly swaddling infants in three layers of clothing
   b. Initiated public health nursing at the Henry Street Settlement
   c. Promoted family-centered care for hospitalized children
   d. Developed infection control procedures in hospitals and foundling homes
2. Which of the following was identified in the chapter as a societal issue affecting maternity and pediatric nursing?
   a. Fewer children are living in poverty.
   b. Violence in the schools has decreased.
   c. Families are the fastest growing group of homeless people.
   d. The number of uninsured American children has decreased.

3. A practice model that uses a systematic approach to identify specific patients and manage patient care is
   a. case management.
   b. the nursing process.
   c. a clinical pathway.
   d. a health maintenance organization.

4. Which statement about family-centered maternity care is correct?
   a. Family-centered care decreases the responsibility of maternity nurses.
   b. Although settings have changed, childbirth is still viewed as a medical event.
   c. Care is adapted to meet the physical and psychological needs of the family.
   d. Maternal-infant bonding is the primary focus of family-centered care.

2

The Nurse's Role in Maternity and Pediatric Nursing

HELPFUL HINT

A fundamentals-of-nursing textbook can provide additional information on professional nursing roles and the nursing process.

THE ROLE OF THE PROFESSIONAL NURSE

Answer as either true (T) or false (F).

1. ______ The professional nurse has a responsibility to provide high-quality care to all clients.
2. ______ Standards of practice describe the level of performance expected of a professional nurse.
3. ______ Maternity nurse practitioners usually assist with childbirth.

Key Concepts

4. List six roles of maternity and pediatric nurses.
   a. ____________________
   b. ____________________
   c. ____________________
   d. ____________________
   e. ____________________
   f. ____________________
5. List the factors that influence learning.

6. Describe the education and services each type of advanced practice nurse is qualified to deliver.
   a. Certified nurse-midwives ______________________________

   b. Nurse practitioners ______________________________

   c. Clinical nurse specialists ______________________________

IMPLICATIONS OF CHANGING ROLES FOR NURSES

1. How does therapeutic communication differ from social communication?

2. When using active listening, the nurse attends to ____________ and ____________.

3. In the situations below, identify the communication block illustrated by the nurse's response. Provide an alternative nursing response.
   a. A child is crying and resisting as the nurse is about to administer an intramuscular injection. The nurse says, "This won't hurt a bit. You will be just fine."

      Communication block: ______________________________

      Alternate response: ______________________________
   b. A pregnant woman, on strict bed rest, tells the nurse, "I don't think I can stand much more of this. I didn't think my pregnancy would be like this." The nurse responds, "Rest up now. You won't get this much rest again in your life."

      Communication block: ______________________________

      Alternate response: ______________________________
4. The primary purpose of critical thinking in nursing is ______________________________

   ______________________________.
5. Identify the five steps in the critical thinking process.
   a. ____________
   b. ____________
   c. ____________
   d. ____________
   e. ____________

Answer as true (T) or false (F).

6. ______ A body posture that facilitates nurse-client communication is talking with the arms crossed over the chest.
7. ______ Cultural differences do not affect communication.
8. ______ Nonverbal behaviors may communicate a more powerful message to a client than spoken words.

THE NURSING PROCESS IN MATERNITY AND PEDIATRIC CARE

1. Describe the difference between a database assessment and a focus assessment.

2. For each broad goal, write at least three outcome criteria that are client focused, use measurable verbs, have a time frame, and are realistic.
   i. Following cesarean birth, the woman will have increased mobility.

   ii. The pregnant woman will have adequate nutrition.

   iii. The child with leukemia will not get an infection.

SUGGESTED LEARNING ACTIVITY

1. Arrange to observe a nurse midwife, nurse practitioner, or clinical nurse specialist. What educational preparation was needed for this advanced practice? What did you find most interesting about this experience?
2. Research the effects of various herbal remedies on pregnant women and on children. What difficulties did you have in obtaining scientific research on the herbal remedies?

CRITICAL THINKING EXERCISES

1. In the clinical setting, select a topic that a client and/or family needs to learn. Use at least four of the principles of teaching and learning in your presentation. Explain how you used each principle in your teaching.

2. Recall a conversation you had with a client. Which therapeutic communication techniques did you use in your dialogue? Give examples from your conversation. What would you do differently to improve your therapeutic communication skills?

REVIEW QUESTIONS

Choose the correct answer.

1. Your friend says she is not sure she wants a doctor to deliver her second baby because she believes doctors are too busy to talk with her when she has check-ups. The best alternative professional for you to suggest is the

   a. maternity nurse practitioner.
   b. certified nurse-midwife.
   c. lay midwife.
   d. clinical nurse specialist.

2. A primary difference between social communication and therapeutic communication is that therapeutic communication is

   a. designed to obtain information in a minimum amount of time.
   b. the only appropriate professional communication.
   c. focused on achieving a relevant goal for the client.
   d. limited to the information necessary for safe care.

3. A pregnant woman tells the nurse, "I'm so confused. My husband wants me to have my tubes tied after the baby comes, but what if something happens to the baby?" The nurse replies, "You are afraid of having permanent contraception before you know if your baby is well." The nurse's response is an example of

   a. directing.
   b. paraphrasing.
   c. summarizing.
   d. pinpointing.

4. A nursing diagnosis differs from a collaborative problem primarily in terms of whether the nurse

   a. can prescribe definitive treatment for the problem.
   b. identifies a client strength or weakness.
   c. determines that an actual or a potential problem exists.
   d. is able to evaluate the client's response to treatment.

3

The Child-Bearing and Child-Rearing Family

HELPFUL HINT

Review stress and coping information in a fundamentals-of-nursing textbook.

MATCHING KEY TERMS

Match the term with the correct definition.

1. ______ coping
2. ______ culture
3. ______ discipline
4. ______ ethnocentrism
5. ______ fatalism
6. ______ nuclear family
7. ______ stress

a. The structure an adult sets for a child's life
b. Belief that events are predestined
c. Efforts directed toward managing or solving various events, problems, or stressors
d. Any situation, positive or negative, requiring adjustment on the part of individuals, families, or groups
e. Family consisting of two generations (parents and children) living together more or less isolated from other close relatives
f. The opinion that the beliefs and customs of one's own ethnic group are superior to those of others
g. The sum of values, beliefs, and practices of a group of people that are transmitted from one generation to the next

THE FAMILY AND NURSING CARE

1. List problems that may be encountered by each of the following types of families.
   a. Dual income

   b. Single parent

   c. Blended

   d. Adoptive

e. Multigenerational

f. Same-sex parents

g. Adolescent parents

h. Families with substance abuse

i. Families with children with special needs

2. In front of each family coping strategy, put "I" if the strategy is internal or "E" if the strategy is external.
   a. _____ role flexibility
   b. _____ optimism
   c. _____ social support system
   d. _____ family problem solving
   e. _____ using humor
   f. _____ seeking information
   g. _____ seeing spiritual meaning in events
   h. _____ joining self-help groups

CULTURAL INFLUENCES ON MATERNITY AND PEDIATRIC NURSING

Explain how characteristics of cultural groups affect nursing communication.

1. Southeast Asians
   a. Voice tone

   b. Eye contact

2. Hispanics—conversational methods

3. African-Americans—language

4. Middle-Easterners
   a. Interpreters

   b. Paternalism

PARENTING

Answer as either true (T) or false (F).

1. ______ An authoritarian parent discusses household rules with the child.
2. ______ Children of authoritarian parents tend to lack self-confidence.
3. ______ Authoritative parents permit compromises about rules.
4. ______ Permissive parents tend to discipline their children inconsistently.

Briefly describe each of the following discipline measures.

5. Redirection

6. Reasoning

7. Time-out

8. Consequences

9. Behavior modification

10. Corporal punishment

SUGGESTED LEARNING ACTIVITIES

1. Interview a classmate who is from a cultural background different from yours. How do your health beliefs differ? How are they similar?

2. Interview a classmate from a similar cultural background. How do your health beliefs differ? How are they similar?

CRITICAL THINKING EXERCISE

The Thomas family is a single-income family consisting of the natural parents and their two sons, ages 4 and 2. The parents are in the process of getting a divorce. The mother will have custody of the boys, and they will move in with her parents so that she will be able to go back to work full-time. The boys will spend every other weekend and one night each week with their father.

1. What stressors may the following experience?

   Father

   Mother

   Children

   Grandparents

2. How can the children be helped through this transition?

REVIEW QUESTIONS

Choose the correct answer.

1. A Muslim woman is admitted to the postpartum unit after delivering a baby girl. Considering the culture needs of this client, which of the following should be included in her plan of care?
   a. including meat with every meal
   b. having only female nurses care for the client
   c. not putting ice in the bedside water pitcher
   d. assessing for herbal use

2. According to Chess and Thomas, children who adapt slowly to new stimuli and express negative reactions are identified as
   a. easy.
   b. difficult.
   c. slow to warm up.

3. The purpose of discipline is to
   a. teach a child how to function effectively in society.
   b. establish the self-fulfilling prophesy.
   c. assert parental control over the child.
   d. transmit the family's culture.

4. An example of a family that is classified as "high risk" is a (an)

   a. traditional family.
   b. single-parent family.
   c. adoptive family.
   d. family headed by adolescents.

5. A nurse reacts with anger because a woman who did not have prenatal care explains that she does not see pregnancy as an illness requiring medical care. The nurse's reaction demonstrates

   a. cultural diversity.
   b. ethnicity.
   c. ethnocentrism.
   d. fatalism.

6. A mother tells the nurse that she puts her 3-year-old son in a time-out chair in a corner for 3 minutes when he misbehaves. She asks the nurse if this is correct. The nurse responds

   a. "You're using time-out correctly."
   b. "You should put the time-out chair in the center of family activity."
   c. "I would increase the time-out to 5 minutes."
   d. "Do you talk about the misbehavior while he's in the chair?"

7. A statement that uses effective reasoning techniques is

   a. "You're not being very nice when you throw toys at your friend."
   b. "I wouldn't throw that toy if I were you."
   c. "I feel embarrassed when you throw toys at someone."
   d. "I won't let you play at your friend's house if you throw toys."

8. An 8-year-old child hit by a car has been in ICU for a week. She has a lengthy recovery ahead. Both parents have been at her side since the injury. They have not been eating properly and look exhausted. An appropriate nursing diagnosis for this family would be

   a. parental role conflict relayed to change in the environment.
   b. fear related to the child's critical condition.
   c. risk for alteration in family health maintenance management related to situational crisis.
   d. risk for impaired home maintenance management related to lack of support.

4

Health Promotion for the Developing Child

HELPFUL HINT

Review growth and development in a developmental psychology textbook.

MATCHING KEY TERMS

Match the terms with the correct definition.

1. ______ cephalocaudal
2. ______ chronologic age
3. ______ developmental age
4. ______ growth spurts
5. ______ heredity
6. ______ learning
7. ______ nutrients
8. ______ proximodistal
9. ______ RDA
10. ______ regression

a. Progression from midline to periphery
b. Age based on functional behavior and ability to adapt
c. Transmission of genetic characteristics
d. Progression from head to toe
e. Appearance of behavior more appropriate at an earlier stage of development
f. Behavior changes that occur as a result of maturation and experience with environment
g. Age in years
h. Brief periods of rapid increase in growth rate
i. Foods that supply the body with elements necessary for metabolism
j. Recommendations for the average amounts of nutrients that should be consumed by healthy people in the United States

TYPES OF PLAY

Match each type of play with its description.

11. ______ dramatic play
12. ______ familiarization
13. ______ symbolic play

a. Use of games and interactions that represent an issue or a concern to be addressed
b. Use of materials associated with health care in creative, playful activities
c. Children act out roles and experiences that happened to them or someone else or that they fear

OVERVIEW OF GROWTH AND DEVELOPMENT

Fill in the blanks.

14. Nurses need to have an understanding of growth and development in order to design care plans that are ________________________.
15. An increase in physical size is referred to as ________________________.
16. Physical change in the complexity of body structures that enables higher-level functioning is known as ________________________.
17. ________________________ is an increase in capabilities resulting from growth, maturation, and learning.
18. Changes in behavior that occur as the result of both maturation and experience with the environment can be termed ________________________.
19. Nurses must be familiar with normal patterns of growth and development so that ________________________ can be detected and treated early.
20. Next to each age write the corresponding stage of growth and development.
    a. 8 years ________________________
    b. 2 years ________________________
    c. 17 years ________________________
    d. 10 months ________________________
    e. 4 years ________________________
    f. 3 weeks ________________________
21. List three parameters used to measure growth in infants and children.
    a. ________________________
    b. ________________________
    c. ________________________
22. An infant's birth weight typically doubles by __________ and triples by __________.
23. ________________________ is an indicator of brain growth.
24. Primary dentition consists of ______________ teeth; permanent teeth number ______________.

PRINCIPLES OF GROWTH AND DEVELOPMENT

Match each pattern of growth and development with its example.

25. ______ cephalocaudal
26. ______ general to specific
27. ______ proximodistal
28. ______ simple to complex

a. An infant responds to abdominal pain by flailing the extremities; the child responds by guarding the abdomen.
b. A toddler uses 2-word sentences; a preschooler tells stories.
c. In the embryo, the trachea develops first, followed by outward development of the bronchial tree.
d. The infant can lift the head before being able to lift the trunk.

Fill in the blanks.

29. Children may regress to earlier developmental levels when they are ______________________________.

30. Define *critical period.*

____.

____.

Answer as either true (T) or false (F).

31. ______ Environmental factors influence growth and development prenatally and after birth.

32. ______ A standard growth curve is appropriate for assessing all children regardless of their racial or ethnic backgrounds.

33. ______ Good nutrition is needed for the normal functioning of growth factor and sex hormones.

34. ______ Only inherited diseases can affect growth and development.

35. ______ Parental attitudes rarely influence growth and development.

THEORIES OF GROWTH AND DEVELOPMENT

Match each stage of Piaget's theory with the example that is characteristic of that stage.

36. ______ sensorimotor
37. ______ preoperational
38. ______ concrete operations
39. ______ formal operations

a. Distinguishes fact from fantasy
b. Exhibits magical thinking
c. Develops sense of object permanence
d. Thinks abstractly

Identify which of Freud's stages of psychosexual development is represented by each of the following.

40. Child explores the world with the mouth: ______________________________

41. Child may initially demonstrate aggression toward the same-sex parent: __________

42. Child develops an adult view of sexuality: ______________________________

43. Child learns to control the elimination processes: __________________________

44. Child typically prefers same-sex friends: ______________________________

Fill in the blanks in the following statements to complete the developmental tasks of Erikson through adolescence.

45. Trust versus ________________.

46. ____ versus shame and doubt.

47. ____ versus guilt.

48. Industry versus ________________.

49. ____ versus role confusion.

Match each level of Kohlberg's theory with its example.

50. ______ preconventional morality
51. ______ conventional morality
52. ______ postconventional morality

a. "I'll take my medicine to make my nurse happy."
b. "I won't hit them because the nurse will yell at me."
c. "I won't blast my radio. It's not fair to the other patients."

THEORIES OF LANGUAGE DEVELOPMENT

Fill in the blanks.

53. Language development closely parallels ______________________ development.
54. Receptive language is the ability to ______________________.
55. Expressive language is the ability to ______________________.

ASSESSMENT OF GROWTH

Fill in the blanks.

56. Why are a child's height, weight, and head circumference plotted on standardized growth charts at every well-child checkup?

    ____

57. Body mass index measures growth and ______________________ in children older than 2 years.

ASSESSMENT OF DEVELOPMENT

Fill in the blanks.

58. List four methods of assessing development.
    a. ______________
    b. ______________
    c. ______________
    d. ______________
59. Name two prescreening tools that have been found to be valid and reliable for detecting developmental delays.
    a. ______________
    b. ______________
60. The Denver Developmental Screening Test II (DDST-II) assesses development in which four functional areas?
    a. ______________
    b. ______________
    c. ______________
    d. ______________

Answer as either true (T) or false (F).

61. ______ Only nurses who have been trained to administer the DDST-II should conduct formal screenings.
62. ______ The DDST-II is similar to an IQ test.
63. ______ Parents should be present during DDST-II screening.
64. ______ When children under 6 years are hospitalized, they should be given the DDST-II.
65. ______ Nurses are able to diagnose developmental delays using the DDST-II.

THE NURSE'S ROLE IN PROMOTING OPTIMAL GROWTH AND DEVELOPMENT

Fill in the blanks.

66. What is anticipatory guidance?

____

67. According to Brazelton, touchpoints are

____

____

THE DEVELOPMENTAL ASSESSMENT

Answer as either true (T) or false (F).

68. ______ Children's developmental needs are the same as their psychosocial needs.
69. ______ When discussing a child's development with parents, it is important to take the family's culture into consideration.
70. ______ Observing a child in a variety of situations can provide information about the child's cognitive development.

Fill in the blanks.

71. Play is often called ______________________.
72. Practice play is also known as ______________________.
73. Symbolic play uses games and interactions to ______________________.
74. Games include ______________________.

Match each type of play with its description.

75. ______ associative
76. ______ cooperative
77. ______ onlooker
78. ______ parallel
79. ______ solitary

a. Independent play
b. Child observing others playing
c. Organized play with group goals
d. Side-by-side play without interaction
e. Group play without group goals

HEALTH PROMOTION

Answer as either true (T) or false (F).

80. ______ Immunizations are effective in decreasing the incidence of childhood infectious diseases.

81. ______ Because all states require immunizations for children attending school, obtaining parental informed consent is not necessary.

82. ______ The preferred site for intramuscular injections in infants is the deltoid.

83. ______ Age-appropriate doses of acetaminophen may be given if the child experiences discomfort following an immunization.

84. ______ When administering more than one injection, the nurse should give the vaccines using separate syringes at different sites.

85. ______ An otherwise healthy child with a low-grade fever can receive immunizations.

86. ______ Because of the threat of bioterrorism, the American Academy of Pediatrics recommends the routine administration of the smallpox vaccine for all children who are not immunocompromised.

Fill in the blanks.

87. The hepatitis B vaccine is never administered in the ________ site regardless of age.

88. In general, children who are immunocompromised should receive neither the ____________ nor the _____________ vaccine.

89. Because of the possibility of anaphylactic reactions, it is essential to have _____________ available while administering immunizations.

Match each nutrient with its function.

90. ______ carbohydrates

91. ______ fats

92. ______ proteins

93. ______ water

94. ______ vitamins/minerals

a. Building and maintaining body tissue
b. Transporting nutrients to, and waste away from, cells
c. Major dietary source of energy
d. Regulating metabolic processes
e. Playing a role in maintaining body temperature

Fill in the blanks.

95. Why is dietary fat intake not restricted in children under age 2 years? ____________

____

96. After age 2 years, fats should comprise no more than ______% of daily calories.

97. Why are milk servings especially important for adolescents? ____________________

____

98. Why is it important to gather data about a hospitalized child's food preferences?

____

99. List three methods of obtaining a dietary history.

    a. ____________

    b. ____________

    c. ____________

100. What is the leading cause of death in children? ____________________________

SUGGESTED LEARNING ACTIVITIES

1. Observe pediatricians or nurse practitioners performing well-child assessments. How did they establish trust with the child and parents? How did they go about assessing the child's growth? How did they assess development? How did they convey their findings to the child's parents? Were they able to work effectively with both the child and the parents?
2. Chart the height, weight, and head circumference of at least three children (an infant, a young child, and a school-age child or adolescent) on a standardized growth chart. Write a brief interpretation of your findings.

STUDENT LEARNING APPLICATIONS

Enhance your learning by discussing your answers with other students.

The Savon's have brought 12-month-old Amy to the pediatrician for a well-baby checkup. They tell you they are concerned because Amy is not as tall as her brother was at 12 months and because she cannot yet walk. You plot her height, weight, and head circumference and find that these measurements fall within the same growth channel as on her previous visits. You have received training in administering the DDST-II. You perform this assessment and find that Amy has no delays. Her immunizations are up to date. From a dietary history, you learn that she is drinking low-fat (2%) milk from a cup.

1. How would you interpret Amy's growth charts for the family?
2. Amy's parents express relief that she "passed the IQ test" when you interpret the results of the DDST-II for them. How would you respond to that?
3. What immunizations are needed at this time?
4. What anticipatory guidance would you give to the Savon family?
5. How would you determine whether the parents' concerns about Amy's growth and development are alleviated?

REVIEW QUESTIONS

Choose the best answer.

1. Cephalocaudal development follows
   a. the pattern of myelinization.
   b. the development of the bronchial tree.
   c. language development.
   d. neuromuscular development.

2. An infant responds to an injection by crying and flailing the extremities, whereas a preschooler responds by rubbing the injection site. This is an example of what pattern of development?
   a. Cephalocaudal
   b. Proximodistal
   c. General to specific
   d. Simple to complex

3. A child's growth and development are affected by
   a. cultural background.
   b. heredity.
   c. socioeconomic status.
   d. all of these.

4. Which of the following theorists described how children learn?
   a. Erikson
   b. Freud
   c. Kohlberg
   d. Piaget

5. Teaching about safety to school-age children should be geared toward their
   a. parents.
   b. chronologic age.
   c. cognitive level of development.
   d. ability to answer questions.

6. Parents of a preschooler are concerned because she wants "to marry" her father and told her mother to "go outside and play in the street and get hit by a car." The nurse realizes that the
   a. family should seek counseling.
   b. preschooler's behavior is normal.
   c. preschooler needs to be seen by a social worker.
   d. parents are not addressing the child's need for initiative.

7. The secondary dietary source of energy is
   a. carbohydrates.
   b. fats.
   c. proteins.
   d. vitamins.

8. An adolescent who has been losing weight will record everything he eats for 3 days. This is an example of
   a. an anthropometric measurement.
   b. cultural influences on diet.
   c. dietary guidelines.
   d. a dietary history.

9. Nurses can prevent childhood injuries by
   a. modeling safety practices.
   b. educating parents through anticipatory guidance.
   c. supporting legislation that advocates safety measures.
   d. all of the above.

10. When children play board games, they learn that taking turns is rewarded and that cheating is not rewarded. This fosters their
    a. cognitive development.
    b. emotional development.
    c. moral development.
    d. physical development.

11. Which of the following pairs of anthropometric data best reflects a child's present nutritional status?
    a. Weight and midarm circumference
    b. Body mass index (BMI) and height
    c. Head circumference and skinfold thickness
    d. Dietary history and 24-hour recall

12. A 12-month-old child's immunization record indicates that only one set of immunizations was given at 2 months. The nurse knows that
    a. the entire series of immunizations must be repeated.
    b. the OPV vaccine should be given now.
    c. it is dangerous to readminister the hepatitis B vaccine.
    d. the DTaP vaccine, and not the dT vaccine, should be given.

5 Health Promotion for the Infant

HELPFUL HINT

Review infant development in a developmental psychology textbook.

MATCHING KEY TERMS

Match the terms with the correct definition.

1. ______ asphyxiation
2. ______ critical milestones
3. ______ developmental milestones
4. ______ egocentrism
5. ______ mistrust
6. ______ object permanence
7. ______ parent-infant attachment
8. ______ pincer grasp
9. ______ sensorimotor stage
10. ______ stranger anxiety
11. ______ trust

a. Benchmarks of development indicating that the child is developing normally
b. Complete absorption with self
c. Emotional foundation on which a healthy personality is built
d. Use of the index finger and thumb to pick up objects
e. State of suffocation that severely compromises oxygen delivery
f. Realization that things continue to exist when out of sight
g. Distress experienced when infant is separated from caregivers
h. Negative resolution of Erikson's first developmental task
i. Developmental milestones that, if not reached, necessitate a full developmental assessment
j. Period in which child uses senses and movement to understand and control the environment
k. Sense of connection between parent and infant

GROWTH AND DEVELOPMENT OF THE INFANT

Next to each activity, write the age at which the behavior generally first appears.

Age Choices

1–2 months 3 months 4–5 months 6–7 months 8–9 months 12 months

12. Begins to obey simple commands ______________________
13. Crying becomes differentiated ______________________
14. Turns from abdomen to back ______________________
15. Smiles in response to others ______________________

16. Birth weight doubles ____________________
17. Can stand alone ____________________
18. Begins to demonstrate stranger anxiety ____________________
19. Is alert for 1.5 to 2 hours ____________________
20. Reflexes dominate behavior ____________________
21. Can breathe when nose is obstructed ____________________
22. Pincer grasp develops ____________________
23. Birth weight triples ____________________
24. Is an obligate nose breather ____________________
25. Has beginning sense of object permanence ____________________

Fill in the blanks.

26. Infants are vulnerable to respiratory infections because of ____________________ and ____________________.
27. During infancy the heart rate ____________________ while the blood pressure ____________________.
28. ____________________transmits additional IgA protection to the infant.
29. At what age does the ability to digest and absorb fats reach adult levels? __________
30. Because infants' renal systems are immature, they are at risk for ______________.

Match each substage of Piaget's sensorimotor stage with its description.

31. ______ reflex activity
32. ______ primary circular reactions
33. ______ secondary circular reactions
34. ______ coordination of secondary schemata

a. Actions become intentional.
b. Begins to have sense of object permanence.
c. Activities become less reflexive and more controlled.
d. Behavior is dominated by reflexes.

Answer as either true (T) or false (F).

35. ______ Depth perception is present at birth.
36. ______ Lack of eye muscle control at 2 months requires evaluation.
37. ______ All newborns should be screened for hearing problems.
38. ______ By 10 months, an infant should respond to his or her name.
39. ______ An infant's social smile is a communication tool.
40. ______ Vocalization is a reflexive activity.
41. ______ Infant sounds become more specific and meaningful by 9 to 15 months

42. Briefly describe how an infant develops a sense of suspicion and mistrust.

____

____

43. How is the parent-infant attachment strengthened?

____

____

44. Why does separation anxiety begin at about 6 to 7 months?

____

____

HEALTH PROMOTION FOR THE INFANT AND FAMILY

Fill in the blanks.

45. Transplacental passive immunity lasts approximately ________ months.
46. Infant formula lacks the ________________ properties and easy ________________ of breast milk.
47. Three examples of mothers who should not breast-feed their infants are those who use __________ drugs, those with untreated __________, and those with __________.
48. Weaning is the transition from breast or bottle feeding to ______________________.
49. If juices are heated before drinking, the ____________________________ is destroyed.

Answer as either true (T) or false (F).

50. ______ Infants typically have 12 teeth by their first birthday.
51. ______ Aspirin is the drug of choice for alleviating teething discomfort.
52. ______ Parents can use a washcloth and a tiny bit of toothpaste to clean their infant's teeth.
53. ______ Bottle mouth caries are preventable.
54. ______ Botulism is associated with infant intake of honey.
55. List four suggestions that may help parents console their infants.
    a. _____________
    b. _____________
    c. _____________
    d. _____________
56. List four suggestions that may help parents reduce their infants' irritability.
    a. _____________
    b. _____________
    c. _____________
    d. _____________

Fill in the blanks.

57. When riding in a car, infants weighing less than 20 pounds should be placed in the back seat in a ________________ -facing car safety seat.
58. Temperature settings on hot water heaters should be no higher than __________ ° F.
59. Gates at the top and bottom of stairs should be in place when the child starts to ____________________.
60. Foods that pose an asphyxiation risk include

____

____

61. Infants should be placed on their ________________ for sleep.

SUGGESTED LEARNING ACTIVITIES

1. Design a safety booklet for parents of infants.
2. Perform a developmental assessment on an infant. Assess fine and gross motor skills, language patterns, and psychosocial interactions. On the basis of your knowledge of infant growth and development, determine whether the infant is functioning at the expected level.

STUDENT LEARNING APPLICATIONS

Enhance your learning by discussing your answers with other students.

Jamal, an 8-month-old infant, is being hospitalized for 2 weeks to receive intravenous antibiotic therapy.

1. What can the nurse do to facilitate parent-infant attachment during this period?
2. How can the nurse deal with Jamal's stranger anxiety?
3. What can the hospital staff do to facilitate the development of trust in Jamal?

REVIEW QUESTIONS

Choose the best answer.

1. According to Piaget, an infant who intentionally shakes a rattle to hear the sound is in what substage?

   a. Reflexive
   b. Primary circular reactions
   c. Secondary circular reactions
   d. Coordination of secondary schemata

2. An 11-month-old infant enjoys picking up pieces of banana one by one with the thumb and index finger and throwing them on the floor. This is an example of

   a. egocentrism.
   b. pincer grasp.
   c. oral activity.
   d. reflexive activity.

3. An infant should turn her eyes and head toward a sound coming from behind her at
   a. birth.
   b. 4 months of age.
   c. 6 months of age.
   d. 10 months of age.

4. An infant will develop a sense of mistrust if he is
   a. adopted.
   b. hospitalized after birth.
   c. consistently ignored.
   d. sent to day care before 2 months of age.

5. Parent-infant attachment
   a. is critical for survival.
   b. is essential for normal development.
   c. involves the infant as an active participant in the process.
   d. is all of the above.

6. The parents of a 3-month-old infant with colic explain that because their daughter does not sleep through the night, they feel very frustrated. The nurse's first action is to
   a. provide information about normal sleep-wake cycles in a 3-month-old infant.
   b. suggest that they practice relaxation techniques.
   c. assure them that they are not bad parents.
   d. demonstrate how to soothe the infant.

7. Which of the following statements suggests that the parent needs more information about infant nutrition?
   a. "I'll change from breast milk to whole milk at about 6 months."
   b. "I'll introduce soft foods at about 5 months."
   c. "I'll add new foods one at a time."
   d. "I'll introduce drinking from a cup gradually."

8. An appropriate "finger food" for an 11-month-old infant is
   a. Cheerios.
   b. lollipops.
   c. popcorn.
   d. raisins.

9. Which of the following statements about immunity and immunizations is true?
   a. Breast-fed infants do not need immunizations until they are weaned.
   b. Infants are prone to infectious diseases because of immature immune systems.
   c. Transplacental passive immunity lasts through the first year of life.
   d. Immunizations offer the infant total protection against infectious diseases.

10. Which of the following infants is at risk for developing lead toxicity?
    a. A 10-month-old whose father crafts stain glass
    b. An 8-month-old living in a newly built house
    c. A 9-month-old whose toys are all made in the United States
    d. A 6-month-old whose cousin living out of town has lead toxicity

6

Health Promotion During Early Childhood

HELPFUL HINT

Review toddler and preschool development in a developmental psychology textbook.

MATCHING KEY TERMS

Match the terms with the correct definition.

1. ______ associative play
2. ______ autonomy
3. ______ caries
4. ______ cooperative play
5. ______ dysfluency
6. ______ irreversibility
7. ______ negativism
8. ______ parallel play
9. ______ physiologic anorexia
10. ______ regression
11. ______ ritualism
12. ______ symbolic play
13. ______ symbolic thought
14. ______ transductive reasoning

a. Return to a behavior characteristic of an earlier stage of development
b. Inability to understand a process in reverse
c. Reasoning from particular to particular
d. Ability to function independently
e. Playing alongside, but not with, others
f. Tooth decay
g. Ability to allow a mental image to represent something that is not present
h. Decreased appetite related to decreased caloric need
i. Group play without goals
j. Need to maintain sameness
k. Disorders in the rhythm of speech in which child knows what to say but is unable to do so
l. Games that represent an issue to be addressed
m. Opposition or resistance to the direction of others
n. Organized play with group goals

GROWTH AND DEVELOPMENT DURING EARLY CHILDHOOD

Fill in the blanks.

15. During early childhood, the average weight gain is ___________ pounds per year.
16. Children reach one half of their adult height between the ages of ___________ and ___________ years.
17. All 20 deciduous teeth are present by age ___________ years.

For each of the following, write T if the behavior first occurs during toddlerhood or P if it first occurs during the preschool years.

18. ______ Learns to walk well
19. ______ May have imaginary friends
20. ______ Handedness clearly established
21. ______ Exhibits negativism as an expression of independence
22. ______ Object permanence firmly established
23. ______ Anterior fontanel closes
24. ______ Gender identity well established
25. ______ May start to use aggressive speech
26. ______ Is in the intuitive substage of Piaget's preoperational stage
27. ______ Thinking characterized by centration and irreversibility
28. ______ Is an avid climber
29. ______ Obeys rules out of self-interest
30. ______ Turns pages of books

Match each characteristic of preoperational thinking with its example.

31. ______ Animism
32. ______ Centration
33. ______ Egocentrism
34. ______ Irreversibility
35. ______ Magical thought

a. Aaron believes the TV is watching him while he sleeps.
b. Beth took the toy truck apart and can't put it back together.
c. Carla's brother is in the hospital. She believes she made him sick because she didn't want to play with him.
d. Diego can follow only one direction at a time.
e. Elgin took Frank's toy and can't understand why Frank is upset.

HEALTH PROMOTION FOR THE TODDLER OR PRESCHOOLER AND FAMILY

Answer as either true (T) or false (F).

36. ______ After age 12 months, low-fat (2%) milk may be given.
37. ______ An appropriate serving size for solid food for the young child is 1 tablespoon of solid food per year of age.
38. ______ It is appropriate to substitute juice for milk.
39. ______ A toddler who eats little solid food but drinks a quart of milk per day is meeting RDAs.
40. ______ Food jags cause physiologic anorexia.
41. When should a child first visit the dentist? ______________________________
42. Why are bedtime rituals important for young children? ______________________________

____

43. Explain the difference between nightmares and night terrors. ________________

____

44. A child learns self-control through ________________ and ________________.

45. List four discipline techniques appropriate for the preschooler.

a. ____________

b. ____________

c. ____________

d. ____________

46. How can parents prevent drownings? ________________________________

____

47. Why is the use of booster seats in the car recommended for preschoolers over 40 pounds?

____

____

48. What should preschoolers be taught to do in the event that their clothes catch on fire?

____

____

49. What do parents need to know about firearm safety?

____

____

50. What is included in teaching children about sexual abuse?

____

____

51. Most children are ready for toilet training by 18 to 24 months. What is the rationale for postponing it until later? ________________________________

52. List four strategies parents can use to decrease the frequency of temper tantrums.

a. ____________

b. ____________

c. ____________

d. ____________

53. How can parents deal with sibling rivalry when a new baby is brought into the household?

____

____

54. How can parents help a child who stutters? ________________________

____

SUGGESTED LEARNING ACTIVITY

Interview the parents of a toddler. Discover how they deal with the child's negativism. How did the parents handle toilet training? Was it difficult or easy? If the child has temper tantrums, how do the parents handle them? Ask the parents what information would have been helpful for them to know before their child entered the "terrible 2s."

STUDENT LEARNING APPLICATIONS

Enhance your learning by discussing your answers with other students.

A mother has brought her 4-year-old son Jonathan into the clinic for a well-child checkup. After the physical examination, she seems uncomfortable and hesitant but eventually tells you that she sometimes finds her son masturbating. She finds this very distressing because of her religious beliefs. She says, "I can't believe my little boy picked up such a filthy habit." She tells you that she has punished Jonathan by not letting him play with the other children in their neighborhood.

1. What is your personal reaction to the mother's story?
2. If you have personal misgivings about her actions or reactions, what could you do to help yourself remain nonjudgmental?
3. How would you explain Jonathan's sexuality to his mother while acknowledging the importance of her religious beliefs?
4. How could you use Kohlberg's theory to help the mother understand Jonathan's ability to distinguish right from wrong?

REVIEW QUESTIONS

Choose the best answer.

1. Which of the following represents a burn safety hazard in a toddler's home?
   a. A steam vaporizer is being used in the child's room.
   b. The fireplace is securely covered with a screen.
   c. Electrical outlets are covered with plastic socket protectors.
   d. The hot water temperature is set at 110° F.
2. Which of these statements indicates that the parents of a toddler need more information about toddler safety?
   a. "We always put her in her car seat, even if we only drive down the street."
   b. "We never let her play outside alone."
   c. "We always put our cleaning supplies on the shelves above the sink."
   d. "One of us stays with her the entire time that she is in the bathtub."

3. During a well-child checkup, a father asks the nurse whether his 3-year-old son, who weighs 33 pounds, can use the car seat belt instead of the child car seat. The nurse's best response is
   a. "He's old enough to use a shoulder harness and lap belt."
   b. "He should continue to use the car safety seat."
   c. "It's time to switch to a booster seat."
   d. "He'll be safest in a rear-facing car safety seat."

4. Which of the following provides a toddler with a sense of security?
   a. Animism
   b. Egocentrism
   c. Negativism
   d. Ritualism

5. Toddlers have temper tantrums because they
   a. have limited language ability.
   b. are not getting enough attention.
   c. are unable to distinguish right from wrong.
   d. have poor parent-child attachments.

6. During a well-child checkup, the nurse notices that a toddler's teeth are brownish and speckled with white. The nurse suspects that the child
   a. does not brush her teeth.
   b. goes to sleep with a bottle of milk.
   c. eats too much candy.
   d. ingests too much fluoride.

7. According to Erikson, preschoolers who are encouraged to try new things and be creative will develop a sense of
   a. autonomy.
   b. initiative.
   c. industry.
   d. integrity.

8. A parent tells the nurse that she is worried because her preschooler has an imaginary friend. The nurse explains that
   a. the parent should enroll in parenting classes.
   b. the child should go to day care 3 days a week.
   c. imaginary friends are not unusual during the preschool period.
   d. the child should see a child psychologist.

9. While 5-year-old Isaac is hospitalized for an appendectomy, he tells the nurse that he is in the hospital because he was bad. The nurse should
   a. suspect child abuse and report it to the authorities.
   b. question the parents about their discipline methods.
   c. explain to the child why he is in the hospital.
   d. ignore the comment.

10. Three-year-old Beth walks out of the kitchen drinking a bottle of dishwashing liquid. After taking the bottle away from Beth, her parents should
    a. call 911.
    b. induce vomiting.
    c. call a Poison Control Center.
    d. give her 4 ounces of milk to drink.

11. A hospitalized 5-year-old thinks that the IV pole is a skinny monster that is going to tie her up. This is an example of
    a. animism.
    b. centration.
    c. egocentrism.
    d. magical thinking.

12. Which of the following suggests that a 20-month-old should not yet begin toilet training?
    a. He says, "Pee-pee," when his diaper is soiled.
    b. His mother is expecting a baby in 3 weeks.
    c. He is able to remove his pants.
    d. He can sit and walk well.

7

Health Promotion for the School-Age Child

HELPFUL HINT

Review school-age development in a developmental psychology textbook.

MATCHING KEY TERMS

Match the terms with the correct definition.

1. ______ caries
2. ______ conservation
3. ______ malocclusion
4. ______ menarche
5. ______ self-care children

a. Misalignment of the teeth
b. Ability to understand that certain properties of objects remain the same despite changes in appearance
c. Children who care for themselves after school
d. Onset of menstruation
e. Tooth decay

GROWTH AND DEVELOPMENT FOR THE SCHOOL-AGE CHILD

Answer as either true (T) or false (F).

6. ______ Throughout the school-age years, boys are consistently taller and heavier than girls.
7. ______ The onset of puberty is signaled by the adolescent growth spurt.
8. ______ Tonsil enlargement in the school-age child is always an abnormal finding.
9. ______ All permanent teeth are in place by age 12 years.
10. ______ A child's racial heritage has no impact on sexual development.
11. Why is active play important for school-age children?

    ____

    ____

12. Why are children more prone to dehydration than adults?

    ____

13. Reversibility allows children in the concrete operational stage to anticipate the results of their ____.
14. Children understand the principle of conservation of ____________________ before they understand conservation of ____________________.

15. Why is collecting stickers an appropriate activity for school-age children?

____

____

16. How do friendships change as school-age children mature?

____

____

17. Why do middle ear infections occur less frequently in school-age children than in younger children?

____

____

18. How do children develop a sense of industry?

____

____

19. How is the developmental task of industry related to self-esteem?

____

____

20. Why are rules important to school-age children?

____

____

Fill in the blanks.

21. Briefly describe why children obey rules in each of the following stages of moral development.
    a. Preconventional, stage 2: ______________________________
    b. Conventional, stage 3: ______________________________
    c. Conventional, stage 4: ______________________________
22. In order for parents' moral teaching to be effective, they must:
    a. be consistent in their ______________ of what the child should do.
    b. be consistent in administering ____________ and ______________.

HEALTH PROMOTION FOR THE SCHOOL-AGE CHILD AND FAMILY

Fill in the blanks.

23. School-age children need how many servings of the following foods each day?
    a. ______ Grains
    b. ______ Vegetables
    c. ______ Fruits
    d. ______ Protein
    e. ______ Dairy

24. A 6-year-old needs about ________ hours of sleep, whereas a 12-year-old needs ________ hours.

25. How can parents foster a sense of responsibility in their children?

____

____

26. List three strategies parents can use to help their child succeed in school.

a. ______________________________

b. ______________________________

c. ______________________________

27. How can nurses act as advocates for self-care children?

____

____

28. What can parents do to prevent childhood obesity? ____________________

____

SUGGESTED LEARNING ACTIVITIES

1. Interview an elementary school teacher. Ask about the common stressors encountered by students in the teacher's class. How does the teacher's perception of student stressors compare with those identified in your textbook? What information does the teacher think school-age children need in order to help them cope more effectively with stress?
2. Choose one of the topics under "Sources of Stress in Children" in your textbook. Design a teaching plan focused on this topic and intended for a group of 8- to 10-year-old children. What makes this topic stressful? How can children in this age group cope with that stressor?

STUDENT LEARNING APPLICATIONS

Enhance your learning by discussing your answers with other students.

Erica, who is 7 years old, missed a week of school because of nausea and vague abdominal pain on waking in the morning. She felt better after her siblings left for school each morning but had temper tantrums when her parents suggested she go to school in the afternoon. She had no symptoms over the weekend. On Monday morning, her symptoms returned, and her parents made an appointment with the pediatric nurse practitioner (PNP). After a thorough physical examination, the PNP made the tentative diagnosis of school refusal.

1. What in Erica's story suggests school refusal?
2. What questions would you ask Erica about her relationships with her parents, teachers, siblings, classmates, and friends to discover the "cause" of her school refusal?
3. Erica's father asks, "What should we do if Erica says she's sick tomorrow?" What suggestions would you give him?
4. Two days later, the father calls to say that Erica told him that she thinks her math teacher "hates" her. How can you help the family and Erica deal with this situation?

REVIEW QUESTIONS

Choose the best answer.

1. The preadolescent growth spurt occurs
   a. earlier in boys than in girls.
   b. earlier in girls than in boys.
   c. at about the same time in boys and girls.

2. Sex education for the 9-year-old child should include information about
   a. anatomy and physiology.
   b. bodily functions.
   c. what to expect during puberty.
   d. all of the above.

3. Children at increased risk for having dental caries include those who
   a. wear braces.
   b. do not wear mouth protectors during sports activities.
   c. use smokeless tobacco.
   d. do any of the above.

4. Children in the intuitive thought stage
   a. form hypotheses.
   b. are able to reverse their thinking.
   c. classify objects into categories.
   d. exhibit egocentrism.

5. Parents should limit school-age children's daily television viewing time to
   a. 1 hour.
   b. 2 hours.
   c. 3 hours.
   d. 4 hours.

6. An appropriate coach for a child's basketball team
   a. has a win-at-all-costs philosophy.
   b. is courteous to children, referees, and other coaches.
   c. divides the children into teams based on age.
   d. demonstrates all of the above.

7. An example of an activity that develops fine motor skills in the school-age child is
   a. rollerblading.
   b. playing the guitar.
   c. playing tag.
   d. swimming.

8. An 8-year-old child typically
   a. problem solves through random guessing.
   b. comprehends historical time.
   c. understands conservation of mass.
   d. cannot appreciate another person's point of view.

9. *Healthy People 2010* objectives for school-age children include which of the following?
   a. Increase the proportion of children with disabilities who spend at least 40% of their time in regular education programs.
   b. Reduce the proportion of children with mental health problems.
   c. Increase the proportion of children over 2 years who consume at least 30% of their calories from fat.
   d. Increase the proportion of children who receive dental sealants on their molar teeth.

10. A child who does not successfully complete the developmental task of industry develops a sense of:
    a. shame and doubt.
    b. guilt.
    c. inferiority.
    d. confusion.

8

Health Promotion for the Adolescent

HELPFUL HINT

Review adolescent development in a developmental psychology text.

MATCHING KEY TERMS

Match the terms with the correct definition.

1. ______ Adolescence
2. ______ Autonomy
3. ______ Egocentrism
4. ______ Identity formation
5. ______ Primary sexual characteristics
6. ______ Puberty
7. ______ Pubescence
8. ______ Reproductive maturity
9. ______ Risk-taking behavior
10. ______ Secondary sex characteristics
11. ______ Sexual maturity rating (SMR)

a. Spermatogenesis in males and menstruation in females
b. Acquisition of psychosocial, sexual, and vocational identity
c. Period before sexual maturity
d. Capacity to be self-governing
e. Transition from childhood to adulthood
f. Internal and external reproductive organs
g. Stages of sexual maturation
h. Behavior that predisposes a person to harm
i. Concern with self
j. Achievement of reproductive maturity
k. Physical characteristics of males and females that have no direct role in reproduction

ADOLESCENT GROWTH AND DEVELOPMENT

Fill in the blanks.

12. Physical maturation in girls occurs with the onset and establishment of ______________________________.
13. Another term for the adolescent growth spurt is ______________________________.
14. In girls, the appearance of ______________ is the first sign of ovarian functioning.
15. Breast enlargement in boys is called ______________________________.
16. An adolescent's chronologic age provides less information about physical development than does ______________________________.
17. In boys, the first sign of pubertal changes is ______________________________.

18. The secretion of sex hormones (______________ in girls and ________________ in boys) stimulates the development of breast tissue, pubic hair, and genitalia.
19. List five effective strategies the nurse can employ when communicating with teens.
    a. ____________________________
    b. ____________________________
    c. ____________________________
    d. ____________________________
    e. ____________________________
20. In adolescent psychosocial development, what is meant by the "moratorium"?
    ____
    ____
21. What functions do the adolescent peer group serve?
    ____
    ____

For questions 22 through 29, identify the period of adolescence (early, middle, or late) during which the described behavior is most likely to occur.

22. Best friends are of the same gender. ______________________________________
23. Adolescents react to an imaginary audience. ________________________________
24. Emancipation from parents is a major issue. ________________________________
25. Adolescents overidentify with glamorous role models. _________________________
26. Conflicts with parents escalate. ____
27. Conformity with peer group becomes less important. __________________________
28. Gang membership brings security. ____
29. This is the most frustrating time for parents. ________________________________

HEALTH PROMOTION FOR THE ADOLESCENT AND FAMILY

Answer as either true (T) or false (F).

30. _____ Common dental problems are gingivitis, malocclusion, and trauma.
31. _____ Adolescents require fewer calories during peak height velocity (PHV).
32. _____ When transporting an avulsed tooth, place it in a container of milk.
33. _____ Because of PHV, adolescents require at least 10 hours of sleep per night.
34. _____ Regular exercise promotes healthy sleep patterns.
35. _____ More teens die from injuries than from all other causes of death combined.
36. _____ Tattooing is considered a health risk.

37. In 2002, the Centers for Disease Control and Prevention found that ________ of all adolescents had been involved in sexual activity.

38. In addition to depression, risk factors for teen suicide include

____

____

39. Complete protection from pregnancy and STDs is achievable only through

____.

Answer as either true (T) or false (F).

40. ______ A teen's cognitive ability affects contraceptive practices.

41. ______ About 40% of teens become pregnant within the first month of intercourse.

42. ______ Ideally, contraceptive education should include both partners.

43. ______ All threats of suicide by an adolescent should be taken seriously.

44. ______ Violence is an innate human behavior.

45. ______ Homicide is the second leading cause of death among teens 15 to 19 years of age.

SUGGESTED LEARNING ACTIVITY

Visit a teen pregnancy center in your community. Find out what services are offered, how teens are selected for the program, how the program is evaluated, and how it is funded. What other health promotion activities does the program provide for teens? Report your findings to your class.

STUDENT LEARNING APPLICATIONS

Enhance your learning by discussing your answers with other students.

You are invited to address a high school parent-teacher meeting to talk about early adolescent health.

1. Which topics would you include on physical health? Why would you include these?
2. What developmental information would you include? Why?
3. Which topics would you include on psychological health? Why?

REVIEW QUESTIONS

Choose the best answer.

1. According to Piaget, most adolescents eventually achieve which stage?
   a. Sensorimotor
   b. Preoperational
   c. Concrete operations
   d. Formal operations

2. In adolescence, sexual activity is usually related to
   a. risk taking.
   b. alcohol and/or substance abuse.
   c. low self-esteem.
   d. all of these.

3. According to Erikson, a person who has not successfully completed the developmental task of adolescence will experience
   a. shame and doubt.
   b. identity.
   c. role confusion.
   d. guilt.

4. Which of the following tools is used to assess sexual maturity?
   a. DDST II
   b. Dubowitz
   c. Tanner
   d. Elkind

5. A hospitalized adolescent has emotional highs followed by emotional lows. The nurse notes that the adolescent
   a. is a substance abuser.
   b. is emotionally labile.
   c. has access to alcohol.
   d. none of the above.

6. Which of the following is a *Healthy People 2010* objective for adolescents?
   a. Increase high school completion.
   b. Reduce physical fighting.
   c. Reduce pregnancies.
   d. All of the above.

7. In boys, PHV occurs during Tanner stages
   a. 1 and 2.
   b. 2 and 3.
   c. 3 and 4.
   d. 4 and 5.

8. Gynecomastia
   a. is always bilateral.
   b. occurs in the majority of adolescent males.
   c. requires surgical intervention
   d. begins in late adolescence.

9

Hereditary and Environmental Influences on Childbearing

HELPFUL HINT

Review the principles of heredity.

MATCHING KEY TERMS

Match the term with the correct definition.

1. ______ allele
2. ______ karyotype
3. ______ monosomy
4. ______ mutation
5. ______ polymorphism
6. ______ polyploidy
7. ______ somatic cell
8. ______ teratogen
9. ______ translocation
10. ______ trisomy

a. Common gene variation
b. Cell with an added set of chromosomes
c. Alternate gene form
d. Variation in a gene affecting function
e. Chromosomes arranged from largest to smallest pairs
f. One extra chromosome present in each body cell
g. All or part of a chromosome attached to another
h. Body cells other than germ cells
i. Cells with only one chromosome
j. Agent that causes or increases the risk for a birth defect

HEREDITARY INFLUENCES

1. Explain how DNA, genes, and chromosomes are related.

2. What is the Human Genome Project?

3. The explosion of knowledge about the genetic basis for disease raises many legal and ethical issues. How can this knowledge affect the following?

   a. Privacy

   b. Self-esteem

c. Level of anxiety

d. Health insurance coverage

4. For each type of single-gene abnormality, describe the conditions necessary for a child to be affected and specify any sex differences.
   a. Autosomal recessive

   b. Autosomal dominant

   c. X-linked recessive

Answer as either true (T) or false (F).

5. ______ Sickle cell disease follows an autosomal recessive pattern of development.
6. ______ Type O blood follows an autosomal dominant pattern of development.
7. ______ All sons of a father with hemophilia will inherit the disease.
8. ______ Turner's syndrome is an example of a numerical abnormality.
9. ______ Fragile X syndrome is the most common form of female mental retardation.

MULTIFACTORIAL DISORDERS

1. Describe two characteristics typical of multifactorial birth defects.

2. What factors influence the risk for the occurrence of a multifactorial disorder?

ENVIRONMENTAL INFLUENCES

1. When should a rubella immunization be administered to a woman of childbearing age?

2. In prescribing drugs for pregnant women, what must the nurse practitioner balance?

3. When a pregnant woman requires an urgent x-ray, her lower abdomen is ____________________.

4. Why should pregnant women avoid saunas and hot tubs?

GENETIC COUNSELING

1. Genetic counseling focuses on the entire ____________________.
2. Genetic counseling is considered ____________________ because the counselor does not tell the client what decision to make.

NURSING CARE OF FAMILIES CONCERNED ABOUT BIRTH DEFECTS

1. How do nurses in the following practices provide care related to genetics?
   a. Women's health nurses

   b. Antepartum nurses

   c. Neonatal nurses

   d. Pediatric nurses

SUGGESTED LEARNING ACTIVITIES

1. In the clinical setting, review charts for women or children who were referred for genetic counseling or genetic studies. Why were they referred? Who participated in the counseling? What were the outcomes? Discuss you findings with your classmates.
2. Using the symbols and examples in your textbook as a guideline, draw a three-generation pedigree of your family tree. Note any traits (normal [e.g., blood type] or abnormal) that you know about each person. What patterns emerge?

REVIEW QUESTIONS

Choose the correct answer.

1. The nurse notes this information on the chromosomal study of an infant with a birth defect: 46, XY. This means that the infant has
   a. abnormal genes in all 46 chromosomes.
   b. a normal male chromosome analysis.
   c. an abnormal female chromosome makeup.
   d. Down syndrome (trisomy 21).

2. The nurse would expect a pregnant African-American woman to be offered genetic testing for which disorder?
   a. Cystic fibrosis.
   b. Tay-Sachs disease.
   c. Rh isoimmunization.
   d. Sickle cell disease.

3. Parents of a child with an abnormal autosomal recessive disorder want to know if the problem is likely to recur if they have another child. The nurse knows that
   a. it is unlikely that they would ever have another child with the abnormality.
   b. each pregnancy has a 1 in 4 (25%) chance of resulting in another affected child.
   c. any pregnancy that occurs before the mother is 40 is not likely to have the defect.
   d. their risk for having another child with the defect cannot be calculated exactly.

4. A woman who is 5 weeks pregnant asks the nurse whether she can take a specific medication to relieve her cold symptoms. The nurse's answer is based primarily on
   a. whether the drug is prescribed or available on an over-the-counter basis.
   b. the severity of the woman's respiratory symptoms.
   c. the pregnancy category of the drug.
   d. how long the woman has had the cold.

5. A pediatric nurse is caring for an infant girl with hemophilia A. The nurse realizes that
   a. both parents must have hemophilia.
   b. the mother is a carrier and the father has hemophilia.
   c. hemophilia is an autosomal dominant trait.
   d. the infant is misdiagnosed.

10

Management of Fertility and Infertility

HELPFUL HINT

A fundamentals-of-nursing textbook can provide additional information on many of the topics covered in the chapter as they relate to the nursing profession.

MATCHING KEY TERMS

Match the term with the correct definition.

1. _______ basal body temperature
2. _______ endometriosis
3. _______ gestational surrogate
4. _______ infertility
5. _______ oligospermia
6. _______ spermicide
7. _______ tubal ligation

a. A chemical that kills sperm
b. Cutting the fallopian tubes to prevent passage of ova and sperm
c. Presence of endometrial tissue outside the uterine cavity
d. Body temperature at rest
e. Inability to conceive after 1 year
f. A woman who carries the embryo of an infertile couple and relinquishes the child
g. Decreased number of sperm in semen

KEY CONCEPTS

1. Why is the typical, or actual, failure rate of a contraceptive more useful than the theoretical failure rate?

2. What are the major side effects of Depo-Provera?

3. When may a perimenopausal woman discontinue contraception?

4. Why should a man have his semen analyzed following vasectomy?

5. How does the hormone implant prevent pregnancy?

6. How do estrogen-progestin oral contraceptives prevent conception?

7. How do progestin-only oral contraceptives prevent conception?

8. What teaching is appropriate in each area related to oral contraceptive use?
   a. Backup contraception

   b. Time of day

   c. Possible pregnancy

   d. Nutrition

   e. Use during lactation

   f. Other medications

9. What annual examinations should the woman have if she takes oral contraceptives?

10. List some types of emergency contraception.

11. Why should women using an IUD be in a mutually monogamous relationship?

12. What teaching is important related to IUD use?

13. What are the two main advantages of barrier methods of contraception?

14. Why is use of spermicide with condoms advisable?

15. What should the woman who uses spermicides be taught about douching?

16. Why is it essential to help the man or woman understand the difference between natural membrane condoms and latex condoms?

17. What are the major problems associated with the female condom?

18. At what times should the woman who uses a diaphragm for contraception have the fit checked?

19. What is the major problem in using natural family planning methods?

20. Complete the following table to describe advantages and disadvantages of each contraceptive method.

	Advantages	Disadvantages
Sterilization		
Hormone injection		
Oral contraception		
Intrauterine device		
Chemical barriers		
Male condom		
Female condom		
Diaphragm		
Natural family planning		

21. List factors that may impair the ability of sperm to fertilize the ovum.

22. List factors that may impair normal erections.

23. List causes of abnormal ejaculation.

24. List factors that may impair function of seminal fluid.

25. List factors that may disrupt the hormonal secretions a woman needs to achieve pregnancy.

26. List factors that may impair normal ovulation.

27. List factors that may impair structure and function of the fallopian tubes.

28. List factors that may obstruct or impair function in the woman's cervix.

29. List factors that may be associated with repeated pregnancy loss.

30. Describe nursing care associated with each of the more common diagnostic tests for infertility.
    a. Semen analysis

    b. Basal body temperature

    c. Postcoital test

    d. Hysterosalpingogram

    e. Endometrial biopsy

31. Describe two complications associated with medications given to induce ovulation.

32. What are some reasons for choosing therapeutic insemination?

33. What precautions lessen the risk that a man will transmit infection or genetic disorders when he donates his sperm?

34. Complete the following table comparing in vitro fertilization (IVF), gamete intrafallopian transfer (GIFT), and tubal embryo transfer (TET).

Procedure	Description	Advantages	Disadvantages
IVF			
GIFT			
TET			

CRITICAL THINKING EXERCISES

1. Have you known of adolescents who had some of the erroneous beliefs discussed in your textbook? Did you have any of these beliefs when you were an adolescent? How might you use age-appropriate counseling to correct the misinformation listed? How would you address the issue of confidentiality?

2. Practice how you might tactfully introduce the subject of contraception to an adolescent, a postpartum woman, and a woman in her mid-40s.

3. You are asked for contraceptive information by a 16-year-old girl, a 28-year-old woman with three children, and a 45-year-old woman with one child. If you could ask only two questions of each woman to help find the best method for her, what questions would be most important? If you had to choose only two types of contraception to offer each, what would they be?

   a. 16-year-old:

b. 28-year-old:

c. 45-year-old:

4. If you could design the perfect contraceptive method, what qualities would it have? Who would use it? How would it be obtained?

5. Oral contraceptives are available without prescription in many countries and may be available on an over-the-counter basis in the United States in the near future. What are the advantages and disadvantages of this?

6. What is your opinion about monetary compensation for a woman who is a surrogate mother and contributes her ovum to the child? What if she is a gestational surrogate and carries the fetus to term but does not contribute a gamete to him/her?

7. Should compensation be different for male sperm donors and females who donate their ovum and carry the fetus? Why?

8. What are your feelings about blastomere analysis to identify genetic defects before implantation of an embryo that results from an assisted reproductive technology procedure? Should an embryo that has an identified defect be implanted? If it is discarded, do you view it as abortion?

9. Should health insurance cover all infertility diagnostic studies and therapy? If not, which ones should not be covered?

10. Should public assistance funds such as Medicaid cover infertility therapy? Why or why not?

REVIEW QUESTIONS

Choose the correct answer.

1. A woman is considering having a tubal ligation after she gives birth to her second child. The nurse should counsel her that
   a. she should wait until several months after birth to be certain that the infant is healthy.
   b. the procedure should be considered permanent and irreversible.
   c. sterilization is an easier procedure to perform after the postpartum period.
   d. she must provide signed informed consent by the sixth month of pregnancy.

2. Postprocedural teaching for a man who has had a vasectomy should include discussion that
   a. urinating may be difficult for several times after the procedure.
   b. a catheterized urine specimen should be obtained in 1 week.
   c. levels of testosterone may fluctuate for the first few months.
   d. another form of contraception should be used until the semen is free of sperm.

3. Which woman would be a good candidate for the hormone contraception?
   a. A 30-year-old woman who thinks she has completed her family
   b. A 22-year-old breastfeeding woman who just gave birth
   c. A 29-year-old woman who has type 2 diabetes secondary to obesity
   d. A 25-year-old woman who takes an anticonvulsant

4. A woman decides to change from the diaphragm to Depo-Provera. Her last menstrual period ended 1 week ago. She should be taught that she should
   a. take the oral contraceptive during this cycle only.
   b. return in 1 week to have the hormone injection.
   c. continue to use the diaphragm for the rest of her cycle.
   d. expect heavier periods than she had when using the diaphragm.

5. How should a woman take oral contraceptives?
   a. On an empty stomach, with a full glass of water
   b. At about the same time each day
   c. Before every episode of intercourse
   d. In the morning and at bedtime

6. Choose the safety teaching related to oral contraceptives.
   a. A barrier method should also be used to protect from infection.
   b. Nausea suggests that stroke may be imminent.
   c. Toxic shock syndrome is more likely to occur when the pill is used.
   d. Increase fluids if urinary frequency or urgency occurs.

7. The intrauterine device is an appropriate contraceptive for the woman who
   a. has unplanned intercourse with several partners.
   b. was recently hospitalized for treatment of a pelvic infection.
   c. is in a mutually monogamous relationship.
   d. has had two ectopic pregnancies.

8. If the IUD strings are longer than usual, the woman should
    a. know that this is expected when the IUD is first inserted.
    b. immediately have a Pap smear to rule out cervical cancer.
    c. take her temperature twice a day for 1 week.
    d. see her physician and use another method of contraception.

9. The major advantage of using a condom for contraception is that it
    a. requires a visit to the health care provider yearly.
    b. reduces transmission of infections.
    c. can be placed several hours before intercourse.
    d. may be incorporated as part of foreplay.

10. When teaching a woman fertility awareness, the nurse should emphasize that the basal body temperature
    a. is the average temperature taken each morning.
    b. should be recorded each morning before any activity.
    c. has a higher degree of accuracy in predicting ovulation than the cervical mucus test.
    d. can be done with a mercury thermometer but not a digital one.

11. At ovulation, the basal body temperature usually
    a. rises abruptly and then falls after 1 or 2 days.
    b. falls and remains low for the last half of the cycle.
    c. is higher during the first half of the cycle than in the last half.
    d. falls slightly at ovulation and is higher during the last half of the cycle.

12. Cervical mucus at ovulation should be
    a. thin and slippery and should stretch to at least 6 cm.
    b. cloudy, with a mild odor, and should stretch to at least 6 cm.
    c. thick, clear, and of a large quantity.
    d. thin and tinged with a small amount of blood.

13. Choose the correct instructions for a man who must provide a semen sample.
    a. After collecting the sample in a condom, refrigerate it until it is transported to the laboratory.
    b. Masturbation is the only way a good sample can be obtained.
    c. Keep the sample near the body, and transport it to the laboratory within 1 hour.
    d. Do not take any regularly scheduled drugs for 3 days before obtaining the sample.

14. A woman who is taking clomiphene citrate (Clomid) calls the infertility clinic and says that she has some nausea each morning and frequency of urination. She suspects that she may be pregnant. The correct nursing response is to
    a. tell her that pregnancy cannot be determined until she misses her next period.
    b. have her come to the clinic promptly for a sensitive pregnancy test.
    c. have her continue taking the drug until she completes this cycle and then have a pregnancy test.
    d. reassure her that her symptoms are commonly seen in women who take this drug.

11

Reproductive Anatomy and Physiology

MATCHING KEY TERMS

Match the terms with the correct definition.

1. ______ linea terminalis
2. ______ nocturnal emissions
3. ______ perineum
4. ______ rugae
5. ______ vulva

a. Imaginary line dividing the upper (false) pelvis from the lower (true) pelvis
b. Involuntary release of seminal fluid from the penis during sleep
c. Small ridges or folds of tissue in the female vagina and on the male scrotum
d. Collective term for all of the female external reproductive organs
e. Posterior part of external female reproductive organs

Match each structure with its function(s). Some letters may be used more than once.

6. ______ acini cells
7. ______ Bartholin's glands
8. ______ corpus cavernosum
9. ______ corpus spongiosum
10. ______ Leydig's cells
11. ______ Montgomery's tubercles
12. ______ myoepithelial cells
13. ______ scrotum
14. ______ Sertoli's cells
15. ______ Skene's glands

a. Enable erection of the penis for coitus
b. Nourish sperm during their formation within the testes
c. Promote lubrication of the vagina for coitus
d. Produce milk from substances extracted from blood
e. Secrete a substance to keep nipples soft during breastfeeding
f. Regulate temperature of testes to promote normal sperm formation
g. Lubricate the female's urethra
h. Secrete testosterone in the male.
i. Discharge milk into the ductal system of the breast

KEY CONCEPTS

1. What mechanism prevents onset of puberty before the proper time?

2. The period of maturation of reproductive organs is called ____________________. It begins at about age _________ years in girls and at about age _________ years in boys.

3. The first outward change of puberty in girls is ______________________________. The first outward change of puberty in boys is ______________________________.

4. Girls usually experience their first menstrual period about __________ years after the first outward change associated with puberty.

5. What factors cause the average male to be taller than the average female at physical maturity?

6. Explain the importance of each type of uterine muscle (myometrial) tissue. Where is each type primarily located?

   a. Longitudinal fibers
      - Importance

      - Location

   b. Interlacing (figure-eight) fibers
      - Importance

      - Location

   c. Circular fibers
      - Importance

      - Location

7. Fertilization normally occurs in the ____.

8. What is the difference in the time when the immature female and male gametes are formed?

9. Describe events in each phase of the ovarian cycle.

   a. Follicular phase

b. Ovulatory phase

c. Luteal phase

10. Describe events in each phase of the menstrual cycle.
    a. Proliferative phase

    b. Secretory phase

    c. Menstrual phase

11. Why might a man who usually wears very tight underwear have a problem with infertility?

REVIEW QUESTIONS

Choose the correct answer.

1. The sex of an infant will be female unless
   a. two X chromosomes are received from the mother.
   b. the short arm of the Y chromosome is received from the father.
   c. conception occurs during the last half of the female reproductive cycle.
   d. the mother's ovary produces testosterone early in pregnancy.

2. The primary purpose of gonadotropin-releasing hormone (GnRH) is to stimulate
   a. development of the woman's breasts for lactation.
   b. growth of pubic and axillary hair.
   c. breakdown of the endometrium in the menstrual flow.
   d. secretion of follicle-stimulating hormone (FSH) and luteinizing hormone (LH) from the anterior pituitary gland.

3. The first outward change of puberty in girls is
   a. rapid growth to reach the adult height and weight.
   b. enlargement and development of the breasts.
   c. onset of menstruation.
   d. increase in clear vaginal secretions.

4. Choose the girl who is most likely to have secondary amenorrhea.
   a. Amanda, 15 years old, who is about 10% above her ideal weight for height
   b. Brittany, 17 years old, who is preparing for competition in a national gymnastic tournament
   c. Chloe, 16 years old, who had her first menstrual period 1 year ago at age 15
   d. Deanna, 16 years old, who had her first signs of puberty at age 10

5. Males are usually taller than females when they reach their adult height because their
   a. growth in height occurs early in puberty and continues for a short time after puberty.
   b. secretion of testosterone delays closure of the epiphyses of the long bones.
   c. puberty changes begin about 2 years later than in the average female.
   d. rapid increase in height begins later in puberty and continues for a longer time.

6. The layer of uterine muscle that is most active during labor is composed of what kind of fibers?
   a. Longitudinal
   b. Interlacing
   c. Circular

7. The layer of uterine tissue that responds to cyclic changes in hormones secreted by the pituitary gland is the
   a. perimetrium.
   b. myometrium.
   c. endometrium.

8. Conditions that cause the fallopian tubes to be narrower than normal may result in
   a. excessive cramping and bleeding during menstruation.
   b. increased likelihood of pregnancy during each cycle.
   c. more rapid propulsion of the ovum through the tube.
   d. implantation of a fertilized ovum within the tube.

9. Extra follicles that remain after ovulation
   a. release their ovum during the last half of the reproductive cycle.
   b. resume maturation during the next reproductive cycle.
   c. may be fertilized during another reproductive cycle.
   d. are never active in another reproductive cycle.

10. Menstruation occurs because the
    a. hormone stimulation from the corpus luteum ceases.
    b. blood vessels in the uterine lining become too long and twisted.
    c. corpus luteum increases estrogen and progesterone production.
    d. ovum has been passed from the woman's body.

11. Milk is manufactured within the __________ of the breast.
    a. lactiferous ducts
    b. alveoli
    c. myoepithelium
    d. Montgomery's tubercles

12. The primary purpose of the cremaster muscle is to
    a. eject milk into the lactiferous ducts of the breasts.
    b. maintain the uterus in an anteflexed position.
    c. keep the testes cooler than the rest of the body.
    d. expel seminal fluids to nourish sperm at ejaculation.

12

Conception and Prenatal Development

MATCHING KEY TERMS

Match the term with the correct definition.

1. ______ autosome
2. ______ conceptus
3. ______ corpus luteum
4. ______ embryo
5. ______ gamete
6. ______ mitosis
7. ______ oogenesis
8. ______ ovulation
9. ______ placenta
10. ______ somatic cell

a. Results of a fertilized ovum
b. Developing baby from week 3 through 8
c. Non–sex chromosome
d. Reproductive cell
e. Ordinary body cell
f. Structure that provides nourishment for developing baby
g. Cells that remain after ovum formation and secrete estrogen and progesterone
h. Formation of female gametes
i. Cell division in body cells
j. Release of the mature ovum from the ovary

KEY CONCEPTS

1. Compare mitosis to meiosis in the following ways:

	Mitosis	**Meiosis**
Type of cell involved		
Number and type of chromosomes in each resulting cell		

2. Compare oogenesis with spermatogenesis in the following ways:

Factor	**Oogenesis**	**Spermatogenesis**
Number and type of chromosomes in each mature gamete		
Number of gametes resulting from each primary cell		
When gametogenesis begins and ends during life		

3. What are the two major occurrences immediately after fertilization?

4. List three reasons why the fundus is the best area for implantation.

5. List the three germ layers and the structures that develop from each.

6. When during prenatal development does each event occur?
   a. Closure of the neural tube

   b. Heart contains four chambers

   c. All abdominal organs are within the abdominal cavity

d. Eyes close

e. Eyes reopen

f. External ear development begins

g. Fetal sex apparent by external genitalia

h. Fetal movements felt by mother

i. Surfactant production begins

7. Describe each of these fetal structures or substances and state their purpose.
   a. Vernix caseosa

   b. Lanugo

   c. Brown fat

   d. Surfactant

8. What is the difference between the fertilization age and the gestational age?

9. Explain how each of the following mechanisms allows the fetus to thrive in the relatively low oxygen environment of the uterus.
   a. Fetal hemoglobin and hematocrit

   b. Relative fetal and maternal blood carbon dioxide levels

10. Describe how passage of maternal IgG antibodies can be either beneficial or harmful to the fetus.
    a. Beneficial

    b. Harmful

11. Explain the function of each placental hormone.
    a. Human chorionic gonadotropin (hCG)

    b. Human placental lactogen (hPL)

    c. Estrogen

    d. Progesterone

12. State the three functions of amniotic fluid.

13. Explain the umbilical cord structures and functions.
    a. Umbilical vein

    b. Umbilical arteries (two)

c. Wharton's jelly

14. Explain factors that cause each of these fetal circulatory shunts to close after birth and the eventual outcome for each.
    a. Foramen ovale
    b. Ductus arteriosus
    c. Ductus venosus

15. Describe monozygotic and dizygotic twinning in the following terms.

	Monozygotic	**Dizygotic**
Number of ova and sperm involved		
Genetic component		
Sex		
Hereditary tendency		
Number of amnions and chorions		

CRITICAL THINKING EXERCISES

1. A woman thinks she is pregnant but begins "spotting" (light vaginal bleeding). Her hCG levels are very low. What is the likely consequence of the low hCG level? Why?

2. What is a likely occurrence if a fetus is born with a lecithin-to-sphingomyelin (L/S) ratio of 1:1?

REVIEW QUESTIONS

Choose the correct answer.

1. An important purpose of seminal fluid is to
   a. digest microorganisms in the female digestive tract.
   b. prevent premature movement of sperm tails.
   c. protect sperm from the acidic vaginal environment.
   d. transport the sperm into the uterine cavity.

2. Fertilization is complete when
   a. fusion of the sperm and ovum nuclei occurs.
   b. a sperm enters the ovum in the fallopian tube.
   c. the fertilized ovum has its first cell division.
   d. the morula fully implants into the uterine lining.

3. The embryo is fully implanted in the uterus on which day after conception?
   a. 3
   b. 6
   c. 10
   d. 15

4. Which fetal circulatory structure carries blood with the highest oxygen concentration?
   a. Umbilical artery
   b. Umbilical vein
   c. Ductus arteriosus
   d. Pulmonary vein

5. What is the significance of a fetal hemoglobin of 13 g/dl and a hematocrit of 39%?
   a. Fetal blood is more likely to clot as it circulates through the placenta.
   b. Greater transfer of carbohydrates will result in rapid fetal growth.
   c. Transfer of harmful substances from the mother to the fetus is lessened.
   d. Anemia reduces the oxygen-carrying capacity of the fetal blood.

13

Physiologic Adaptation to Pregnancy

MATCHING KEY TERMS

Match the term with the correct definition.

1. ______ amenorrhea
2. ______ chloasma
3. ______ hyperemia
4. ______ multigravida
5. ______ physiologic anemia of pregnancy
6. ______ striae gravidarum

a. A woman who has been pregnant more than once
b. Mask of pregnancy
c. Excess of blood in a part of the body
d. Irregular reddish streaks caused by tears in connective tissue; "stretch marks"
e. Fall in hematocrit that occurs because plasma volume expands more than red blood cell volume
f. Absence of menstruation

KEY CONCEPTS

1. When during pregnancy does each of these markers in fundal height occur?
   a. Uterus can first be palpated above the symphysis pubis.

   b. Fundus can be palpated about halfway between symphysis pubis and umbilicus.

   c. Fundus is at level of umbilicus.

   d. Fundus is at xiphoid process.

2. What is the cause of each of the following changes in the cervix during pregnancy?
   a. Chadwick's sign

   b. Goodell's sign

c. Mucous plug

d. Bloody show

3. What is the possible result of each of the following changes in the vagina during pregnancy?
   a. Increase in vascularity

   b. Growth of connective tissue

   c. Secretion of increased amounts of glycogen

4. Why is progesterone essential in pregnancy?

5. Progesterone is produced first by the ____________ and then by the ____________.
6. Why does ovulation cease during pregnancy?

7. What breast changes occur during pregnancy?

8. Describe changes in maternal heart sounds that may occur during pregnancy. When do the heart sound changes occur? Describe common changes in heart sounds.

9. Complete the table to describe changes in the pregnant woman's blood. Consult a manual of laboratory tests or medical-surgical text for nonpregnant values, if needed.

Component	**Nonpregnancy Level**	**Pregnancy Level**	**Change**
Plasma volume			
Red blood cell volume			
Leukocytes			
Fibrinogen			

10. What is "supine hypotensive syndrome"? What signs and symptoms might a woman with this syndrome display? What should the nurse do to prevent or relieve it?

11. Why does the pregnancy-induced change in fibrinogen levels have a protective effect yet also increase risk?

12. What nasal changes are common during pregnancy? What causes them?

13. What two factors contribute to a woman's sense of dyspnea?

14. Why are pregnant women more likely to develop gallstones?

15. Why does the pregnant woman's bone mass stay stable even though the fetus requires calcium for skeleton development?

16. What changes in carbohydrate metabolism and the production, utilization, and breakdown of insulin occur during pregnancy? Why do the changes occur? How does the woman's body normally respond to these changes?

17. Describe edema that is expected during pregnancy and why it occurs. When should it be reported?

18. List the presumptive, probable, and positive indications of pregnancy. What is the difference among the three classifications?

19. List some reasons for a false-negative pregnancy test.

20. At what point in gestation is it possible to hear fetal heart sounds with the following tools?

    a. Doppler

    b. Fetoscope

21. Use Nagele's rule to calculate estimated dates of delivery (EDDs) for each of these dates representing last normal menstrual period dates.

    a. February 4

    b. August 2

22. Why is pregnancy risk assessment not a one-time evaluation?

23. What routine urine testing is done during prenatal visits?

24. How do each of the following differ when a woman has a multifetus pregnancy?
    a. Uterine size

    b. Fetal movements

    c. Weight gain

25. Describe significant maternal changes that occur in a multifetus pregnancy.
    a. Blood volume

    b. Cardiac workload

    c. Respiratory workload

    d. Blood vessel compression

    e. Ureter compression

    f. Bowels

26. What teaching is appropriate for each common discomfort of pregnancy?
    a. Nausea and vomiting

    b. Heartburn

    c. Backache

d. Urinary frequency

e. Varicosities

f. Hemorrhoids

g. Constipation

h. Leg cramps

27. What should the pregnant woman be taught about the following practices during pregnancy? How would you explain this to a woman if you were the nurse?

    a. Over-the-counter drugs

    b. Tobacco

    c. Illegal drugs

    d. Hot tubs and saunas

    e. Douching

    f. Exercise

    g. Use of a seat belt

CRITICAL THINKING EXERCISES

1. Why might spasm of the uterine spiral arteries cause the pregnant woman's blood pressure to rise abnormally? (See also Chapter 12.)

2. Assess a pregnant woman's blood pressure in each of the following ways. Allow at least 2 minutes between readings. Compare the systolic and diastolic blood pressures. Compute the mean arterial pressure (MAP) for each reading.

   a. Lateral recumbent position

   b. Sitting with arm supported

   c. Sitting with arm dependent

   d. Standing

   e. Diastolic pressure at sound muffling (Korotkoff's fourth phase)

   f. Diastolic pressure at disappearance of sounds (Korotkoff's fifth phase)

3. Compare a prenatal clinic's documentation forms for initial and subsequent antepartal visits to the recommended assessments listed in the text. What is that clinic's usual recommended frequency for follow-up prenatal visits?

4. Talk with nurses at a local prenatal clinic to determine which different cultural groups they typically serve. Ask them how they incorporate cultural beliefs and values into care.

CASE STUDY

Katherine is making her first antepartum visit on August 15. She has a 2-year-old son who was delivered at 40 weeks, a 5-year-old daughter delivered at 38 weeks, and 7-year-old twin daughters delivered at 35 weeks. She had a spontaneous abortion 3 years ago at

10 weeks. Her last menstrual period was April 5. Her fundal height is at the level of the umbilicus. She denies any major complaints and states that her health has been good.

1. Determine Katherine's gravida and para. Describe her obstetric history with the TPAL acronym.

2. What is Katherine's EDD?

3. What is Katherine's gestation on the day of her first visit?

4. Compare the present fundal height to the gestation of her pregnancy. If there is a discrepancy, what are some possible causes for it?

5. What factors may have influenced Katherine to delay her first antepartum visit?

6. What diagnostic studies should the nurse anticipate?

REVIEW QUESTIONS

Choose the correct answer.

1. A pregnant woman expects to give birth to her first baby in about 1 week. She asks the nurse if she has a bladder infection because she urinates so much, even though urination causes no discomfort. The nurse should explain to her that
   a. urinary tract infections are most common just before birth, so she should have a urine specimen tested.
   b. her fetus is probably lower in her pelvis, putting more pressure on her bladder.
   c. limiting her fluid can reduce the number of times she must interrupt her activity to urinate.
   d. the fetal growth has probably stopped and she should expect to start labor in a few days.

2. A woman having physiologic anemia of pregnancy has a hemoglobin and hematocrit level of at least
   a. 10 g/dl and 30%.
   b. 10.5 g/dl and 33%.
   c. 11 g/dl and 35%.
   d. 12 g/dl and 38%.

3. Slight respiratory alkalosis during pregnancy enhances
   a. growth of fetal arteries within the placenta.
   b. the fall in systolic and diastolic blood pressures.
   c. maternal metabolism of food and nutrients.
   d. transfer of fetal carbon dioxide to maternal blood.

4. A pregnant woman is prone to urinary tract infection primarily because
   a. a large volume of fetal wastes must be excreted by her kidneys.
   b. nutrients that enhance bacterial growth are excreted by her kidneys.
   c. the volume of urine excreted is reduced and its specific gravity is high.
   d. reduced blood flow to the urinary tract allows wastes to accumulate.

5. A pregnant woman complains that both of her thumbs hurt at times. Neither thumb is inflamed or discolored. The nurse should explain to the woman that
   a. she probably injured her hand and does not recall doing so.
   b. an undiagnosed fracture may have healed improperly.
   c. osteoarthritis often has its onset during pregnancy.
   d. increased tissue fluid is causing compression of a nerve.

6. A pregnant woman has a blood glucose screening at 26 weeks' gestation. The result is 128 mg/dl. The nurse should expect that
   a. no additional glucose testing will be needed.
   b. insulin injections will be needed by 30 weeks' gestation.
   c. oral drugs may be prescribed to lower her glucose level.
   d. more testing is needed to determine additional therapy.

14

Psychosocial Adaptations to Pregnancy

MATCHING KEY TERMS

Match the term with the correct definition.

1. ______ ambivalence
2. ______ couvades
3. ______ introversion
4. ______ mimicry
5. ______ narcissism
6. ______ role transition

a. conflicting emotions
b. changing from one pattern of behavior to another
c. Inward concentration
d. Preoccupation with self
e. Copying the behaviors of others
f. pregnancy-related rituals experienced by some prospective fathers

KEY CONCEPTS

1. List the typical maternal responses for each trimester of pregnancy.
   a. First

   b. Second

   c. Third

2. What changes occur that make the fetus seem real to the pregnant woman?

3. How might sexual interest and activity change during pregnancy? What factors may increase or decrease interest in either of the couple?

4. How does the woman's perception of the baby change during pregnancy?

   a. First trimester

   b. Second trimester

   c. Third trimester

5. What is the significance of quickening in the woman's developing relationship with her fetus?

6. Why might grief have a place during a desired and normal pregnancy?

7. Describe the four maternal tasks of pregnancy, according to Rubin.

   a. ____________________________

   b. ____________________________

   c. ____________________________

   d. ____________________________

8. Describe the three developmental processes that the expectant father goes through during pregnancy.

   a. ____________________________

   b. ____________________________

   c. ____________________________

9. Describe three major factors that influence grandparents' responses to pregnancy and birth.

   a. ____________________________

   b. ____________________________

   c. ____________________________

10. Describe ways to ease the adaptation of siblings to the birth of an infant.

    a. Toddlers

    b. Preschoolers

c. School-age children

d. Adolescents

11. How may each of these factors influence a woman's psychosocial adaptation to pregnancy?

   a. Young age

   b. Absence of a partner

   c. Multiparity

12. How may health beliefs differ for pregnant clients from the following cultures?

   a. Hispanics

   b. Native Americans

   c. Southeast Asians

   d. Muslims

   e. Africans

13. What do each of these factors have to do with a woman's choice to take childbirth classes?

   a. Income

   b. Desire to participate

c. Fear

14. List content typically covered in early pregnancy classes.
    a. First trimester

    b. Second trimester

15. List three important precautions for exercise classes during pregnancy.
    a. ______________________________
    b. ______________________________
    c. ______________________________
16. What are important topics to cover related to cesarean birth preparation in each type of class?
    a. Cesarean birth preparation class

    b. Vaginal birth after cesarean (VBAC) class

CRITICAL THINKING EXERCISES

1. Talk to a pregnant woman about her psychological reactions to pregnancy. Compare her reactions with typical responses listed in the text.

2. Talk with expectant fathers about when their baby first became real to them.

3. Observe interactions of the nursing staff with a woman who did not have prenatal care. Do you note any differences from the interactions with women who have had prenatal care?

4. What are the major cultural groups you encounter in the clinical setting? What specific practices or beliefs can you identify that are unique to each group?

5. You may have to help a woman correct her labor breathing or breathe with her while she is in labor, so you must know it well. Practice the breathing techniques until you are comfortable with them. Then teach them to a friend or family member.

6. Try the breathing techniques during a stressful situation. For example, take a cleansing breath when you begin your next nursing test. Breathe slowly as you take the test. Did it help reduce your stress?

7. Prepare a birth plan that you would like, identifying any special preferences you would like to include in a birth experience.

CASE STUDY

Sara is a 17-year-old girl who is making her first visit to the prenatal clinic at 24 weeks' gestation with her first pregnancy. She admits that this pregnancy was not planned and that she has little contact with the baby's father. She quit school during her senior year of high school because she is embarrassed about her situation. She has gained 20 pounds and feels that she is unattractive and fat. She is the oldest of six children and lives at home with her parents.

1. What factors may be involved in Sara's delay in seeking prenatal care?

2. What two priority nursing diagnoses are apparent by Sara's situation?

3. What conflicts are likely between Sara and the clinic staff (physicians and nurses)?

4. What services besides prenatal care is Sara likely to need because of her situation?

5. What long-term consequences are more likely because of Sara's pregnancy at this time in her life? Why?

REVIEW QUESTIONS

Choose the correct answer.

1. A woman who is 12 weeks pregnant begins wearing maternity clothes. This is most likely an example of

   a. introversion.
   b. mimicry.
   c. narcissism.
   d. fantasy.

2. Choose the maternal behavior that best describes role playing during pregnancy.

   a. The woman shifts from saying, "I am pregnant" to "I am having a baby."
   b. The woman begins calling her fetus by a name rather than "it."
   c. The woman tries to care for infants while an experienced mother watches.
   d. The woman becomes less absorbed in her own needs and focuses on the fetus.

3. The nurse can best help a man assume his role as a parent by

   a. encouraging him to attend prenatal visits with the woman and ask questions.
   b. referring him to prenatal discussion groups for expectant fathers.
   c. advising the woman to limit discussions of her symptoms during early pregnancy.
   d. enrolling him in childbirth classes to involve him actively in the birth.

4. Choose the most likely reaction of an 8-year-old to his mother's pregnancy.

   a. Embarrassment or shame at his mother's appearance
   b. Inability to sense the reality of the infant
   c. Desire to role-play his big-brother status
   d. Interest in learning about the developing baby

5. The nurse is teaching a Laotian woman about self-care during pregnancy. The nurse can best determine if she learned the information by

   a. asking the woman to indicate what teaching she did and did not understand.
   b. observing for the woman's eye contact with the nurse during teaching.
   c. recognizing that nodding while being taught indicates understanding.
   d. having the woman restate the information that is taught.

6. The primary benefit of a preconception class is to

   a. reduce the risk of having a baby with a birth defect.
   b. begin the pregnancy in an optimal nutritional state.
   c. limit the number of unplanned pregnancies in the community.
   d. encourage the couple to have their baby at that facility.

7. The primary benefit of perinatal education is to help

   a. reduce the likelihood that parents will have problems with their infant.
   b. women have a satisfying, medication-free childbirth.
   c. parents become active in health maintenance during pregnancy and birth.
   d. enhance the chance that prospective parents will return to a hospital.

15

Nutrition for Childbearing

MATCHING KEY TERMS

Match the term with the correct definition.

1. ______ gynecologic age
2. ______ heme iron
3. ______ kilocalorie
4. ______ lactovegetarian
5. ______ lacto-ovovegetarian
6. ______ ovovegetarian
7. ______ pica
8. ______ nonheme iron
9. ______ nutrient density
10. ______ vegetarian
11. ______ vegan

a. Ingestion of nonfood substance
b. Measure of the energy value of foods
c. Quality of the protein, vitamins, and minerals per 100 calories
d. Number of years since onset of menstruation
e. Iron form most usable by body; obtained from meat, poultry, or fish
f. Iron form less usable by body; obtained from plants
g. One who eats no animal products
h. One whose diet is primarily plant foods and who avoids animal foods
i. Vegetarian who includes milk products in diet
j. Vegetarian who includes eggs in diet
k. Vegetarian who includes milk and eggs in diet

KEY CONCEPTS

1. List three major consequences associated with inadequate prenatal weight gain.

2. List three major consequences associated with excessive prenatal weight gain.

3. List suggested pregnancy weight gains for each category.
   a. Normal prepregnancy weight

   b. Prepregnancy BMI <19.8

c. Prepregnancy BMI 26-29

d. Prepregnancy BMI >29

4. A general guideline for pregnancy weight gain is ______ pounds (______ kg) during the first trimester and ______ pounds (______ kg) per week thereafter.
5. List the kilocalorie content for the following food types.
   a. Carbohydrates ______/g
   b. Protein ______/g
   c. Fat ______/g
6. After early pregnancy, the woman should take in about ______ kcal/day more than her usual intake.
7. Daily prepregnancy protein needs average ______ g. Protein need during pregnancy is ______ g daily.
8. Name the four fat-soluble vitamins.

9. List some high-calcium foods other than dairy foods.

10. Why is routine vitamin-mineral capsule supplementation risky?

11. The recommended fluid intake during pregnancy is ______ glasses (______ ounces each) daily. Which fluids should be limited?

12. What is the recommended number of servings from each food pyramid group for pregnant women?
    a. Whole grains

    b. Vegetables and fruits

    c. Dairy foods

d. Protein foods

e. Fats, oils, concentrated sugars

13. Explain the influence of "hot" and "cold" (or "yin" and "yang") on the diet of some pregnant women.

14. Describe the childbearing diet preferences typical of Southeast Asian women.
    a. Foods encouraged

    b. Foods discouraged

    c. Postpartum changes

    d. Nutrients commonly deficient in diet

    e. Increasing nutrient intake with traditional foods

15. Describe the childbearing diet preferences typical of Hispanic women.
    a. Influence of "hot" and "cold" theory

    b. Common foods

    c. Common problem areas in the diet

16. Describe eligibility aspects of the WIC (Women, Infants and Children) program.

17. Which nutrients are usually lacking in diets of adolescents?

18. Describe nursing approaches that enhance the likelihood that an adolescent will follow a nutritional diet during pregnancy.

19. Explain how a vegetarian woman can meet needs of pregnancy for each nutrient listed.

   a. Protein

   b. Calcium

   c. Vitamin B_{12}

20. List nursing teaching that helps the pregnant woman manage nausea and vomiting.

21. What nutritional problems may the multipara have?

22. What additional nutritional needs does the woman with a multifetal pregnancy have?

23. What nutritional needs do women in each of these situations have?

   a. Substance abuse

   b. Smoking

   c. Alcohol abuse

24. How may each of these drugs interfere with nutrition during pregnancy?
    a. Marijuana

    b. Heroin

    c. Cocaine

    d. Amphetamine

25. What problems may occur in each of these lactating mothers?
    a. Dieter

    b. Adolescent

    c. Vegan

    d. One who avoids dairy products

26. What are the recommendations for each of these substances during lactation?
    a. Alcohol

    b. Caffeine

    c. Fluid intake

CRITICAL THINKING EXERCISES

1. Select a cultural group prevalent in your clinical agency. Ask the women if there are any foods that are encouraged or forbidden by their culture during pregnancy and

the reasons for each. Ask them how long they have been in the United States and how this influences their food choices.

2. Determine what non-English diet pamphlets and teaching materials are available at your clinical facility.
3. Use a pediatric textbook or growth chart to solve this problem related to a young adolescent's weight gain during pregnancy.

   Prepregnancy height: 64 inches (162 cm)
   Prepregnancy weight: 105 pounds (47.7 kg)
   Expected normal weight gain over 40 weeks: ____ pounds (____ kg)
   Expected weight gain for pregnancy: ____ pounds (____ kg)
   Total desired weight gain during pregnancy: ____ pounds (____ kg)

4. Call your local WIC program and tell them you are a nursing student. Ask about services they provide, eligibility criteria, and the number of women and children served in your area. If possible, observe a counseling session.
5. Complete a 24-hour diet history on yourself. Determine whether you meet recommended daily allowances (RDA) and what, if any, changes you should make.
6. Ask pregnant or postpartum women if they are aware of food cravings or aversions during pregnancy. What nutritional consequences might result from those you find?

CASE STUDY

Carmen Lopez is a 23-year-old Latina who is pregnant with her third baby. She is being seen for the first time in the clinic. Her other two children are 1 and 2 years old. Her last menstrual period was 15 weeks ago. She is 63 inches tall and weighs 152 pounds, 15 pounds more than her prepregnant weight. Her hemoglobin is 10.5 g/dl. She says she "can't drink milk" but prefers to drink colas. Carmen is married and her husband works as a gardener.

1. What is Carmen's top-priority nutrition-related problem?

2. What nutritional problems are likely during this pregnancy? What foods help manage these problems?

3. What cultural aspects should the nurse consider?

REVIEW QUESTIONS

Choose the correct answer.

1. The recommended total weight gain for a 15-year-old of normal weight for height should be about
   a. 12 pounds.
   b. 20 pounds.
   c. 35 pounds.
   d. 45 pounds.
2. Poor weight gain during early pregnancy is associated with
   a. pregnancy-induced hypertension.
   b. small-for-gestational-age infants.
   c. preterm labor and birth.
   d. high risk for postpartum hemorrhage.

3. To reduce the incidence of neural tube defects such as spina bifida, women of childbearing age are recommended to consume
   a. 0.4 mg folic acid per day in foods and supplements.
   b. 300 extra calories near the expected conception date.
   c. 60 mg of supplemental iron, in addition to high-iron foods.
   d. two added servings of foods high in vitamin C.

4. Choose the correct nursing teaching about a woman's iron supplement during pregnancy.
   a. Take the iron 30 minutes before the first food of the day.
   b. Taking the iron with dairy foods will reduce the gastric side effects.
   c. Stools are somewhat loose and are lighter brown than usual.
   d. A food high in vitamin C may enhance absorption of iron.

5. A calcium supplement is best taken
   a. with high-iron foods.
   b. at bedtime.
   c. with meals.
   d. upon arising.

6. When teaching an adolescent about nutrition during pregnancy, the nursing approach should
   a. focus on the girl's responsibility to her fetus.
   b. provide as many choices as possible from nutritious foods.
   c. ask the girl to limit snacking and fast foods.
   d. explain how a good pregnancy diet will promote her health.

7. The main risk to a woman who practices pica during pregnancy is
   a. inadequate intake of essential nutrients.
   b. rapid absorption of nutrients such as iron.
   c. reduced fluid intake because of ice consumption.
   d. nonacceptance of the practice by caregivers.

8. Choose the correct nursing approach regarding caffeine use during pregnancy.
   a. Teach that caffeine has not been shown to be a risk.
   b. Limit total intake of caffeine-containing drinks to four daily.
   c. Discuss sources of caffeine in addition to coffee and tea.
   d. Drink one additional glass of plain water for each caffeine-containing drink.

9. A non–breast-feeding woman is anxious to lose weight after birth. Which nursing education is most appropriate?
   a. She may begin dieting immediately since she is not breast-feeding.
   b. She should consume a minimum of 1800 calories each day to maintain energy.
   c. She should take her prenatal vitamin-mineral supplement while dieting.
   d. She should wait at least 3 weeks before beginning a diet.

16

Prenatal Diagnostic Tests

MATCHING KEY TERMS

Match the term with the correct definition.

1. ______ alpha-fetoprotein (AFP)
2. ______ amniocentesis
3. ______ biophysical profile
4. ______ chorionic villus sampling (CVS)
5. ______ lecithin/sphingomyelin ratio
6. ______ neural tube defect
7. ______ surfactant
8. ______ ultrasonography

a. Imaging technique that uses high-frequency sound waves to visualize internal body structures
b. Substance secreted by mature fetal lungs
c. Congenital defect of the spinal cord
d. Method of evaluating fetal status
e. Tissue obtained from fetal side of the developing placenta
f. Ratio used to determine fetal lung maturity
g. Withdrawing amniotic fluid for laboratory examination
h. Fetal protein used to screen for specific abnormalities

KEY CONCEPTS

1. List typical purposes for an ultrasound examination during the
   a. first trimester

   b. second and third trimesters

2. In which type of ultrasound examination is a full bladder needed, transvaginal or transabdominal? What is the reason?

3. Under what circumstances is an accurate gestational age especially important? How is it assessed by ultrasonography? When is the gestational age determination most accurate?

4. What conditions are suggested by alpha-fetoprotein levels that are
   a. low

   b. high

5. What is triple-marker screening and what is its purpose? What follow-up tests may be needed?

6. Chorionic villus sampling (CVS) is done as early as _______ weeks of pregnancy.
7. List four risks of CVS.

8. List purposes for amniocentesis during the
   a. second trimester

   b. third trimester

9. What lecithin-sphingomyelin (L/S) ratio suggests fetal lung maturity? In what maternal disorder may this ratio not be associated with fetal lung maturity?

10. What is the purpose of testing phosphatidylglycerol (PG) and phosphatidylinositol (PI) in the amniotic fluid?

11. Mid-trimester amniocentesis results are known in about _______ weeks.
12. What is the purpose of a vibroacoustic stimulation test (VST)?

13. The basic principle of the contraction stress test is to observe the response of the ___________________ to the stress of _____________________.

14. What two methods are used to cause uterine contractions when doing a contraction stress test?

15. Describe possible results and implications of a contraction stress test.

16. The biophysical profile assesses which five fetal parameters?

17. What is the significance of oligohydramnios?

CRITICAL THINKING EXERCISES

Test your knowledge of nonstress tests. Using Figures 16-8 A and B in the text, answer the following questions about each strip.

Figure 16-8 A:

a. Baseline fetal heart rate?

b. Time duration of each strip?

c. Number of accelerations?

d. Number of decelerations?

e. Beats per minute and duration of the accelerations?

f. Reactive? Why or why not?

Figure 16-8 B:

a. Baseline fetal heart rate?

b. Time duration of each strip?

c. Number of accelerations?

d. Number of decelerations?

e. Beats per minute and duration of the accelerations?

f. Reactive? Why or why not?

CASE STUDIES

1. Joann is a primigravida with pregnancy-induced hypertension in her 35th week of pregnancy. She is scheduled for amniocentesis this morning.
   a. Why is she having the test?

   b. What preprocedure and postprocedure care is indicated?

2. Betty is an insulin-dependent diabetic in her 32nd week of pregnancy. She is scheduled for a nonstress test.
   a. Why is she having the test?

   b. What findings suggest that the fetus is healthy?

   c. How often is this test likely to be performed?

REVIEW QUESTIONS

Choose the correct answer.

1. The fetal heartbeat should be visible on ultrasound by the
   a. 4th week following the last menstrual period.
   b. 8th week following the last menstrual period.
   c. 12th week following the last menstrual period.
   d. 20th week following the last menstrual period.

2. Fewer fetal movements than expected suggest possible
   a. intrauterine fetal growth retardation.
   b. inaccurate gestational age dating.
   c. rapid intrauterine fetal maturation.
   d. reduced placental perfusion with fetal hypoxia.

3. Choose appropriate client teaching related to maternal serum alpha-fetoprotein (MSAFP) analysis.
   a. Abnormal MSAFP levels should be followed by more specific tests.
   b. High MSAFP levels are usually associated with chromosome abnormalities.
   c. Having MSAFP testing will eliminate the need to do an ultrasound examination.
   d. The initial MSAFP testing will be done at 12 weeks of gestation.

4. Choose the correct client teaching following amniocentesis.
   a. Drink 1 to 2 quarts of clear fluid to replace fluid taken in the procedure.
   b. Resume all normal activities when desired.
   c. Report persistent contractions, vaginal bleeding, or fluid leaking.
   d. Eat a diet with increased iron for the 2 days after amniocentesis.

5. A woman who is assessing fetal movements each day should notify her health care provider if
   a. more than 6 movements are felt during a 30- to 60-minute period.
   b. fewer than 12 fetal movements occur during the day.
   c. the movement pattern changes very little from day to day.
   d. fetal movements are more frequent during the evening than in the morning.

17

Giving Birth

MATCHING KEY TERMS

Match the term with the correct definition.

1. ______ amniotomy
2. ______ attitude
3. ______ crowning
4. ______ EDD
5. ______ engagement
6. ______ ferning
7. ______ molding
8. ______ nitrazine paper
9. ______ nuchal cord
10. ______ para
11. ______ station

a. Measurement of descent of the fetal presenting part
b. Estimated date of delivery
c. Descent of widest fetal presenting part to zero station
d. Number of pregnancies that end after 20 weeks' gestation
e. Change in the shape of the fetal head during birth
f. Relationship of fetal body parts to one another
g. Umbilical cord around the fetal neck
h. Artificial rupture of the amniotic sac
i. Used for assessment of pH to detect ruptured membranes
j. Appearance of the fetal presenting part at the vaginal opening
k. Characteristic appearance of dry amniotic fluid when viewed under a microscope

KEY CONCEPTS

1. Explain why each characteristic of uterine contractions is important during birth.
   a. Coordination

   b. Involuntary

   c. Intermittent

2. Describe differences in how the upper and lower uterus contract during labor. Why is it important that the upper and lower parts of the uterus have different contraction characteristics?

3. Why should the nurse regularly check the woman's bladder during labor?

4. What maternal and fetal conditions may reduce fetal tolerance for the intermittent interruption in placental blood flow that occurs during contractions?

5. What are the changes in fetal lung fluid during pregnancy, during labor, and after birth?

6. What are the two powers of labor? When during labor do they come into play?

7. Why are the sutures and fontanels of the fetal head important during birth?

8. Describe the most common variations in
   a. fetal lie

   b. fetal attitude

   c. fetal presentation

9. Draw the three variations of a breech presentation. Which one is most common?

10. What fetal anatomic reference point is used for each presentation or position?
    a. Vertex

    b. Face

    c. Breech

11. How can nursing measures help increase a woman's sense of control during labor?

12. How do each of these factors affect the onset of labor?
    a. Fetal hormone production
    b. Change in maternal progesterone and estrogen relationship

13. Describe common premonitory signs of labor. Are there differences between a nullipara and a parous woman?

14. Describe each mechanism of labor and its significance.
    a. Descent
    b. Engagement
    c. Flexion
    d. Internal rotation
    e. Extension
    f. External rotation
    g. Expulsion

15. Why must the fetal head and shoulders undergo rotation within the pelvis?

16. What are the three labor phases within stage I? What cervical dilation marks each phase?

17. How do average durations of labor vary between nulliparas and multiparas for first and second stages of labor?

18. List four signs that suggest that the placenta has separated.

19. Why is it important that the uterus remain firmly contracted after birth?

20. Complete the chart about the characteristics of normal labor.

	First Stage	Second Stage	Third Stage	Fourth Stage
Duration Nullipara:				
Multipara:				
Cervical Dilation Latent phase:				
Active phase:				
Transition phase:				
Uterine Contractions Latent phase:				
Active phase:				
Transition phase:				
Discomfort				
Maternal Behaviors				

21. The two nursing priorities when a woman enters a birth center are to determine ____________________ and ____________________.
22. When should the nurse *not* perform a vaginal examination? Why?

23. List important nursing assessments after the membranes rupture. Describe normal and abnormal assessments, as appropriate.

24. Why is it important to place a small pillow under one hip if the mother must lie on her back?

25. What maternal vital signs may indicate problems?
    a. Blood pressure

    b. Temperature

26. Describe basic comfort measures the nurse can provide during labor.

27. Immediate nursing care of the newborn includes supporting __________ and __________ function and placing ____________________.
28. Nursing care of the mother during the fourth stage of labor focuses on observing for _____________ and relieving _______________.
29. Discuss the relationship between a full bladder and postpartum hemorrhage.

CRITICAL THINKING EXERCISES

1. Place a tennis ball in a sock. Slowly push it out of the cuff to get the idea of cervical effacement and dilation.

2. In performing a vaginal examination during labor, the nurse collects the following information:
   a. Cervix is open 4 cm and its length is about 0.5 cm.
   b. The presenting part is rounded and hard. A triangular depression on the presenting part has three linear depressions leading from it. Clear fluid flows from the vagina as the fetus moves during the examination.

   What is the correct interpretation of these findings?

3. During your clinical experience, note what effects fetal presentation and position have on the woman's comfort and the progress of labor.

4. Review the routine permits used in the intrapartal area at your birth facility.

5. During your clinical experience, use Leopold's maneuvers to identify fetal presentation, position, and engagement.

CASE STUDY

Erin is an 18-year-old primigravida who calls the intrapartum unit because she thinks she may be in labor.

1. What information should the nurse obtain to help determine if Erin is in true labor?

The nurse decides that Erin may be in true labor and tells her to come to the birth center. On arrival, Erin says she thinks her "water broke."

2. What is the priority nursing care at this time?

3. What tests might the nurse use to verify that Erin's membranes have indeed ruptured?

The nurse determines that Erin's contractions are every 5 minutes, of moderate intensity, and last 40 seconds. The fetal heart rate is 135 to 145, and it accelerates when the fetus moves. Amniotic fluid is light green with small white flecks in it. Vaginal examination reveals that the cervix is dilated 5 cm and is completely effaced. The fetal presenting part is hard and round, and a small triangular depression on the head can be felt in Erin's right posterior pelvis.

4. What stage (and phase, if applicable) of labor is Erin in?

5. How should the fetal heart rate be interpreted?

6. Is the amniotic fluid normal?

7. What is the fetal presentation and position?

Erin complains of back discomfort during each contraction.

8. What interventions might make this discomfort more tolerable?

After 4 hours of labor in the birth center, Erin's cervix is completely dilated and effaced, and the fetal station is +1. Erin feels the need to push during some contractions.

9. What is the safest way to advise Erin to push?

10. When should Erin be positioned for birth?

Erin gives birth to a boy. The nurse notes the following on the baby at 1 minute: heart rate 138, loud vigorous crying, spontaneous movement and flexion of the extremities, and pink skin color except for bluish color of the hands and feet.

11. What Apgar score will be assigned to the baby?

12. What are the priority nursing measures for the infant in relation to
    a. respiration

    b. temperature regulation

Erin is now in the fourth stage of labor. She and her husband are getting acquainted with their baby, Derrick.

13. During what time period does the fourth stage involve?

14. What nursing assessments are needed to observe for hemorrhage?

15. What are appropriate pain relief methods during the fourth stage?

REVIEW QUESTIONS

Choose the correct answer.

1. When assessing a laboring woman's blood pressure, the nurse should
   a. inflate the cuff at the beginning of a contraction.
   b. check the blood pressure between two contractions.
   c. expect a slight elevation of the blood pressure.
   d. position the woman on her back with her knees bent.

2. A woman is admitted in active labor. Her leukocyte count is 14,500. Based on this information, the nurse should
   a. assess the woman for other evidence of infection.
   b. inform the nurse-midwife of the results promptly.
   c. use isolation techniques to limit spread of infection.
   d. record the expected results in the woman's chart.

3. The most appropriate time for the nurse to encourage a laboring woman to push is during
   a. the interval between contractions.
   b. first-stage labor.
   c. second-stage labor.
   d. whenever she feels the need.

4. The abbreviation LOA means that the fetal occiput is
   a. on the examiner's left and in the front of the pelvis.
   b. in the left front part of the mother's pelvis.
   c. anterior to the fetal breech.
   d. lower than the fetal breech.

5. Choose the most reliable evidence that true labor has begun.
   a. Regular contractions that occur every 15 minutes.
   b. Change in the amount of cervical thinning.
   c. Increased ease of breathing with frequent urination.
   d. A sudden urge to do household tasks.

6. The nurse should note how long the interval between contractions lasts because
   a. maternal cells restore their glucose levels during the interval.
   b. a very short interval requires earlier administration of analgesia.
   c. most exchange of fetal oxygen and waste products occurs then.
   d. the interval becomes longer as cervical dilation increases.

7. What is the primary benefit of the stress of labor to the newborn?
   a. It stimulates breathing and elimination of lung fluid.
   b. It increases alertness and enhances parent-infant bonding.
   c. It speeds peristalsis to eliminate meconium quickly.
   d. It enhances tolerance of microorganisms from others.

8. Choose the abbreviation that represents the fetal presentation and position that is most favorable for vaginal birth.
   a. LOA
   b. RMP
   c. LST
   d. ROP

9. A station of +1 means that the
   a. maternal cervix is open 1 cm.
   b. mother's ischial spines project into her pelvis 1 cm.
   c. fetus is unlikely to be born vaginally because the pelvis is small.
   d. fetal presenting part is 1 cm below the mother's ischial spines.

10. Bloody show differs from active vaginal bleeding in that bloody show
    a. quickly clots on the perineal pad.
    b. is dark red and mixed with mucus.
    c. flows freely from the vagina during vaginal examination.
    d. decreases in quantity as labor progresses.

11. A laboring woman abruptly stops her previous breathing techniques during a contraction and makes low-pitched grunting sounds. The priority nursing action is to
    a. ask her if she needs pain medication.
    b. turn her to her left side.
    c. assess contraction duration.
    d. look at her perineum.

12. A woman's membranes rupture during a contraction. The priority nursing action is to
    a. assess the fetal heart rate.
    b. note the color of the discharge.
    c. check the woman's vital signs.
    d. determine whether the fluid has a foul odor.

13. When palpating labor contractions, the nurse should
    a. use the palm of one hand while palpating the lower uterus.
    b. avoid palpating during the period of maximum intensity.
    c. place the fingertips over the fundus of the uterus.
    d. limit palpation to three consecutive contractions.

14. When doing Leopold's maneuvers, the nurse palpates a hard round object in the uterine fundus. A smooth, rounded surface is on the mother's right side, and irregular movable parts are felt on her left side. An irregularly shaped fetal part is felt in the suprapubic area and is easily moved upward. How should these findings be interpreted?
    a. The fetal presentation is cephalic, the position is ROA, and the presenting part is engaged.
    b. The fetal presentation is cephalic, the position is LOP, and the presenting part is not engaged.
    c. The fetal presentation is breech, the position is RST, and the presenting part is engaged.
    d. The fetal presentation is breech, the position is RSA, and the presenting part is not engaged.

15. When doing the fourth Leopold maneuver, the nurse determines that the cephalic prominence is on the same side as the fetal back. How should this assessment be interpreted?
    a. The fetus is in a breech presentation with the head extended.
    b. The fetus is in a face presentation with the head extended.
    c. The fetus is in a transverse lie with the face toward the mother's back.
    d. The fetus is in a cephalic presentation with the head well flexed.

16. When auscultating the fetal heart rate, the nurse notes a rate of 86 and a soft sound. The appropriate nursing action is to
    a. chart this expected fetal heart rate.
    b. notify the physician of the abnormal fetal heart rate.
    c. determine the woman's current labor status.
    d. assess the mother's radial pulse.

17. The nurse notes the following contraction pattern:

Beginning of Contraction	**End of Contraction**
11:15:00	11:15:40
11:20:00	11:20:45
11:24:00	11:24:50
11:28:30	11:29:10
11:33:00	11:33:35

Choose the correct documentation for the pattern.
    a. Contractions every 4-5 minutes; duration 40-50 seconds.
    b. Contractions every 5 minutes; duration 35-40 seconds.
    c. Contractions every 3-5 minutes; duration 30-50 seconds.
    d. Contractions every 3-4 minutes; duration 30-40 seconds.

18. A woman who is having her third baby planned epidural analgesia for labor and birth. However, her labor was so rapid that she did not have the epidural. What is the best nursing approach in this case?
    a. Congratulate her on having a labor that was quicker than expected.
    b. Use open-ended questions to clarify her true feelings about the experience.
    c. Tactfully explain why a nonepidural labor and birth is actually better.
    d. Explain that it is often difficult to time epidural analgesia for labor.

19. A woman having her first baby has been observed 2 hours for labor but is having false labor contractions. Choose the most appropriate teaching before she returns home.
    a. "It is unlikely that your labor will be fast, so you can stay home until your water breaks."
    b. "If your water breaks, you can wait until contractions are 5 minutes apart or closer."
    c. "As long as the baby is active, there is no hurry to return to the birth center."
    d. "Your contractions will usually be 5 minutes apart or closer for 1 hour if labor is real."

18

Intrapartum Fetal Monitoring

MATCHING KEY TERMS

Match the term with the correct definition.

1. ______ amnioinfusion
2. ______ hypoxia
3. ______ nuchal cord
4. ______ nadir
5. ______ tocolytic
6. ______ uterine resting tone
7. ______ transducer

a. Translates fetal heart motion into electrical signals
b. Cord around the fetal neck
c. Reduced oxygen to the blood
d. Lowest point
e. Infusion of saline into the amniotic cavity to reduce cord compression or wash out meconium
f. Muscle tension when the uterus is not contracting
g. Drug that reduces uterine muscle contractions

KEY CONCEPTS

1. List the five factors that affect fetal oxygenation.

2. Explain how each of these factors influences the fetal heart rate.
   a. Autonomic nervous system

   b. Baroreceptors

   c. Chemoreceptors

   d. Adrenal glands

   e. Central nervous system

3. Explain how each factor can reduce fetal oxygenation. How would you explain each in simple terms to a woman in labor?
   a. Maternal hypotension
   b. Maternal hypertension
   c. Maternal hypoxia
   d. Hypertonic uterine activity
   e. Placental disruptions
   f. Umbilical cord blood flow compression
   g. Fetal bradycardia or tachycardia

4. List the advantages and limitations of the two methods of intrapartal fetal assessment: auscultation with palpation of contractions and electronic fetal monitoring.

	Auscultation With Palpation	**Electronic Fetal Monitoring**
Advantages		
Limitations		

5. What must the nurse consider when evaluating intrauterine pressures from a solid catheter versus a fluid-filled catheter?

6. Define these terms that describe the fetal heart rate.
   a. Normal

b. Bradycardia

c. Tachycardia

d. Short-term variability

e. Long-term variability

7. List factors that may decrease short-term and long-term variability.

8. Why is variability an important component of fetal heart pattern evaluation?

9. Describe each fetal heart rate periodic change, list possible causes, and note whether the change is reassuring or nonreassuring and the basic actions to take if nonreassuring.

Periodic Change	Appearance on Strip	Possible Causes	Reassuring or Nonreassuring (With Nursing Actions)
Accelerations			
Early decelerations			
Late decelerations			
Variable decelerations			

10. Describe methods that may be used during labor to clarify the fetal condition.

11. The normal fetal scalp pH is ______ to ______. Use a medical-surgical nursing text to compare to the normal adult pH.

12. List possible nursing interventions to identify and/or correct the cause of a nonreassuring fetal monitor pattern.
    a. Identifying the cause

    b. Increasing placental perfusion

    c. Increasing maternal oxygen saturation

    d. Reducing umbilical cord compression

13. List two uses for amnioinfusion.

CRITICAL THINKING EXERCISES

1. Look at fetal monitor strips in your clinical facility. Identify the following about each.
    a. Baseline rate

    b. Presence of variability (short and/or long term)

    c. Periodic changes

    d. Contraction frequency, duration, and intensity

    e. Nursing interventions for nonreassuring patterns

    f. Fetal responses to nursing interventions

2. Your friend is 7 months pregnant and is uncertain about whether she wants to have electronic fetal monitoring. Develop a plan to explain the pros and cons of each method of fetal surveillance during labor.

REVIEW QUESTIONS

Choose the correct answer.

1. Firm contractions that occur every 3 minutes and last 100 seconds (1 minute, 40 seconds) may reduce fetal oxygen supply because they
   a. cause fetal bradycardia and reduce oxygen concentration.
   b. activate the fetal sympathetic nervous system.
   c. limit time for oxygen exchange in the placenta.
   d. suppress the normal variability of the fetal heart.

2. The expected response of the fetal heart rate to active fetal movement is
   a. suppression of normal short-term variability for 15 seconds.
   b. acceleration of at least 15 beats per minute for 15 seconds.
   c. increase in long-term variability by 15 beats per minute.
   d. acceleration followed by a 15-second deceleration of the heart rate.

3. The nurse notes a pattern of variable decelerations to 75 bpm on the fetal monitor. The initial nursing action is to
   a. reposition the woman.
   b. administer oxygen.
   c. increase the intravenous fluid infusion.
   d. stimulate the fetal scalp.

4. The woman who uses cocaine is more likely to have which pattern on the electronic fetal heart monitor?
   a. Tachycardia.
   b. Periodic accelerations.
   c. Variable decelerations.
   d. Late decelerations.

5. The tocotransducer should be placed
   a. in the suprapubic area.
   b. in the fundal area.
   c. over the xiphoid process.
   d. within the uterus.

6. Choose the important precaution when a fluid-filled catheter is used to monitor the uterine contractions during labor.
   a. The tip of the catheter must be at the same level as the transducer.
   b. The fluid that fills the catheter must be warmed to room temperature.
   c. Understand that pressures within the fluid-filled catheter are higher than those in the solid catheter.
   d. Fluid-filled catheters cannot be used when a spiral electrode is applied.

7. The nurse notes a pattern of decelerations on the fetal monitor that begins shortly after the contraction and returns to baseline just before the contraction is over. The correct nursing response is to
   a. give the woman oxygen by face mask at 8 to 10 L/min.
   b. position the woman on her opposite side.
   c. increase the rate of the woman's intravenous fluid.
   d. continue to observe and record the normal pattern.

19

Pain Management for Childbirth

MATCHING KEY TERMS

Match the term with the correct definition.

1. _____ agonist
2. _____ analgesia
3. _____ anesthesia
4. _____ antagonist
5. _____ endorphin
6. _____ pain tolerance

a. Blocking effect of a drug
b. Loss of sensation with or without loss of consciousness
c. Maximum pain one is willing to endure
d. Relief of pain without loss of consciousness
e. Causing a physiologic effect
f. Natural substance similar to morphine

KEY CONCEPTS

1. Explain how childbirth pain may differ from other pain.

2. How can excessive pain reduce fetal oxygenation?

3. How is labor affected when the fetus is in an occiput posterior (OP) position?

4. List four categories of nonpharmacologic techniques that can be used during labor.

5. Give an example of both direct and indirect effects of maternal drugs on the fetus.

6. What is the purpose of giving a test dose before doing an epidural block? What would be signs of problems after the test dose, and what causes these signs?

7. What causes these adverse reactions to epidural block analgesia/anesthesia? What may be done to prevent or correct each?
   a. Headache

   b. Hypotension

   c. Bladder distention

   d. Prolonged second-stage labor

8. In which regional anesthesia method is it *desirable* to obtain cerebrospinal fluid (CSF)? Why?

9. Complete the following table on intrapartal pain relief methods.

Technique	Advantages	Disadvantages	Adverse Effects	Nursing Care
Systemic analgesics				
Epidural block				
Local infiltration				
Pudendal block				
Subarachnoid block				
General anesthesia				

10. List methods to relieve pain of a postspinal headache.

11. Under what two circumstances should butorphanol (Stadol) or nalbuphine (Nubain) *not* be given to a woman in labor?

CRITICAL THINKING EXERCISES

1. Make a plan to help a woman deal with the anxiety and fear that may accompany labor. Use the experience of a woman you have helped to care for or that of a friend or relative or your own experience when making your plan.
2. Talk to an anesthesia clinician in your clinical facility about how staff compensate for the normal changes of pregnancy when giving anesthesia.

CASE STUDY

Alice is a 16-year-old primigravida in the latent phase of first-stage labor. She did not attend prepared childbirth classes. She is very anxious and tense, crying during each contraction. Her cervix is dilated to 3 cm, station –1, effacement 90%, and the membranes are ruptured (fluid is clear). Her baseline vital signs are pulse 92, respirations 24, and blood pressure 120/70. FHR is 126-136 with average variability. Her 17-year-old husband is at her side but seems very frustrated and helpless. Her parents live out of town.

1. What assumptions must the nurse be careful to avoid when caring for Alice?

2. What initial nursing interventions are appropriate to help Alice cope with her contractions?

3. Can Alice be taught breathing techniques at this time? If so, how should the nurse approach the teaching?

4. Are analgesics desirable for Alice at this time? Why or why not?

Alice progresses to 6-cm cervical dilation, effacement 100%, and fetal station 0. Maternal and fetal vital signs remain stable. Alice wants "something stronger" for the pain.

5. What pharmacologic options are possible for Alice, based on the information given?

Alice receives epidural block analgesia.

6. What nursing care is essential related to the block? Why?

Alice gives birth to a 6-pound 2-ounce girl. Apgar scores are 7 at 1 minute and 9 at 5 minutes.

7. What are appropriate nursing measures related to Alice's epidural while Alice is in the recovery area?

REVIEW QUESTIONS

Choose the correct answer.

1. Firm sacral pressure is likely to be most helpful in which situation?
   a. Rapid labor and birth.
   b. Fetal occiput posterior position.
   c. Oxytocin induction of labor.
   d. If analgesics should be avoided.

2. A woman receives meperidine (Demerol) during labor. Because this analgesic is being used, the nurse should have on hand
   a. butorphanol (Stadol).
   b. lidocaine (Xylocaine).
   c. nalbuphine (Nubain).
   d. naloxone (Narcan).

3. When stocking a cart for epidural analgesia, the most important nursing action is to
   a. add additional bags of intravenous normal saline.
   b. place anticoagulant drugs to allow rapid access.
   c. verify that no epidural drugs have preservatives.
   d. provide an indwelling catheterization tray.

4. The physician orders meperidine (Demerol) 35 mg and hydroxyzine (Vistaril) 25 mg low IV push for a laboring woman. The appropriate nursing action is to
   a. remind the physician that hydroxyzine is not given IV.
   b. give the meperidine IV and the hydroxyzine deep IM.
   c. dilute the two drugs before giving them slow IV push.
   d. give the drugs as ordered by the physician.

5. The appropriate nursing action for a woman who has a postspinal headache is to
   a. keep her bed in a semi-Fowler's position.
   b. encourage intake of fluids that she enjoys.
   c. have her ambulate at least every 4 hours.
   d. restrict intake of high-carbohydrate foods.

6. A woman having her first baby is trying to use breathing techniques during labor, but she has difficulty concentrating. She is 3-cm dilated, 80% effaced, and the station is 0. What nursing measure can best help her?
   a. Encourage her to change to a different breathing pattern.
   b. Have a family member other than her husband coach her.
   c. Give her a very small dose of narcotic that is ordered PRN.
   d. Help her find a specific point in the room on which to focus.

7. A woman must have general anesthesia for planned cesarean birth because of previous back surgery. The nurse should therefore expect to administer
   a. naltrexone (Trexan).
   b. an oral barbiturate.
   c. ranitidine (Zantac).
   d. promethazine (Phenergan).

20

Nursing Care During Obstetrical Procedures

MATCHING KEY TERMS

Match the term with the correct definition.

1. _____ chignon
2. _____ dystocia
3. _____ iatrogenic
4. _____ oligohydramnios

a. Newborn scalp edema caused by a vacuum extractor
b. Abnormally small quantity of amniotic fluid
c. Difficult or prolonged labor
d. Adverse condition resulting from treatment

KEY CONCEPTS

1. List the potential complications of amniotomy.

2. List nursing considerations necessary prior to and after an amniotomy.

3. List three nursing measures following use of prostaglandin E_2 to ripen the cervix and the rationale for each.

4. Describe fetal and maternal nursing assessments associated with oxytocin infusion. What are signs of problems?

5. List nursing interventions if fetal or maternal assessments are not reassuring when oxytocin induction or augmentation of labor is being done.

6. Explain the purpose of each aspect of care for the woman having external version.

   a. Nonstress test

b. Ultrasound

c. Tocolytic drug

d. Rh immune globulin

e. Fetal heart rate monitoring

f. Uterine activity monitoring

7. Describe nursing care associated with a forceps- or vacuum extractor–assisted birth. What is the rationale for each?

8. List the major risks associated with an episiotomy.

9. Describe techniques that may reduce the need for an episiotomy.

10. Explain why cesarean birth is not necessarily easy for the newborn.

11. Explain the rationale for each intervention associated with cesarean birth.
    a. Medication such as famotidine administered.

    b. Placing a wedge under one hip

    c. Complete blood cell count, coagulation studies, blood type, and crossmatch

    d. Antibiotic

    e. Indwelling catheter

CRITICAL THINKING EXERCISES

1. Observe a cesarean birth and compare the sequence of events with those of vaginal birth. What are the similarities and differences?

2. What measures do you see the nursing staff taking to keep the emphasis on the birth experience rather than on surgery when a woman has cesarean birth?

3. Write a simply worded explanation that you might give to a woman immediately after birth about why you are placing a cold pack on her perineal area. How would you explain the change to warm packs the next day?

4. A woman gave birth to her first baby, a 9-pound boy. Low forceps with a mediolateral episiotomy were required. List three nursing diagnoses or collaborative problems that would be expected during the first 12 hours postpartum and appropriate nursing measures for each.

Nursing Diagnosis or Collaborative Problem	Nursing Interventions

CASE STUDY

Linda is a gravida 3, para 2, at 42 weeks' gestation. She is scheduled for oxytocin induction of labor. Her first two pregnancies ended at 39 and 40 weeks, and the babies weighed 8 pounds 13 ounces, and 9 pounds 11 ounces.

1. What is the probable reason for Linda's induction?

2. What tests might be performed before her induction?

Linda's initial assessments are normal and the fetal heart rate is reassuring. She is having an occasional light contraction, but no regular contractions.

3. How should the nurse set up the oxytocin infusion? What is the rationale for these precautions?

After 3 hours, Linda's cervix is dilated to 3 cm, effacement is 80%, and the fetal station is –1. Contractions are every 4 to 5 minutes, lasting 45 seconds, and of moderate intensity. The FHR is 132-148. The physician decides to perform an amniotomy.

4. What nursing measures are appropriate before and after the amniotomy?

5. Should there be any change in the oxytocin infusion at this time? Why or why not?

Linda's labor progresses and she is having contractions every 2 to 3 minutes, 75 to 90 seconds' duration, and firm. FHR is 130-140. She is dilated to 7 cm, effacement is 90%, and fetal station is –1.

6. Should there be any change in her oxytocin infusion at this time? Why or why not?

Despite adequate contractions, Linda's cervical dilation does not progress beyond 7 cm and she will have a cesarean birth.

7. What nursing measures are appropriate for the planned birth?

Linda delivers a 10-pound 3-ounce girl by low transverse cesarean birth.

8. What nursing care is appropriate for Linda while in the recovery phase?

REVIEW QUESTIONS

Choose the correct answer.

1. After the physician performs an amniotomy, the fluid is dark green with a mild odor and the FHR is 130-140. The most appropriate nursing care is to
   a. take the woman's temperature hourly until delivery.
   b. monitor the fetus more closely for nonreassuring signs.
   c. tell the woman that she cannot have anything by mouth.
   d. observe the woman closely for hypotension.

2. Choose the correct setup for oxytocin induction of labor.
   a. Oxytocin is mixed with an electrolyte solution and delivered as a single infusion.
   b. Oxytocin is mixed with normal saline to equal 10 ml and given slow IV push.
   c. Oxytocin is begun at a rapid rate; its rate is decreased as labor progresses.
   d. Oxytocin is given as a secondary infusion and is controlled by an infusion pump.

3. A method to prepare the cervix for induction of labor the following day is
   a. prostaglandin preparations.
   b. fetal fibronectin.
   c. oral oxytocin tablets.
   d. amniotomy.

4. Choose the nursing assessment finding that is most likely to occur with hypertonic uterine contractions.
   a. foul-smelling amniotic fluid.
   b. contraction interval of 90 seconds.
   c. fetal heart rate of 80 to 100 bpm.
   d. maternal pulse of 80 to 90/minute.

5. A woman has external version to change her fetus' position from breech to cephalic. Choose the post-procedure nursing observation that would indicate she should not be released to go home.
   a. FHR is 135-145 with average variability.
   b. Occasional mild, brief contractions occur.
   c. Maternal temperature is 99.2° F and pulse is 90.
   d. Vaginal discharge is a pale and watery fluid.

6. Parents of a newborn born with a forceps-assisted vaginal birth ask about small reddened areas on the infant's cheeks. The nurse should tell them that the areas
   a. are temporary and will disappear.
   b. are typical of all vaginal births.
   c. will be reported to the physician.
   d. may lead to a serious infection.

7. A urinary catheter should be readily available when a woman has a forceps-assisted birth because
   a. emergency cesarean birth may be required.
   b. edema reduces the woman's sensation to void after birth.
   c. a full bladder reduces available room in the pelvis.
   d. a large median or mediolateral episiotomy is likely.

8. During the recovery period after low forceps birth with a median episiotomy, the nurse should
   a. assess for purulent drainage from the episiotomy.
   b. apply cold packs to the perineal area promptly.
   c. expect a larger quantity of lochia rubra drainage.
   d. limit oral intake to ice chips until transfer to a room.

9. Choose correct preoperative teaching before planned cesarean birth.
   a. Oral intake will be limited to clear fluids for 12 hours before surgery.
   b. Intravenous fluids are usually continued for 2 days after birth.
   c. The woman will be asked to take deep breaths and cough regularly after birth.
   d. The nurse will help her ambulate to the restroom to urinate within 4 hours of birth.

10. The best method to prevent hemorrhage after cesarean birth is to
   a. provide regular analgesia to enhance urination.
   b. reposition the woman from side to side.
   c. observe vital signs for falling blood pressure.
   d. assess the uterine fundus regularly for firmness.

21

Postpartum Adaptations

MATCHING KEY TERMS

Match the term with the correct definition.

1. ______ attachment
2. ______ bonding
3. ______ catabolism
4. ______ en face
5. ______ engrossment
6. ______ entrainment
7. ______ fingertipping
8. ______ fundus
9. ______ involution
10. ______ Kegel exercises
11. ______ puerperium
12. ______ REEDA
13. ______ taking-in

a. Method to increase tone of muscles in the vaginal and urinary meatal area
b. Part of the uterus above the openings of the fallopian tubes
c. Conversion of living cellular substances to simpler compounds
d. Acronym that helps assess wound healing (redness, edema, ecchymosis, discharge, approximation)
e. Period from childbirth until return of the reproductive organs to their prepregnancy states
f. Retrogressive changes that return the reproductive organs to their prepregnancy states
g. First phase of maternal adaptation
h. Longer-term development of affection between the infant and significant other
i. Movement of the newborn in rhythm with adult speech
j. Position that facilitates eye-to-eye contact between parent and newborn
k. Development of an emotional tie to the infant
l. Initial touch characteristic between mother and newborn
m. Intense fascination between father and newborn

KEY CONCEPTS

1. Describe postpartum changes in the
   a. uterine muscle

   b. uterine muscle cells

   c. uterine lining

2. Describe the changes in lochia and when these occur.

3. Describe the effect of breast-feeding on
   a. uterine involution

   b. sexual intercourse

4. What is the significance of bradycardia during the early postpartum period?

5. What makes any pregnant and postpartum woman at risk for venous thrombosis? What factors increase this risk?

6. How does the leukocyte level change during the early postpartum period? How would a normal leukocyte level for a postpartum woman be interpreted for a nonpregnant woman?

7. Explain how a full bladder at birth can lead to postpartum hemorrhage.

8. Describe the influence of these hormones on lactation.
   a. Estrogen

   b. Progesterone

   c. Prolactin

   d. Oxytocin

9. Discuss which postpartum mothers would be appropriate candidates for Rho(D) immune globulin and rubella vaccine.

10. Describe the proper technique to massage a soft fundus. How should the nurse expel clots?

11. Complete the chart below for postpartum assessments.

Assessment	What to Assess and Expected Findings	Deviations From Normal, Cause, and Nursing Actions
Fundus		
Lochia		
Bladder		
Perineum		
Vital signs		
Breasts		
Lower extremities		

12. Write out in simple terms how you would teach a woman about each of these postpartum comfort measures.
    a. Cold packs
    b. Perineal care
    c. Topical medications
    d. How to sit
    e. Sitz baths

13. Describe additional nursing assessments and care for the woman who gave birth by cesarean.
    a. Respiratory

    b. Abdomen

    c. Intake and output

14. What teaching should you provide the postpartum woman to prevent constipation?

15. List signs and symptoms that the postpartum woman should report to her physician or nurse-midwife.

16. Describe the processes of bonding and attachment. Note the similarities and differences in these processes.

17. Describe progression of maternal touch.

18. Describe progression of maternal verbal behaviors.

19. Complete the table by describing maternal behaviors in the three phases of maternal adaptation. How can nurses help mothers meet their needs in each phase?

Phase	**Maternal Behaviors**	**Nursing Considerations**
Taking-in		
Taking-hold		
Letting-go		

20. Describe postpartum blues. What is the best response to them?

21. How can the nurse help the new father adapt to his role?

22. How should the nurse respond to the parent who is disappointed in the sex of the newborn?

23. What nursing measures can help the mother of twins attach to her babies?

24. New parents may not recognize signals from the infant that he or she has had enough stimulation and now needs to rest. What signals should the nurse teach parents to recognize?

CRITICAL THINKING EXERCISES

1. You may note that some postpartum women have a urine output that is greater than their oral fluid intake. Should you be concerned? Why or why not?

2. Ask a nurse on the gynecology surgery unit what the usual time is for a woman to first urinate after surgery (if a catheter is not used). How does this time interval compare to when a postpartum woman is expected to first urinate?

3. Write a narrative nurse's note to document expected findings for a postpartum woman 12 hours after birth.

4. If you are a parent, did you or your partner experience separation grief because of the demands of employment? How did you deal with it?

5. During clinical practice, observe the reactions of siblings to a new infant. What steps do you see parents take to reassure the older child that he or she is still loved?

6. What cultural practices related to childbirth do you see in your clinical setting? Does the nursing staff support these? Discuss specific cultural practices with new parents of a different culture than your own.

CASE STUDY

Nita is a multipara who vaginally delivered twin boys 4 hours ago. One weighed 6 pounds and the other weighed 5 pounds 6 ounces. She is admitted to the mother-baby unit after an uneventful recovery. Your initial assessment reveals the following data: temperature 37.6° C (97.9° F), pulse 60, respiration 20, blood pressure 110/70; fundus slightly soft and located to the right of the umbilicus; lochia moderate; midline episiotomy intact with slight edema.

1. What is your interpretation of these data?

2. What is your first intervention? Why?

3. What should you immediately teach Nita?

Nita's vital signs 8 hours after birth are blood pressure 112/80, temperature 37.2° C (99° F), pulse 52, respiration 18.

4. Are any nursing interventions needed based on these vital signs? What is the rationale for your judgment?

Nita plans to breast feed her twins. She successfully breast fed her other two children. However, she says, "I want to breast feed, but I really have a lot of cramping when I nurse. I don't remember having that with the other two children."

5. What is the nurse's best response?

6. Why is Nita having more cramping than with her other two infants?

7. What intervention can help this problem?

Nita is worried about constipation because she had the problem after her previous births and has been constipated during the last months of this pregnancy.

8. What interventions and teaching can help Nita avoid constipation?

Nita will receive Rh immune globulin (RhoGAM) and rubella vaccine before discharge.

9. Under what circumstances are these drugs given?

10. What precautions should the nurse teach Nita? Why?

On a home visit 2 days postpartum, the nurse assesses Nita's fundus as firm, midline, and −1.

11. Are these assessments normal? Why or why not? If they are not normal, is there an explanation?

12. What should the nurse expect to find in the lochia flow?

Nita's episiotomy is slightly reddened along the suture line, the edges are closely approximated, and there is no edema, bruising, or drainage.

13. Do these data support the supposition that the episiotomy is healing properly? Why or why not? What nursing actions are appropriate?

REVIEW QUESTIONS

Choose the correct answer.

1. When checking a woman's fundus 24 hours after cesarean birth of her third baby, the nurse finds her fundus at the level of her umbilicus, firm, and in the midline. The appropriate nursing action related to this assessment is to
   a. document the normal assessment.
   b. determine when she last urinated.
   c. limit her intake of oral fluids.
   d. massage her fundus vigorously.

2. A woman who is 18 hours postpartum says she is having "hot flashes" and "sweats all the time." The appropriate nursing response is to
   a. report her signs and symptoms of hypovolemic shock.
   b. tell her that her body is getting rid of unneeded fluid.
   c. notify her nurse-midwife that she may have an infection.
   d. limit her intake of caffeine-containing fluids.

3. A woman who is 3 hours postpartum has had difficulty urinating. She finally urinates 100 ml. The initial nursing action is to
   a. insert an indwelling catheter.
   b. have her drink additional fluids.
   c. assess the height of her fundus.
   d. chart the urination amount.

4. When teaching the postpartum woman about Peripads, the nurse should tell her that
   a. she can change to tampons when the initial perineal soreness goes away.
   b. pads having cold packs within them usually hold more lochia than regular pads.
   c. blood-soaked pads must be returned in a plastic bag to the hospital after discharge.
   d. the pads should be applied and removed in a front-to-back direction.

5. A young mother is excited about her first baby. Choose the best teaching to help her obtain adequate rest after discharge.
   a. Plan to sleep or rest any time the infant sleeps.
   b. Do all housecleaning while the infant sleeps.
   c. Cook several meals at once and freeze for later use.
   d. Tell family and friends not to visit for the first month.

6. Choose the best independent nursing action to aid episiotomy healing in the woman who is 24 hours postpartum.
   a. Antibiotic cream applications to the area.
   b. Warm sitz baths taken four times per day.
   c. Maintaining cold packs to the area at all times.
   d. Checking the leukocyte level.

7. To prevent breast engorgement, the nurse should teach the nonlactating postpartum woman to
   a. maintain loose-fitting clothing over her breasts.
   b. pump the breasts briefly if they become painful.
   c. limit fluid intake to suppress milk production.
   d. wear a well-fitting bra or breast binder constantly.

8. A woman who is 4 hours postpartum ambulates to the bathroom and suddenly has a large gush of lochia rubra. The nurse's first action should be to
   a. determine if the bleeding slows to normal or remains large.
   b. observe vital signs for signs of hypovolemic shock.
   c. check to see what her previous lochia flow has been.

d. identify the type of pain relief that was given when she was in labor.

9. To help the postpartum woman avoid constipation, the nurse should teach her to
   a. avoid intake of foods such as milk, cheese, or yogurt.
   b. take a laxative for the first 3 postpartum days.
   c. drink at least 2500 ml of noncaffeinated fluids daily.
   d. limit her walking until the episiotomy is fully healed.

10. Choose the sign or symptom that the new mother should be taught to report.
   a. Occasional uterine cramping when the infant nurses.
   b. Oral temperature that is 37.2° C (99° F) in the morning.
   c. Descent of the fundus one fingerbreadth each day.
   d. Reappearance of red lochia after it changes to serous.

11. Twelve hours after birth, a mother lies in bed resting. Although she will be discharged in another 12 hours, she does not ask about her baby or provide any care. What is the probable reason for her behavior?
   a. She is still in the taking-in phase of maternal adaptation.
   b. She shows behaviors that may lead to postpartum depression.
   c. She is still affected by medications given during labor.
   d. She may be dissatisfied with some aspect of the newborn.

12. A new father is reluctant to "spoil" his newborn when she cries by picking her up. The best nursing response is to
   a. teach him that she will eventually stop crying if he waits.
   b. take the baby to the nursery to allow the parents to rest.
   c. pick the baby up and rock her until she sleeps again.
   d. tell the father that the baby cries to communicate a need.

13. A newborn is rooming in with his teenage mother, who is watching TV. The nurse notes that the baby is awake and quiet. The best nursing action is to
   a. pick the baby up and point out his alert behaviors to the mother.
   b. tell the mother to pick up her baby and talk with him while he is awake.
   c. focus care on the mother, rather than the infant, so she can recuperate.
   d. encourage the mother to feed the infant before he begins crying.

14. The best nursing encouragement for parents to care for their infant is to
   a. stay out of the room for as long as possible.
   b. have the grandmother nearby as a backup.
   c. give positive feedback when they provide care.
   d. correct their performance whenever they make a mistake.

22

The Normal Newborn: Adaptation and Assessment

MATCHING KEY TERMS

Match the term with the correct definition.

1. ______ asphyxia
2. ______ bilirubin
3. ______ brown fat
4. ______ jaundice
5. ______ lanugo
6. ______ neutral thermal environment
7. ______ strabismus
8. ______ surfactant

a. Slippery fluid that reduces surface tension in lung alveoli
b. Tissue designed for newborn heat production
c. Surroundings in which the infant can maintain a stable temperature with minimal oxygen consumption and a low metabolic rate
d. Fine hair covering the fetus
e. Bilirubin staining of the skin and sclerae
f. Low blood oxygen and high blood and tissue carbon dioxide
g. "Crossed" eyes
h. Unusable component of hemolyzed erythrocytes

Listed below are conditions that may be found when the newborn is assessed. Match the condition with the part(s) of the body where it would be observed. Note if it is found only in males or only in females. Star those that are abnormal variations.

9. ______ candidiasis
10. ______ pseudomenstruation
11. ______ jaundice
12. ______ engorgement
13. ______ choanal atresia
14. ______ cephalhematoma
15. ______ syndactyly
16. ______ preauricular sinus
17. ______ hydrocele
18. ______ subconjunctival hemorrhage
19. ______ caput succedaneum
20. ______ lanugo
21. ______ Epstein's pearls
22. ______ hymenal tag
23. ______ polydactyly
24. ______ developmental hip dysplasia
25. ______ spina bifida
26. ______ cataract
27. ______ hypospadias
28. ______ vernix caseosa

a. Head
b. Mouth
c. Skin
d. Genitalia
e. Spine
f. Ear
g. Eye
h. Nose
i. Breast
j. Hands and feet
k. Hip

KEY CONCEPTS

1. Explain how each factor helps the newborn initiate respirations.
   a. Chemical

   b. Thermal

   c. Mechanical

2. Why is adequate functional residual capacity in the lungs important?

3. Number the following events in the correct order of occurrence.
   a. _____ Increased blood oxygen level
   b. _____ Respirations initiated
   c. _____ Fibrosis of the ductus venosus
   d. _____ Increased pressure in the left side of the heart
   e. _____ Increased blood carbon dioxide level
   f. _____ Surfactant action keeps alveoli open
   g. _____ Foramen ovale closes
   h. _____ Ductus arteriosus constricts
4. List characteristics that predispose newborns to heat loss.

5. Describe each method by which the newborn can lose heat. Which ones can also be methods of heat gain?

6. How does brown fat help the newborn maintain a near-constant temperature? Under what circumstances may newborns have inadequate brown fat, and why?

7. Explain the relationship between oxygenation, body temperature, glucose stores, and bilirubin levels in the newborn.

8. Compare the normal values for fetal and adult erythrocytes, hemoglobin, and hematocrit.

9. How would you explain the prophylactic neonatal vitamin K injection to new parents?

10. Describe each newborn stool as you would explain it to a new parent. When should parents expect the first meconium stool? What differences in stools should parents expect if their infant is breast-fed versus formula fed?
    a. Meconium stools

b. Transitional stools

c. Milk stools

11. What glucose level on a screening test requires further follow-up?

12. Which infants are at risk for hypoglycemia? Why?

13. Describe how each of the following factors can contribute to high newborn bilirubin levels. Which may be correctable with nursing interventions?
    a. Red blood cell quantity and lifespan

    b. Liver immaturity

    c. Intestinal factors

    d. Time of first feeding

    e. Birth trauma

    f. Fatty acid production

14. When does jaundice become pathologic rather than physiologic?

15. How does each of these problems result in jaundice? What is the usual treatment for each?

    a. Poor intake

    b. True breast milk jaundice

16. Compare extracellular water distribution in the newborn and the adult.

17. What limitations does the newborn have in terms of

    a. Handling excess fluid

    b. Compensating for inadequate fluid

18. What factors make the newborn vulnerable to infection that might not be a problem for an older infant or child?

19. Each of the following antibodies protects the newborn from what pathogens? Which one(s) are received from the mother?

    a. IgG

    b. IgM

    c. IgA

20. Describe the two periods of reactivity. What are the nursing implications associated with each?

21. Describe the six behavioral states seen in the newborn.

22. What are the two immediate newborn assessments after birth?

23. Complete the following table.

Head Variation	Cause(s)	Characteristic Features	Parent Teaching
Caput succedaneum			
Cephalhematoma			

24. Explain the possible significance of each neonatal assessment.
    a. Two-vessel umbilical cord

    b. Simian line

    c. Hair tuft on lower spine

    d. Ears below the level of the canthi of the eye

    e. Drooping of one side of the mouth

25. Complete the table below on newborn measurements.

Measurement	Average for Full-Term Infant	Possible Causes for Deviations
Weight		
Length		
Head circumference		
Chest circumference		

26. List the normal ranges for term neonatal vital signs. Describe the correct assessment technique for each.
   a. Pulse rate
   b. Respiratory rate
   c. Blood pressure
   d. Temperature
      - Rectal
      - Axillary

27. List signs that suggest neonatal respiratory distress.

28. List signs that suggest neonatal hypoglycemia.

29. Describe normal assessments of female and male genitalia.

30. State possible significance of each skin variance. Note if any special care is needed.
    a. Ruddiness

    b. Green-brown discoloration of skin and vernix

    c. Red, blotchy areas with white papules in center

    d. Blue-black marks over the sacral area

    e. Flat, purplish area that does not blanch with pressure

    f. Light-brown spots

31. What facial marks may be present if the infant had a nuchal cord?

CRITICAL THINKING EXERCISES

1. During clinical practice, note steps taken to conserve the newborn's body heat. Identify which method of loss each is designed to interrupt.

2. Use a medical dictionary or laboratory manual to distinguish between indirect and direct bilirubin tests. How would each help identify possible causes of jaundice in the newborn?

3. What is the protocol for neonatal blood glucose screening at your clinical facility?

4. Find infants whose gestational age assessments were LGA or SGA. Look at the mothers' charts to determine possible causes. Check the infants' charts to identify nursing assessments and care that were different (or in more depth) for these infants during the early hours after birth. Did any problems develop related to their being LGA or SGA?

5. Perform a gestational age assessment on an infant. Ask a classmate to assess the infant separately. Compare your scores and discuss reasons for any differences. Do the same with a staff nurse. Be careful not to stress the infant.

6. Identify different periods of reactivity in infants. Note the response of mothers to the different periods. Determine their understanding of each period of reactivity and teach them as needed.

7. Identify habituation and self-consoling activities in infants. Determine what stimuli caused the habituation.

CASE STUDIES

You are admitting a newborn and performing a gestational age assessment. The infant weighs 6 pounds, 10 ounces; her length is 19 inches; her head circumference is 13 inches. You obtain this information on the assessment: fully flexed position; 0° wrist angle; 90°-100° angle on arm recoil; 90° popliteal angle; elbow reaches sternum when extending arm across the chest; lower leg at 90° angle when flexing thigh onto abdomen. Skin is dry and cracking and no blood vessels are visible through the skin. No lanugo is present. Sole creases cover the entire foot. Areola is 4 mm and ear cartilage is stiff. Clitoris and labia minora are completely covered by the labia majora.

1. Using Figure 22-23, circle the above information on the neuromuscular and physical maturity scale. What is your total score for both?

2. Determine the approximate weeks of gestation.

3. Using Figure 22-23, plot the infant's weight, length, and head circumference. (You will have to convert from English to metric measures.) Determine if she is SGA, AGA, or LGA.

4. Based on your assessments, does the nurse need additional care for this infant? Why or why not?

REVIEW QUESTIONS

Choose the correct answer.

1. When doing an admission assessment on a term newborn, the nurse notes that the lung sounds are slightly moist. The skin color is pink except for acrocyanosis. Pulse is 156 and respirations are 55 and unlabored. The appropriate nursing action is to
   a. notify the pediatrician of the abnormal lung sounds.
   b. continue to observe the infant's respiratory status.
   c. recheck the high respiratory and pulse rates in 30 minutes.
   d. keep the infant in the newborn nursery until stable.

2. A newborn has a hemoglobin of 24 and a hematocrit of 71%. The nurse should anticipate
   a. temperature instability.
   b. high calcium levels.
   c. delayed breast-feeding.
   d. greater than normal jaundice.

3. Becoming cold can lead to respiratory distress primarily because the infant
   a. needs more oxygen than he or she can supply to generate heat.
   b. breathes more slowly and shallowly when hypothermic.
   c. reopens fetal shunts when the body temperature reaches 36.1° C (97° F).
   d. cannot supply enough glucose to provide fuel for respirations.

4. The primary purpose of surfactant is to
   a. maintain normal blood glucose levels.
   b. keep lung alveoli partly open between breaths.
   c. inhibit excess erythrocyte production.
   d. stimulate passage of the first meconium stool.

5. The foramen ovale closes because the
   a. arterial pressures in the lungs are higher than in the body.
   b. presence of slight hypoxia and acidosis cause constriction.
   c. blood flow through it is redirected through the liver.
   d. pressure in the left atrium is higher than in the right.

6. Brown fat is used to
   a. maintain temperature.
   b. facilitate digestion.
   c. metabolize glucose.
   d. conjugate bilirubin.

7. The infant of a diabetic mother is prone to hypoglycemia because
   a. liver conversion of glycogen to glucose is sluggish.
   b. excess subcutaneous fat reduces blood flow to tissues.
   c. high insulin production rapidly metabolizes glucose.
   d. vulnerability to infections increases metabolic stress.

8. The primary difference between physiologic and pathologic jaundice is the
   a. number of fetal erythrocytes that are broken down.
   b. type of feeding method chosen by the mother.
   c. location of the yellow areas on the newborn's skin.
   d. time of onset and rate of rise in bilirubin levels.

9. The nurse can help prevent many cases of jaundice in the breast-fed infant by
   a. encouraging extra water between each nursing session.
   b. teaching the mother how to encourage regular and adequate nursing.
   c. placing the infants under phototherapy prophylactically.
   d. advising mothers of suitable formulas to use if it occurs.

10. Infection in the newborn often has subtle signs because

    a. body temperature rises slowly in response to pathogens.
    b. passive antibodies from the mother fight infection early.
    c. high urine output causes a lower body temperature.
    d. leukocyte response and inflammatory signs are immature.

11. A hungry infant is crying vigorously. The best initial intervention is to

    a. immediately give formula until the infant is satisfied.
    b. place the infant in a quiet, dark area, wrapped tightly.
    c. console the infant before the mother tries to feed it.
    d. encourage the parents to engage their infant in eye-to-eye contact.

12. A 9 pound 11 ounce infant was born vaginally. The labor nurse reports that there was shoulder dystocia at birth but that Apgar scores were 8 at 1 minute and 9 at 5 minutes. The nurse should do a focus assessment for

    a. hip dysplasia.
    b. head molding.
    c. clavicle fracture.
    d. abnormal cord vessels.

13. The nurse notes that the infant's feet are turned inward. The appropriate nursing action is to

    a. apply a splint to the feet and lower legs.
    b. notify the pediatrician or nurse-practitioner.
    c. explain to the parents that this is typical for intrauterine position.
    d. determine if the feet can be moved to a normal, straight position.

14. While performing an admission assessment on a term newborn, the nurse notes poor muscle tone and slight jitteriness. The appropriate nursing action is to

    a. assess the infant's blood glucose level.
    b. stop the assessment and wrap the infant tightly in blankets.
    c. check the mother's chart for narcotics given late in labor.
    d. give supplemental oxygen by face mask.

15. While making a home visit to a mother and newborn on the second day after birth, the nurse notes that the infant's skin color is yellowish to the midsternal level. The most important action is to

    a. teach the mother to nurse the infant at least every 2-3 hours.
    b. explain that jaundice after birth is common and will resolve without treatment.
    c. ask the mother if she has been feeding the infant supplemental formula.
    d. notify the pediatrician or nurse-practitioner of the early, intense jaundice.

16. Choose the nursing observation that is most important if the nurse notes a two-vessel umbilical cord.

    a. Urine output.
    b. Onset of jaundice.
    c. Respiratory rate.
    d. Heart rhythm.

17. An infant's gestational age assessment reveals that her weight is SGA. This means that

    a. she was born before 37 completed weeks of gestation.
    b. her weight falls between the 10th and 90th percentile.
    c. she has a low birth weight in relation to her length.
    d. her weight is lower than expected for her gestation.

18. When weighing an infant, the nurse places a covering on the scale tray to
    a. avoid causing multiple startle (Moro) reflexes when weighing.
    b. ensure that conductive heat loss from the infant is minimal.
    c. compensate for negative weight balance to ensure correct weight.
    d. avoid contaminating the nurse's hands with blood or other body substances.

19. Which newborn reflex can help the new mother learn to breast-feed?
    a. Tonic neck.
    b. Rooting.
    c. Palmar grasp.
    d. Moro.

20. The nurse notes slight resistance when first inserting a rectal thermometer to take a newborn's first temperature. The best nursing action is to
    a. notify the infant's pediatrician.
    b. rotate the thermometer to the left while inserting.
    c. listen for the presence of bowel sounds.
    d. check for rectal patency using the fifth digit.

21. The best location for an infant's glucose determination is the
    a. great toe of either foot.
    b. nondominant heel.
    c. midline of the heel.
    d. lateral surface of the heel.

23

The Normal Newborn: Nursing Care

COMMON CONCERNS OF STUDENTS WHEN TEACHING PARENTS

Students without newborn experience often worry about their ability to teach new parents. Concerns include lack of experience, fear of giving inaccurate information, and dealing with experienced mothers. However, there are many methods to increase knowledge and confidence to make parent teaching one of the most enjoyable aspects of nursing.

Resources

Take advantage of available resources for increasing your knowledge of infant care. In addition to reading nursing textbooks, visit college and hospital libraries for journal articles about newborn nursing care. Parent education materials available on the maternity unit provide easy-to-read, quick information.

Seek out resource people who can help. Most nurses enjoy sharing their knowledge. Listen as they work with parents to learn teaching approaches and answers to common parent questions. Talk to the lactation educator to learn more about breast-feeding. Attend parent classes on infant care and feeding.

Make use of audiovisual materials for parent education. Watching a video with parents helps the student and parents learn and provides a starting place for clarifying parent questions.

Repetitive Teaching

Students have the opportunity to repeat teaching because all parents need the same basic information. Material that is at first new quickly becomes familiar with repeat practice. Students soon become polished and even develop creative new ways to present information.

Experienced Mothers

What does one teach the mother having her fourth (or eighth) baby? Begin by assessing the mother's knowledge. If her youngest child is older than 1 or 2 years, she has probably forgotten some of the details of infant care. Briefly review the material that is routinely given to first-time mothers to discover any gaps in the experienced mother's knowledge. For example, the mother of girls may need information about care of the penis if she has a boy.

As you teach, acknowledge the mother's past experience. For example, you may say, "I'm sure you know much of this information, but let's check this list to see if anything has changed or you think of any questions." Insert phrases like, "As you remember . . ." or "And you probably know about . . . ." This recognizes the mother's knowledge but allows her to refresh her memory.

Some mothers hesitate to ask about topics they feel the nurse might expect them to know. Reviewing all material allows the mother to ask questions without feeling foolish. Providing a warm and accepting environment helps her feel it is "safe" to ask questions.

Ask the mother about her opinions and about problems she had in the past. For example, "What is the most difficult part of caring for a new baby, in your experience?" Not only does this provide an opportunity for discussion, but you may learn from the mother's experience!

Sometimes the mother is more concerned about her other children than the new baby. She may wonder how they will feel about the newborn, and how she can meet the needs of each child when she is so tired. Use therapeutic communication techniques to act as a "sounding board" as she sorts out priorities and makes plans.

Experienced Nurse-Parents

Nursing students who are parents may rely on personal experience in parent teaching. However, personal experiences should seldom be shared with clients. The clients want to talk about their own experiences and may not feel that the nurse's experiences apply in their situation. In addition, information about infant care changes. Nurses who rely on their own parenting experiences may pass along incorrect information or information that conflicts with that taught by the birth center.

KEY CONCEPTS

1. What is the correct order for suctioning an infant's airway with the bulb syringe? Why?

2. Why is it particularly important that the infant's head be dried promptly?

3. What added assessments and interventions should the nurse do if an infant has a subnormal temperature?

4. What type of heat loss can occur in each situation?

   a. Placing the newborn on a cold, unpadded scale

   b. Using a cold stethoscope to listen to breath sounds

   c. Placing the infant's crib by a window on a snowy day

d. Partially drying the infant's hair after the bath

e. Placing the infant's crib near an air conditioner vent

5. A newborn who is large for gestational age (LGA) has a low blood glucose on the first screening and will have repeat glucose screenings for about the next 8 hours. Explain in simple terms, as you would explain to parents, the reason for feeding the newborn promptly and for repeat screenings.

6. When should the initial bath be given to a newborn?

7. What are the two primary nursing observations after circumcision?

8. What circumcision problems should parents be taught to report?

9. List signs that suggest infection at the umbilical cord. What measures can prevent cord infection?

10. What is the primary method of identifying the newborn and mother (or other support person)?

11. List five general signs of newborn infection.

12. Explain why these medications are typically given to newborns.

    a. Vitamin K

b. Erythromycin eye ointment

c. Hepatitis B immunization

13. Do infants of mothers having hepatitis B need any additional medication? Why?

14. Compare advantages and disadvantages of each type of postdischarge follow-up for mothers and infants.

	Advantages	**Disadvantages**
Home visits		
Telephone counseling		

CRITICAL THINKING EXERCISES

1. Newborn circumcision is a controversial topic. Take common reasons for having the procedure done on a newborn and refute each. Do the same for reasons for not having circumcision done.

2. What screening tests are routinely done at your clinical facility? What information is given to parents about testing?

3. Use a pediatric or clinical nursing skills text to compare techniques for giving an intramuscular injection to an infant, a toddler, a preschool child, and a school-aged child. How do precautions differ? What needle sizes are appropriate for each age group? What are the maximum injection volumes for each?

4. What security measures are used at your clinical facility to prevent infant abduction? Ask several parents who have previously been taught security measures to restate these measures. How well do they recall them?

5. Does your clinical facility offer follow-up care, such as warm lines or home visits, for new parents? Ask staff members about its effectiveness.

REVIEW QUESTIONS

Choose the correct answer.

1. An infant's axillary temperature is 35.9° C (96.6° F). The priority nursing action is to
   a. recheck the infant's temperature rectally.
   b. have the mother breast feed the infant.
   c. place the infant in a radiant warmer.
   d. chart the normal axillary temperature.

2. To care for the uncircumcised penis, parents should be taught to
   a. retract the foreskin with each diaper change.
   b. wash under the foreskin as far as it has separated.
   c. use an emollient cream to hasten foreskin separation.
   d. avoid putting soap on the foreskin before separation.

3. A nursing student has been caring for a woman and her newborn all morning. The student takes the infant to the nursery for screening tests prior to discharge. When the infant is returned to the mother, the correct procedure is to
   a. have the mother read her printed band number and verify that it matches the infant's.
   b. ask the mother to state her name and the name of her infant.
   c. call out the mother's full name before leaving the infant with her.
   d. return the infant with no special procedure since the student knows both mother and infant.

4. The correct site for injection of hepatitis B immunization for a newborn is the
   a. subcutaneous tissue of the thigh.
   b. dorsogluteal muscle.
   c. deltoid muscle.
   d. vastus lateralis muscle.

5. A new mother should be taught to support her baby's head when holding the infant because
   a. doing so will promote better eye contact and bonding.
   b. the baby's muscles are too weak to support the heavy head.
   c. it allows better guidance of the head toward the breast.
   d. less regurgitation of gastric contents will occur.

6. A new mother anxiously summons the nurse to her baby's room because she sneezed twice. A brief assessment shows nothing unusual. The appropriate teaching is that
   a. lint from the clothes or blankets probably tickled the baby's nose.
   b. multiple sneezes are characteristic of the second period of reactivity.
   c. the baby may be developing a cold, so the pediatrician will be notified.
   d. sneezing may indicate sensitivity to the drugs given to the mother during labor.

7. Choose the normal circumcision assessment.
   a. Slipping of the Plastibell onto the shaft of the penis.
   b. Oozing of blood from the site after a Gomco circumcision.
   c. Delay in urination for 12 to 16 hours.
   d. Development of a dry yellow crust on the site.

8. Choose the correct parent teaching about cord care.
   a. Fold the diaper below the cord to speed drying.
   b. Expect the cord to detach in no more than 7 days.
   c. Tub baths are safe as soon as the cord detaches.
   d. Skin near the cord site may be red until it detaches.

24

Newborn Feeding

MATCHING KEY TERMS

Match the term with the correct definition.

1. ______ foremilk
2. ______ hindmilk
3. ______ mastitis
4. ______ milk-ejection reflex

a. Contraction of myoepithelial cells to eject milk into ducts
b. Breast inflammation
c. Thirst-quenching milk
d. Higher-fat milk

KEY CONCEPTS

1. Determine the number of calories per day needed by an infant weighing 8 pounds. Then calculate the number of ounces of breast milk or formula (each having 20 calories per ounce) the infant needs daily. What are the infant's daily fluid needs?

2. Describe changes in composition and appearance of colostrum, transitional milk, and mature milk. When do the changes occur?

3. Complete the following table to contrast breast milk and cow's milk. What are the effects of the differences on newborns?

Component	**Breast Milk**	**Cow's Milk**
Proteins		
Fats		
Vitamins		
Minerals		
Other substances, such as antibodies		

4. Describe the purposes of prolactin and oxytocin in breast-feeding. What can enhance or interfere with their secretion?

5. What care can help the mother who has flat or inverted nipples?

6. Describe differences in breast fullness.
   a. Soft

   b. Filling

   c. Engorged

7. Describe each of these hand positions for breast feeding. Which is preferred?
   a. "C" position

   b. Scissors position

8. Describe differences between nutritive and nonnutritive suckling. How does infant swallowing sound?

9. What should the mother be taught about removing the infant from the breast?

10. During the first few weeks, babies usually breast feed about every ________ to ________ hours. They should eat about _______ times a day.

11. How does breast feeding help resolve jaundice? Why should breast-feeding be frequent?

12. When is the best time to administer medications to a breast-feeding mother in order to decrease the amount of the drug being transferred to the baby?

13. In what maternal conditions is breast feeding not advised?

14. What should the mother be taught about storage of breast milk?
    a. Containers

    b. Temperature

    c. Thawing frozen milk

15. Describe use and precautions associated with each type of formula.
    a. Ready-to-use

    b. Concentrated liquid

    c. Powdered

16. Explain what a new mother should be taught about each of these aspects of formula feeding.
    a. Frequency

    b. Propping the bottle

    c. Microwaving formula

CRITICAL THINKING QUESTIONS

1. Ask women you care for during clinical what their reasons were for choosing their method of feeding. Were any of their reasons based on cultural influences?

2. Make a teaching plan to help mothers with these breast-feeding problems.
   a. Engorgement
   b. Sore nipples
   c. Flat or inverted nipples
   d. Sleepy baby or one who falls asleep soon after nursing begins

3. A mother tells you that she does not think she has enough milk for her baby. How can you guide her?

4. If your clinical experience includes postpartum clinic or home visits, ask breast-feeding mothers if they have encountered problems since they were discharged. If they have stopped breast feeding, why? Have any of the women forgotten information that was taught when they were in the birth center?

CASE STUDY

Margaret is breast feeding for the first time. She seems awkward in handling her baby and says that the baby is not feeding well. The baby cries frequently while Margaret tries to feed her.

1. What is the first nursing action to take in this situation?

2. What additional nursing actions can help Margaret?

After your nursing actions, the infant latches on to the breast and begins suckling vigorously. Margaret begins to relax. She says, "I thought this would be easy, but it isn't."

3. What basic teaching is appropriate for Margaret?

After about 3 minutes, Margaret asks, "Shouldn't I change breasts now? I don't want to have sore nipples."

4. What teaching is appropriate about nursing duration and frequency?

5. What should you tell her about caring for her breasts?

Margaret successfully completes her first breast feeding. She asks, "The baby seemed to suck a lot, but how do I know she is getting enough to eat?"

6. What infant signs or behaviors can you teach Margaret to look for that indicate adequate milk intake?

REVIEW QUESTIONS

Choose the correct answer.

1. A new mother wants to nurse her infant only 5 minutes at each breast to avoid sore nipples. Choose the appropriate teaching.
   a. Limiting time during the early days can lessen trauma to the nipples and allow them time to toughen.
   b. Limiting time can cause frequent infant hunger because the baby does not receive richer milk.
   c. Limiting time at the breast does not reduce sore nipples but does reduce engorgement.
   d. Limiting time at the breast delays the transition from colostrum to transitional and true milk.

2. A new mother wants to breast feed but also to feed her infant formula occasionally. The nurse should teach her to
   a. avoid using any bottles the first month to establish her milk supply.
   b. make a clear choice to feed by one method or the other to avoid nipple confusion.
   c. limit formula feeding to once each day until her milk supply is well established.
   d. alternate formula and nursing to allow the infant to become accustomed to both.

3. A woman has had a baby at 29 weeks of gestation. She tells the nurse that she cannot breast feed because the baby is so small and early. The nurse should tell her that
   a. she will be able to establish lactation when the baby is strong enough to nurse.
   b. special formulas are actually better for preterm infants than her breast milk.
   c. infections are more likely to occur if the infant takes stored breast milk.
   d. she can use a breast pump to maintain lactation until nursing is possible.

4. A breast-feeding mother is reluctant to take a prescribed analgesic because she doesn't want to pass it to the baby. The nurse should teach her that
   a. less medication will reach the baby if she takes it after a feeding.
   b. limiting the duration of feedings when she needs medication will reduce transfer to the baby.
   c. it is best to avoid all medications during nursing, including analgesics.
   d. formula feeding while she needs analgesics may be best for the baby.

5. The maximum length of time formula should be kept after preparation is
   a. 12-18 hours.
   b. 18-24 hours.
   c. 24-48 hours.
   d. 48-72 hours.

6. A new mother is worried because her 1-day-old baby is only taking 3/4 ounce of formula at most feedings. The nurse should teach her that
   a. her baby should be taking 2 to 3 ounces at each feeding by the next day.
   b. the amount the baby is taking at each feeding is normal at this time.
   c. the baby might take more if a different formula is used.
   d. the nipple may be too firm for the baby to suck easily.

25

The Childbearing Family With Special Needs

MATCHING KEY TERMS

Match the term with the correct definition.

1. ______ crack
2. ______ egocentrism
3. ______ fetal alcohol syndrome
4. ______ methadone
5. ______ opiate
6. ______ withdrawal syndrome

a. Interest centered on self rather than on others
b. Symptoms seen when an individual who is addicted to a specific drug abstains
c. Fetal disorders associated with maternal alcohol use
d. Substance containing opium or any of its derivatives
e. Highly addictive form of cocaine
f. Long-acting drug to substitute for heroin or morphine

KEY CONCEPTS

1. Explain how pregnancy impacts the adolescent's
   a. development of independence
   b. education
   c. employment opportunities
2. What pregnancy risks are higher for adolescents than for adults?
3. List complications the mature pregnant woman is more likely to encounter.
   a. Genetic

b. Preexisting disorders

c. Obstetric complications

4. What problems is the mature mother likely to encounter in terms of the following?
   a. Fatigue

   b. Support of friends or family

5. Why do substances ingested by the mother tend to have a more pronounced effect on her fetus than on her?

6. Complete the chart below related to fetal and neonatal effects of maternal substance use.

	Fetal Effects	**Neonatal Effects**
Tobacco		
Alcohol		
Cocaine		
Marijuana		
Heroin		

7. Why might the birth center staff screen a woman for cocaine if she is admitted in preterm labor and having intense contractions?

8. What therapeutic management is necessary for a pregnant woman that desires to stop her use of heroin during the pregnancy?

9. List antepartal signs associated with drug abuse.
   a. Behaviors
   b. Physical appearance
   c. Obstetrical history
   d. Emotional reaction to pregnancy

10. What signs might the woman have during the intrapartum period if she has recently ingested these drugs?
    a. Cocaine
    b. Heroin

11. What special concerns exist if the infant has facial or genital anomalies?

12. Why is grief an essential aspect of attachment to an infant with an anomaly?

13. Why is it important that both fathers and mothers be supported in the grief aspects of having a baby with an anomaly or of perinatal loss?

14. Describe the risks to an abused pregnant woman and her fetus.

15. Describe each phase of the violence cycle.

CRITICAL THINKING EXERCISES

1. If you care for a teenage mother, discuss the involvement of the infant's father and the grandmother in infant care. What evidence of the "honeymoon phase" did you see? What are the future plans of the young mother (and father, if involved)? Are their plans realistic? Why or why not?

2. What does your state require if either the mother or the infant shows evidence of drug abuse in toxicology screens?

3. Talk with your hospital's emergency department about their experiences with battered women. Do they note any differences in abuse when a woman is pregnant?

REVIEW QUESTIONS

Choose the correct answer.

1. The best way for the nurse to evaluate the quality of a pregnant adolescent's diet is to
   a. ask her how well she eats in a non-threatening manner.
   b. assume it is inadequate and give her advice.
   c. ask her to describe what she ate the previous day.
   d. have her record everything she eats for 1 week.

2. Correct advice for women who ask about using alcohol during pregnancy is that it is
   a. safest if taken during the last trimester.
   b. best to avoid during the first 12 weeks.
   c. unknown if there is any fetal harm from its use.
   d. important to avoid it entirely throughout pregnancy.

3. When first presenting an infant with an anomaly to parents, the nurse should
   a. have the physician initially discuss the causes of the anomaly, if known.
   b. emphasize the most normal aspects of the infant before showing them the anomaly.
   c. wait until the mother has had time to recuperate from the stress of labor.
   d. limit their time with the infant the first time they see him or her.

4. A woman who had a stillborn infant at 37 weeks of gestation angrily asks the nurse why her physician didn't "take the baby early." The nurse should understand that the mother's behavior
   a. is unusual when stillbirth occurs at this late gestation.
   b. suggests discord between the woman and her partner.
   c. should be expected as part of the normal grieving process.
   d. reflects intense guilt about her own self-care in pregnancy.

5. The main goal when caring for battered women is to
   a. emphasize that they have the right not to be hurt.
   b. help them better identify their role in the family.
   c. encourage them to ask their partners about counseling.
   d. limit their ability to return to the abusive partner.

26

The Pregnant Woman With Complications

MATCHING KEY TERMS

Match the term with the correct definition.

1. ______ cerclage
2. ______ dystocia
3. ______ euglycemia
4. ______ kernicterus
5. ______ seroconversion
6. ______ maceration
7. ______ lipogenic substance

a. Substance that stimulates production of fat
b. Development of antibodies in response to infection or immunization
c. Normal blood glucose levels
d. Difficult or prolonged labor
e. Encircling the cervix with sutures
f. Bilirubin accumulation within the brain that may cause damage
g. Degeneration of a fetus retained in the uterus after its death

KEY CONCEPTS

1. Define spontaneous abortion.

2. Complete the table on types of spontaneous abortions.

	Clinical Manifestations	Therapeutic Management
Threatened		
Inevitable		
Incomplete		
Complete		
Missed		
Recurrent		

3. Describe altered laboratory studies seen in DIC.

4. Write a simply worded response that you might use if a woman expresses the feeling that she did something to cause her spontaneous abortion.

5. What is the possible significance of sudden shoulder pain during early pregnancy?

6. What teaching is needed for the woman having methotrexate therapy for an early ectopic pregnancy?

7. List the typical signs and symptoms of a hydatidiform mole.

8. What is the relationship between hydatidiform mole and cancer? What precautions related to cancer detection are taken after evacuation of the mole?

9. List foods that should be emphasized for a woman who experienced a bleeding complication of pregnancy (at any gestation). How would you explain simply the need for these foods?

10. Complete the chart below to compare placenta previa with abruptio placentae.

	Placenta Previa	**Abruptio Placentae**
Placenta location		
Character of bleeding		
Presence of pain		
Uterine activity		
Diagnosis		
Therapeutic management		

11. List nursing teaching associated with home care when a woman has placenta previa.

12. What is the relationship between cocaine use and abruptio placentae?

13. Why is the amount of external bleeding in abruptio placentae not a reliable indicator of the true amount of blood loss?

14. List early and late signs of hypovolemic shock.

15. List nursing measures and their rationales to promote maternal and fetal oxygenation in hemorrhagic disorders.

16. Describe how generalized vasospasm of preeclampsia affects each organ and how these effects are manifested.
    a. Kidneys

    b. Liver

    c. Brain

    d. Lungs

    e. Placenta

17. What is the primary difference between the expected edema of pregnancy and that of preeclampsia?

18. What is the significance of epigastric pain in a woman with preeclampsia?

19. List signs of magnesium toxicity.

20. What is the antidote for magnesium toxicity?

21. What feature distinguishes chronic hypertension from pregnancy-induced hypertension?

22. What conditions are necessary for the woman to receive anti-Rho(D) immune globulin? What does each mean?

    a. Rh of the woman

    b. Rh of the fetus or newborn

    c. Indirect Coombs' test (woman)

    d. Direct Coombs' test (newborn)

23. How can ABO incompatibility occur?

24. List the four classic signs of diabetes.

    a. ____________
    b. ____________
    c. ____________
    d. ____________

25. Why is maintenance of a normal blood glucose level before and during early pregnancy particularly important?

26. What are the effects of maternal vascular involvement on the fetus/newborn of a diabetic mother?

27. Do insulin needs increase, decrease, or remain stable during these times? Why?
    a. First trimester

    b. Second and third trimesters

    c. Labor

    d. Postpartum

28. When would the physician want a pregnant woman to have an oral glucose tolerance test?

29. Why is it important to give a pregnant woman who has diabetes as many choices as possible?

30. What steps minimize insulin leakage from the injection site?

31. Why is it recommended that a woman who has hypoglycemia avoid sucrose or unrefined sugar, such as candy?

32. List early signs and symptoms of congestive heart failure.

33. Janet is a 26-year-old woman who is 30 weeks' pregnant with her first baby. She has rheumatic heart disease. She had to stop working at her desk job at 20 weeks of pregnancy because of fatigue. She has no problems when sitting quietly, but tasks such as making her bed or gathering laundry to wash cause her to have slight chest pain and a rapid heartbeat. She complains that she always feels tired. What class of heart disease do her symptoms suggest?

34. What anticoagulant is recommended if one is needed during pregnancy? Why?

35. Why are labor and the immediate postpartum period especially dangerous for a woman who has heart disease?

36. A woman who is 32 weeks' pregnant and has class II heart disease visits the antepartal clinic for a routine visit. You find that she has gained 7 pounds since her last visit. Is her weight gain normal? What possibilities should you consider?

37. Why is it important to take folic acid before and during pregnancy?

38. Why does maternal sickle cell crisis make fetal death more likely?

39. Describe the signs of sickle cell crisis.

40. List pregnancy-associated risks for the woman who has systemic lupus erythematosus.

41. Why is drug management of the woman who has epilepsy difficult during pregnancy?

42. Describe the four stages in the course of HIV infection.

43. Complete the table to learn more about viral infections during pregnancy.

Infection	Maternal Effects	Fetal and Neonatal Effects	Prevention	Treatment
Cytomegalovirus				
Rubella				
Varicella zoster				
Herpes viruses				
Parvovirus B-19				
Hepatitis B				

44. At what point is the person said to have acquired immunodeficiency syndrome?

45. Which drug is recommended for HIV-infected pregnant women to prevent viral transmission to the fetus?

46. What nursing care is appropriate for the HIV-infected pregnant woman?

47. Complete the table to learn more about nonviral infections during pregnancy.

Infection	Maternal Effects	Fetal and Neonatal Effects	Prevention	Treatment
Toxoplasmosis				
Group B streptococci				
Tuberculosis				

CRITICAL THINKING EXERCISES

1. Examine your own feelings about induced abortion. Are your feelings different for early and later abortions? Can you care for a woman who is having induced abortion?

2. Ask staff nurses at your clinical facility about their experiences with women who have hyperemesis gravidarum. Do you detect any preset beliefs about the disorder among the nurses?

3. Review client charts to determine whether they had a glucose challenge test and their response to it. What follow-up was done if their blood level was 140 mg/dl or higher?

4. Examine your attitudes toward people with HIV. Are you fearful of them? Did you have to confront this fear before entering nursing school? How do you feel about pregnant women who have HIV? Are your feelings for "innocent" victims, such as infants, different from feelings for those who acquired the infection through unsafe sexual intercourse or intravenous drug use?

CASE STUDIES

Patricia is a 17-year-old gravida 1, para 0 at 34 weeks of gestation who is visiting her doctor for a routine prenatal visit. When weighing Patricia, the nurse finds that she has gained 8 pounds in the past month.

1. What is the main objective after this initial assessment?

2. What is the most important question or problem that must be solved during Patricia's prenatal visit?

3. What are the nurse's priority assessments? Why?

The nurse obtains a clean-catch urine specimen from Patricia and takes her vital signs (T 37° C [98.6° F], P 82, R 20, BP 146/90) and the FHR (144-150). Deep tendon reflexes are normal (2+), and no clonus is present.

4. What testing would you expect to be done on the urine specimen? Why?

5. What information might the nurse need from previous prenatal visits and why?

6. What questions should the nurse ask Patricia while assessing her?

Patricia's physician diagnoses mild preeclampsia and will initially manage Patricia at home.

7. What findings would lead the physician to the diagnosis of mild preeclampsia?

8. Why do you think the physician is recommending home management at this time?

9. What teaching is essential regarding Patricia's home care?

Debra is a 22-year-old gravida 1, para 0, who has had type I (insulin-dependent) diabetes for 6 years. Her last menstrual period was 12 weeks ago.

10. How will Debra's diabetes be affected by her pregnancy?

11. What changes will she most likely have to make in her diabetes management because she is pregnant?

12. What routine assessments will be made at each prenatal visit?

13. What additional tests will Debra need as her pregnancy progresses?

14. How may Debra's fetus be affected by her diabetes?

15. What nursing management during labor should be expected?

16. What newborn problems should the nurse anticipate?

17. What added care will Debra's infant need?

REVIEW QUESTIONS

Choose the correct answer.

1. Choose the primary distinction between threatened and inevitable abortion.
   a. Presence of cramping.
   b. Rupture of membranes.
   c. Vaginal bleeding.
   d. Pelvic pressure.

2. A woman is admitted to the emergency department with a possible ectopic pregnancy. Choose the sign/symptom that should be immediately reported to her physician.
   a. Low level of β-hCG.
   b. Hemoglobin of 11.5; hematocrit of 34%.
   c. Light vaginal bleeding.
   d. Pulse increase from 78 to 100 bpm.

3. When caring for the woman who had a hydatidiform mole evacuated, the clinic nurse should primarily
   a. reinforce the need to delay a new pregnancy for 1 year.
   b. ask the woman if she has any cramping or bleeding.
   c. observe return of her blood pressure to normal.
   d. palpate the uterus for return to its normal size.

4. The woman who is receiving methotrexate for an ectopic pregnancy should be cautioned to avoid
   a. driving or operating machinery.
   b. eating raw vegetables or fruits.
   c. using latex condoms for intercourse.
   d. taking vitamins with folic acid.

5. A woman who is 34 weeks' pregnant is admitted with contractions every 2 minutes, lasting 60 seconds, and a high uterine resting tone. She says she had some vaginal bleeding at home, and there is a small amount of blood on her perineal pad. The priority action of the nurse is to
   a. establish if she is in labor by performing a vaginal examination.
   b. ask her if she has had recent intercourse or a vaginal examination.
   c. evaluate the maternal and fetal circulation and oxygenation.
   d. determine whether this is the first episode of pain she has had.

6. Nursing teaching for the woman who has hyperemesis gravidarum should include
   a. adding favorite seasonings to foods while cooking.
   b. eating simple foods such as breads and fruits.
   c. lying down on the right side after eating.
   d. eating creamed soup with every meal.

7. The nurse makes the following assessments on a woman who is receiving intravenous magnesium sulfate: FHR 148-158; P 88; R 10; BP 158/96. The priority nursing action is to
   a. increase the rate of the magnesium infusion.
   b. maintain the magnesium infusion at the current rate.
   c. slow the rate of the magnesium infusion.
   d. stop the magnesium infusion.

8. When providing intrapartal care for the woman with severe preeclampsia, priority nursing care is to
   a. maintain the ordered rate of anticonvulsant medications.
   b. promote placental blood flow and prevent maternal injury.
   c. give intravenous fluids and observe urine output.
   d. reduce maternal blood pressure to the prepregnancy level.

9. Clonus indicates that the
   a. central nervous system is very irritable.
   b. renal blood flow is severely reduced.
   c. lungs are filling with interstitial fluid.
   d. muscles of the foot are inflamed.

10. The feature that distinguishes preeclampsia from eclampsia is the
    a. amount of blood pressure elevation.
    b. edema of the face and fingers.
    c. presence of proteinuria.
    d. onset of convulsions.

11. Which woman should receive $RH_o(D)$ immune globulin after birth?
    a. Rh-negative mother; Rh-positive infant; positive direct Coombs' test.
    b. Rh-positive mother; Rh-negative infant; negative direct Coombs' test.
    c. Rh-negative mother; Rh-positive infant; negative direct Coombs' test.
    d. Rh-positive mother; Rh-positive infant; positive direct Coombs' test.

12. The test used to screen for gestational diabetes is the
    a. glycosylated hemoglobin test.
    b. glucose challenge test.
    c. oral glucose tolerance test.
    d. postprandial glucose test.

13. The best evaluation for the client goal of accurate insulin administration is that she will
    a. repeat the taught steps of the technique.
    b. accurately withdraw, mix, and inject insulin.
    c. have normal fasting and postprandial glucose levels.
    d. state that she understands the teaching given.

14. Rheumatic heart disease is usually preceded by which infection?
    a. Streptococcal pharyngitis.
    b. Syphilis.
    c. Pneumococcal pneumonia.
    d. Chlamydial vaginitis.

15. The primary fetal risk when the mother has any type of anemia is
    a. neonatal anemia.
    b. elevated bilirubin.
    c. limited infection defenses.
    d. reduced oxygen delivery.

16. Intrapartum nursing care for a woman who has sickle cell disease focuses on
    a. maintaining oxygenation and preventing dehydration.
    b. controlling pain and avoiding unnecessary movement.
    c. preventing excess exertion and limiting visitors.
    d. increasing calorie intake and avoiding internal monitoring.

17. When caring for a pregnant woman with systemic lupus erythematosus, the clinic nurse must especially observe for development of
    a. urinary tract infections.
    b. excessive weight gain.
    c. elevated blood pressure.
    d. reduced blood glucose.

18. Reduction in congenital rubella is best accomplished by
    a. avoiding contact with young children when infections are prevalent.
    b. taking prophylactic antibiotics during the second half of pregnancy.
    c. testing the rubella titer at the first prenatal visit to determine immunity.
    d. immunizing susceptible women at least 3 months before they become pregnant.

19. The pregnant woman who becomes infected with chickenpox should be taught to report promptly
    a. cough or dyspnea.
    b. severe skin itching.
    c. joint pain.
    d. increased urination.

20. Choose the appropriate infant care teaching for the woman who gave birth by cesarean because of active herpes.
    a. Do not breast-feed the infant until all lesions are healed.
    b. Thoroughly wash your hands before handling the infant.
    c. Wear a mask when breast-feeding or holding the infant close.
    d. No special precautions are needed when caring for the infant.

21. Correct injection technique for infants of mothers who are known carriers of hepatitis B virus is to
    a. avoid all intramuscular injections until 1 month of age.
    b. dilute intramuscular injections with added normal saline.
    c. mix all injections the infant will need in a single syringe.
    d. delay all injections until the infant has been bathed.

22. The nurse should expect the HIV-infected pregnant woman to receive
    a. antibiotics.
    b. protease inhibitors.
    c. zidovudine.
    d. acyclovir.

23. Expected drug treatment for a pregnant woman who has tuberculosis is
    a. acyclovir and zidovudine.
    b. isoniazid and rifampin
    c. cefotaxime and vancomycin
    d. ampicillin and gentamicin

27

The Woman With an Intrapartum Complication

MATCHING KEY TERMS

Match the term with the correct definition.

1. ______ abruption placentae
2. ______ hydramnios
3. ______ placenta accreta
4. ______ shoulder dystocia
5. ______ tocolytic

a. Delayed or difficult birth of the shoulders after the head has emerged
b. Premature separation of a normally implanted placenta
c. Excessive volume of amniotic fluid
d. Placenta that is abnormally adherent to the uterine muscle
e. Medication to stop preterm or hypertonic labor contractions

KEY CONCEPTS

1. What are three characteristics of effective uterine activity?

2. Complete the following table to compare the characteristics of hypotonic and hypertonic labor dysfunction.

	Hypotonic Dysfunction	**Hypertonic Dysfunction**
Contraction characteristics		
Uterine resting tone		
Phase of labor when it is most common		
Therapeutic management		

3. What two measurers may be used to stimulate labor that slows down after it is established?

4. What is the central principle of nursing actions when dysfunctional labor is a result of ineffective maternal pushing?

5. Why are upright positions good for women who have ineffective second-stage pushing?

6. List nursing measures to promote normal labor when maternal pushing is ineffective for each reason listed.

   a. Fear of injury

   b. Exhaustion

7. Why are upright maternal positions best to relieve persistent occiput posterior positions?

8. List four intrapartal problems that are more likely if a woman has a multifetal pregnancy.

9. What are the expected rates for dilation and fetal descent for the following?

   a. Nulliparas

   b. Parous women

10. List nursing measures for a woman having prolonged labor and for her fetus.

11. List nursing measures that may be used when a woman has precipitate labor.
    a. Promoting fetal oxygenation

    b. Promoting maternal comfort

12. What factors may make a woman think her membranes have ruptured when they have not?

13. A client will be discharged with ruptured membranes at 32 weeks' gestation. Write a summary of client teaching in simple terms that you might use.

14. List side effects that may occur with beta-adrenergic drugs such as terbutaline. What drug should be available to reverse serious adverse effects of beta-adrenergic drugs, and what is its classification?

15. How do these drugs stop preterm labor? Give an example of each.
    a. Prostaglandin synthesis inhibitors

    b. Calcium antagonists

16. What are the primary nursing assessments related to each of these tocolytic drugs?
    a. Terbutaline

    b. Magnesium sulfate

    c. Indomethacin

    d. Nifedipine

    e. Corticosteroids

17. What are the two variations of prolapsed cord?

18. What are the two objectives if umbilical cord prolapse occurs or is suspected?

19. Describe three variations of uterine rupture.

20. Why is it important that the nurse not push on the uncontracted uterine fundus after birth? What is the correct procedure?

21. Why may amniotic fluid embolism result in disseminated intravascular coagulation?

22. If a pregnant woman suffers trauma, why should medical and nursing care focus on her stabilization before fetal stabilization?

23. A woman at 32 weeks' gestation has had a car accident. Her vital signs are stable, and the fetal heart rate is 150-160. What should the nurse suspect if the woman's uterus seems to be enlarging? What is the correct action?

CRITICAL THINKING EXERCISES

1. During clinical practice, observe and discuss with nurses what measures they use for women having back labor.

2. Practice the positions listed for back labor so you will be familiar with them during clinical practice.

3. If you had to be on bed rest for preterm labor, possibly for 6 weeks, what adjustments would you and your family have to make to achieve that recommendation? What would be the single most important obstacle to adhering to bed rest in your life? What type of quiet activities could you do while maintaining bed rest?

CASE STUDIES

Ann Craig is admitted at 33 weeks' gestation saying that she thinks her "water broke." This is her fourth pregnancy. Two of her infants were preterm, born at 32 and 27 weeks' gestation, and she has had one elective abortion. She has had regular prenatal care since 6 weeks' gestation.

1. What are the most important additional assessments that the nurse should make?

The nurse notes that a small amount of cloudy fluid is draining from Ann's vagina. A Nitrazine paper turns blue-black in color, and a fern test is positive. Maternal vital signs are T 37.2° C (99° F), P 86, R 22, BP 132/80. The fetal heart rate is 162-170 and has average variability. Ann occasionally has a contraction lasting 20 to 30 seconds.

2. What data from the above assessments are most relevant?

3. What is the main judgment you would make from these data? What is the basis for that judgment?

4. Would you perform a vaginal examination at this point? Why or why not?

Shawna is an 18-year-old primigravida admitted to the birth center at 27 weeks' gestation in probable preterm labor. Her membranes are intact. The physician writes these orders:

- NPO except ice chips
- Complete blood count
- Catheterized urine for routine analysis and culture and sensitivity
- IV fluids: Ringer's lactate at 200 ml/hr for 1 hour, then 125 ml/hr
- Routine fetal monitoring and maternal vital signs

5. Which of these orders has priority? Why?

6. What position is appropriate for Shawna? Why?

Shawna will receive magnesium sulfate for tocolysis.

7. What nursing observations are essential related to magnesium sulfate? Why?

Contractions stop, and Shawna will begin taking oral terbutaline before she is discharged.

8. What teaching is appropriate related to home use of this drug?

9. What additional teaching is important before Shawna is discharged?

REVIEW QUESTIONS

Choose the correct answer.

1. A woman is having hypotonic labor and is very frustrated because this is her third trip to the birth center. What nursing measure is most appropriate for her?
   a. Do not allow any oral intake.
   b. Start oxytocin at a low rate.
   c. Offer her a warm shower or bath.
   d. Reassure her that her problem is common.

2. A woman has shoulder dystocia when giving birth. The nurse should expect
   a. immediate forceps delivery.
   b. application of suprapubic pressure.
   c. oxytocin labor augmentation.
   d. turning into a hands-and-knees position.

3. While in bed, a good position for the woman laboring with a twin pregnancy is
   a. supine.
   b. hands and knees.
   c. knee-chest.
   d. side-lying.

4. Choose the primary nursing measure to promote fetal descent.
   a. Remind the woman to empty her bladder every 1 to 2 hours.
   b. Assist fetal head rotation while doing a vaginal examination.
   c. Have the woman push at least three times with each contraction.
   d. Promote intake of glucose-containing fluids during labor.

5. An infant weighing 8 pounds 10 ounces is born vaginally. Shoulder dystocia occurred at birth. Because of this problem, the nurse should assess the infant for
   a. head swelling that does not extend beyond the skull bone.
   b. inward turning of the feet and/or legs.
   c. creaking sensation when the clavicles are palpated.
   d. limited abduction of one or both hips.

6. A woman is fully dilated, and the fetal station is 0. The fetus is in a right occiput posterior position. Choose the optimal maternal position for pushing.
   a. Squatting.
   b. Left side-lying.
   c. Hands and knees.
   d. Semisitting.

7. A woman is having very rapid labor with her fourth child. What nursing measure is most appropriate to help her manage pain?
   a. Offer meperidine (Demerol) when she reaches 5 cm cervical dilation.
   b. Keep her in an upright position until full cervical dilation.
   c. Avoid vaginal examinations during the peak of a contraction.
   d. Coach her to use breathing techniques with each contraction as it occurs.

8. Choose the nursing assessment that most clearly suggests intrauterine infection.
   a. Fetal heart rate of 145-155.
   b. Cloudy amniotic fluid.
   c. Maternal temperature of 37.8° C (100° F).
   d. Increased bloody show.

9. A woman telephones the labor unit and says she has been having back discomfort all day. She is at 32 weeks' gestation. The nurse should tell the woman that she
   a. is having discomfort that is typical of late pregnancy.
   b. should come to the hospital if she has increased vaginal drainage.
   c. can increase her fluid intake to reduce Braxton-Hicks contractions.
   d. should come to the hospital for further evaluation.

10. A woman is receiving magnesium sulfate to stop preterm labor. The essential nursing assessment related to this drug is
    a. for frequency and duration of uterine contractions.
    b. hourly vital signs, heart sounds, and lung sounds.
    c. for presence of fetal movements with contractions.
    d. vaginal examination for cervical dilation, effacement, and station.

11. A few minutes after a woman's membranes rupture during labor, the fetal heart rate drops from an average of 140 to 75-80 bpm. The nurse should immediately
    a. call via telephone the physician and report the decreased fetal heart rate.
    b. assess for other signs that indicate chorioamnionitis.
    c. perform a vaginal examination and palpate for prolapsed cord.
    d. insert an indwelling catheter to keep the bladder empty.

12. A woman telephones the labor unit saying that she has recent onset of pain between her shoulder blades that is worse when she breathes in. The nurse should
    a. ask her if she has had a recent upper respiratory infection.
    b. explain that the growing fetus reduces space to breathe.
    c. have her palpate her uterus for frequent contractions.
    d. tell her that she should come to the hospital promptly.

13. Choose the nursing assessment that most clearly suggests hypovolemia.
    a. Urine output of 20-25 ml/hr.
    b. Fetal heart rate of 155-165.
    c. Blood pressure of 108/84.
    d. Maternal heart rate of 90-100.

28

The Woman with a Postpartum Complication

MATCHING KEY TERMS

Match the term with the correct definition.

1. ______ atony
2. ______ embolus
3. ______ hematoma
4. ______ hypovolemia
5. ______ psychosis
6. ______ thrombus

a. Blood clot within a vessel
b. A clot, usually a thrombus, forced into smaller vessels by the blood circulation
c. Less-than-normal muscle tone
d. Decreased volume of circulating fluid
e. Localized collection of blood
f. Mental state in which a person's ability to recognize reality is impaired

KEY CONCEPTS

1. What is the time difference between early and late postpartum hemorrhage? What quantity of blood loss constitutes postpartum hemorrhage?

2. What is the most common cause of early postpartum hemorrhage? Describe the pathophysiology of this cause of hemorrhage.

3. How will the nurse recognize uterine atony?

4. What is the correct nursing action if uterine atony is discovered?

5. What signs typically distinguish postpartum hemorrhage caused by uterine atony from that caused by lacerations of the birth canal?

6. How do the signs and symptoms of a hematoma differ from those of uterine atony or a bleeding laceration?

7. Describe the body's reaction to hypovolemia and the clinical signs the nurse might detect.

   a. Compensatory

   b. Failure of compensatory mechanisms

8. What discharge teaching related to late postpartum hemorrhage is essential?

9. Why are pregnant and postpartum women prone to develop venous thrombosis?

10. Complete the following chart on venous thrombosis. Include preventive measures.

	Signs and Symptoms	**Medical and Nursing Management**
Superficial venous thrombosis		
Deep vein thrombosis		

11. What laboratory studies should the nurse expect if the woman is on heparin anticoagulation? If the woman is on warfarin anticoagulation?

12. List client teaching related to long-term anticoagulation.

13. What are the signs and symptoms of pulmonary embolism?

14. Define *puerperal infection*.

15. What anatomic features of the woman's reproductive tract make infection there potentially serious?

16. What changes of uncomplicated childbirth further increase a woman's risk for reproductive tract infection? What are her protective factors?

17. What is the significance of a distended, boardlike abdomen in a woman who has metritis? Are other assessments needed? What action should the nurse take?

18. List signs and symptoms of wound infection.

19. What liquids can help acidify urine? Why is this helpful in preventing or treating urinary tract infection?

20. Why is it important that the breast-feeding mother with mastitis empty her breasts completely?

21. How does septic pelvic thrombophlebitis differ from thrombophlebitis?

22. What is the key difference between postpartum "blues" and postpartum depression?

23. Describe the characteristics of each category of postpartum psychosis.

CRITICAL THINKING EXERCISES

1. During clinical practice, review the charts of postpartum women. List all factors that put them at higher risk for infection and the type of infection that would probably occur based on these factors. How should your nursing care change according to their risk for infection and/or the site of the infection?

2. Use the information in Chapter 15 to plan a diet for a breast-feeding woman who had a postpartum hemorrhage without blood replacement.

CASE STUDY

Jana is a gravida 1, para 1, who had a vaginal birth of a 9-pound baby 1½ hours ago. Her fundus has remained firm, midline, and 1 fingerbreadth below the umbilicus. She has not yet voided. Vital signs are stable, and she is afebrile. She received 2 tablets of hydrocodone with acetaminophen (Vicodin) for perineal pain 30 minutes after birth. She now requests "something stronger" for pain because the previous analgesic has been ineffective.

1. What are some possible explanations for the ineffectiveness of the analgesic?

2. Does the nurse need more information? If so, what?

The nurse checks Jana's vital signs 30 minutes later. Her blood pressure is near its previous levels, but her pulse is slightly higher. Her fundal height, firmness, and lochia amount are unchanged. Her perineum is intact and has a small amount of edema. The nurse replaces the ice pack to the perineum that has been in place since Jana's recovery period began.

3. Are any other interventions warranted? If so, what are they and why are they appropriate?

REVIEW QUESTIONS

Choose the correct answer.

1. The nurse notes that a woman has excess lochia 2 hours after vaginal birth of an 8-pound baby. The priority nursing action is to
   a. catheterize her to check urine output.
   b. check her blood pressure, pulse, and respirations.
   c. assess the firmness of her uterus.
   d. notify her physician or nurse-midwife.

2. Choose the signs and symptoms that suggest concealed postpartum hemorrhage.
   a. Rectal pain accompanied by a rising pulse.
   b. Cramping accompanied by a steady trickle of blood.
   c. Soft uterine fundus and a falling blood pressure.
   d. Heavy lochia accompanied by tachypnea and dyspnea.

3. One hour after a woman gives birth vaginally, the nurse notes that her fundus is firm, 2 fingerbreadths above the umbilicus, and deviated to the right. Lochia rubra is moderate. Her perineum is slightly edematous, with no bruising; an ice pack is in place. The priority nursing action is to
   a. chart the expected assessments.
   b. have the woman empty her bladder in the bathroom.
   c. change the perineal ice pack to a warm pack.
   d. increase the rate of the oxytocin infusion.

4. What drug should be readily available when a woman is on heparin therapy?
   a. Vitamin K.
   b. Methylergonovine.
   c. Ferrous sulfate.
   d. Protamine sulfate.

5. The nurse's initial response to a suspected pulmonary embolism should be to
   a. start a second IV line of hypotonic solution.
   b. raise the head of the bed and administer oxygen.
   c. insert a catheter to monitor urine output.
   d. lower the head of the bed and elevate the legs.

6. A woman has an 8 pound 9 ounce baby after an 18-hour labor that required a low-forceps delivery. Her membranes were ruptured for 15 hours. Based on these facts, client teaching should emphasize
   a. reporting foul-smelling lochia.
   b. delaying intercourse for at least 6 weeks.
   c. eating a diet that is high in iron.
   d. losing weight over at least a 6-month period.

7. Postpartum teaching related to urinary health should emphasize
   a. drinking any type of fluid whenever thirsty.
   b. allowing the bladder to fill to promote emptying.
   c. cleansing the perineum in a front-to-back direction.
   d. eating two servings of acidic fruits or vegetables each day.

8. The best position for a woman who has postpartum endometritis is
   a. left lateral.
   b. Trendelenburg.
   c. supine.
   d. Fowler's.

9. A breast-feeding woman develops mastitis. She tells the nurse that she will just feed her baby formula instead of breast feeding. The best nursing response is that
   a. emptying the breast is important to prevent an abscess.
   b. a tight breast binder or bra will help reduce engorgement.
   c. she should continue to drink extra fluids while weaning.
   d. breast-feeding can continue when her temperature is normal.

10. A woman who has a postpartum bipolar psychosis is most likely to demonstrate
   a. intermittent feelings of letdown or frustration with the baby and her life.
   b. gradual reduction of interest in her surroundings and family.
   c. hyperactivity and poor judgment alternating with tearfulness and guilt.
   d. delusions that her baby is dead or will be kidnapped by a stranger.

29 The High-Risk Newborn: Problems Related to Gestational Age and Development

MATCHING KEY TERMS

Match the term with the correct definition.

1. ______ bronchopulmonary dysplasia
2. ______ containment
3. ______ necrotizing enterocolitis
4. ______ pulse oximetry
5. ______ retinopathy of prematurity

a. Damage to blood vessels by oxygen use that may cause blindness
b. Method to determine level of blood oxygen saturation
c. Inflammatory condition of the intestines
d. Pulmonary condition due to prolonged use of supplemental oxygen
e. Method to increase comfort in infants by swaddling

Classify each of these newborn physical characteristics as (a) preterm, (b) term, or (c) postmature. Some letters may be used more than once.

6. ______ underdeveloped flexor muscles
7. ______ abundant hair on the head
8. ______ loose skin
9. ______ little or no lanugo
10. ______ poor muscle tone
11. ______ long fingernails
12. ______ visible blood vessels on the abdomen
13. ______ long, thin body
14. ______ creases cover the entire sole
15. ______ alert and wide-eyed
16. ______ no subcutaneous fat
17. ______ dry and peeling skin
18. ______ “frog-leg” position
19. ______ meconium staining
20. ______ abundant vernix caseosa
21. ______ full areola 5 to 10 mm
22. ______ thick ear cartilage

23. ______ soft, flexible ears
24. ______ labia majora covers clitoris and minora

KEY CONCEPTS

1. Explain newborn classifications of gestational age and birth weight.
   a. Preterm

   b. Low birth weight

   c. Very low birth weight

   d. Extremely low birth weight

   e. Intrauterine growth–restricted

2. Distinguish periodic breathing from apneic spells.

3. Why is the prone position not advised for normal newborns but good for the preterm infant?

4. Why is proper hydration important to maintain good respiratory status?

5. Describe the four major disadvantages the preterm infant has in regulating temperature.
   a. ______________________________
   b. ______________________________
   c. ______________________________
   d. ______________________________
6. List common measures to help the preterm infant maintain thermoregulation.

7. What factors make fluid and electrolyte balance difficult in the preterm infant?

8. Describe measures to evaluate fluid status in the preterm infant.

9. List signs of dehydration and overhydration.

10. What factors typically increase a preterm infant's risk for infection?

11. What are the possible reasons why a preterm infant will need intravenous or gavage feedings?

12. List four methods to identify intestinal complications.
    a. ________________________________
    b. ________________________________
    c. ________________________________
    d. ________________________________

13. What is the purpose of giving an infant a pacifier when gavage feeding?

14. What advantages do nursing and breast milk have for the preterm infant?

15. What signs suggest development of respiratory distress syndrome?

16. What are the two complications of oxygen therapy that may be manifested in preterm infants?

17. What are the two possible consequences for a postmature fetus?

18. Why is the postmature infant likely to have problems with the following?
    a. Hypoglycemia

    b. Thermoregulation

    c. Hyperbilirubinemia

19. What is the difference between symmetrical and asymmetrical intrauterine growth restriction?

20. What are some possible complications of birth for an LGA infant?

CRITICAL THINKING EXERCISES

1. During clinical practice, assess the gestational age of infants you care for and plot their weight, length, and head circumferences on a chart to classify them as SGA, AGA, or LGA. Identify those that have intrauterine growth restriction and what type of IUGR exists (symmetrical or asymmetrical).

2. Note sources of environmental stress in the newborn nursery (for either normal or sick infants). How might these stresses be reduced while maintaining supervision of the babies?

CASE STUDY

Kaylee was born 2 weeks ago at 30 weeks' gestation. Her mother had placenta previa. Continued bleeding along with persistent contractions required a cesarean birth. Kaylee weighed 3 pounds 10 ounces (1642 g) at birth. She had surfactant therapy and mild respiratory distress but did not require mechanical ventilation. She is no longer receiving supplemental oxygen. Her present weight is 3 pounds 7 ounces (1558 g), after a low weight of 3 pounds 4 ounces (1474 g). She is being fed breast milk by a combination of gavage with bottle or breast feeding.

1. What are the three priority nursing diagnoses likely in this scenario? What factors support the nursing diagnoses?

2. What nursing interventions can help Kaylee's parents feel that she is indeed *their* baby?

REVIEW QUESTIONS

Choose the correct answer.

1. To promote drainage of lung secretions in the preterm infant, the nurse should
   a. position the infant in a head-down position.
   b. frequently change the infant's position.
   c. keep the infant in a supine position with the head elevated.
   d. place a small roll under the infant's neck and shoulders.

2. After discharge teaching to the parents of a preterm infant, the nurse evaluates understanding of the information when the parent states
   a. "I don't have to worry about feeding my baby at night if he/she is asleep."
   b. "The car seat I used for my other children will work with this baby."
   c. "My baby will probably start walking later than my other children."
   d. "My baby will take less care than my other children when they were newborns."

3. The purpose of containment in care of the preterm infant is to
   a. simulate the enclosed uterine environment when stressful procedures must be done.
   b. gradually reduce the percentage of supplemental oxygen needed to prevent hypoxia.
   c. recover fluid lost by insensible means and return it to the infant.
   d. limit the formula given by gavage feedings as the infant starts nipple feeding.

4. Discharge teaching for the parents of an infant with bronchopulmonary dysplasia should emphasize
   a. that recurrent grunting and retractions are common.
   b. the importance of providing enzyme formula supplements.
   c. careful handling to prevent pulmonary hemorrhage.
   d. managing equipment for oxygen supplementation.

5. Nursing care that reduces the risk for periventricular or intraventricular hemorrhage includes
   a. assessing for abnormal heart rhythms or murmurs.
   b. minimal and gentle handling of the infant.
   c. limiting the duration of parental visits.
   d. examining the eyes at 4 weeks and 8 weeks.

6. What intervention should be expected for the postmature infant during the first 8 to 12 hours after birth?
   a. Blood glucose determinations.
   b. Placement under phototherapy.
   c. Surfactant replacement.
   d. Blood transfusions.

7. The mother of a preterm infant weighing 1200 g is worried because her baby does not seem to respond to her. The nurse's best response is that
   a. she should stroke her baby as well as talk to him.
   b. infants this young cannot sense the presence of others.
   c. her baby is too immature to tolerate much stimulation.
   d. the baby will respond to her better just before feeding.

30

The High-Risk Newborn: Acquired and Congenital Conditions

MATCHING KEY TERMS

Match the terms with the correct definition.

1. ______ asphyxia
2. ______ bilirubin encephalopathy
3. ______ neonatal abstinence syndrome
4. ______ persistent pulmonary hypertension
5. ______ transient tachypnea of the newborn

a. Brain damage resulting from deposits of bilirubin
b. Vasoconstriction of the infant's pulmonary vessels after birth
c. Insufficient oxygen and excess carbon dioxide in the blood
d. Condition of rapid respirations caused by inadequate absorption of fetal lung fluid
e. Signs exhibited by the newborn exposed in utero to maternal substance abuse

KEY CONCEPTS

1. What is the difference between primary and secondary apnea? Which is more ominous? Why?

2. Compare these newborn respiratory complications.

	Transient Tachypnea of the Newborn	**Meconium Aspiration Syndrome**	**Persistent Pulmonary Hypertension**
Cause(s)			
Manifestations			
Therapeutic management			
Nursing considerations			

3. What is the relationship among bilirubin, jaundice, kernicterus, and bilirubin encephalopathy?

4. Why is phototherapy begun at lower bilirubin levels if the infant is preterm rather than full-term?

5. Formulate a simple explanation about phototherapy to give to parents of a jaundiced newborn. Include in your explanation why the treatment is needed, how it works, and what precautions are needed to prevent injury.

6. What is the purpose of an exchange transfusion?

7. Determine which neonatal infection(s) each of these statements refers to (see Table 30-1, Common Infections in the Newborn.)

   a. Infection is preventable through immunization.

   b. This is typically manifested by white patches in mouth that resemble milk curds.

   c. Mental retardation is associated with the infection.

   d. Antibiotics may be given to high-risk mothers in labor or to an infant after birth.

   e. Antibiotic prophylaxis given soon after birth can prevent blindness.

   f. Maternal antiviral treatment during pregnancy can reduce transmission to infant.

8. List factors that make newborns more vulnerable to sepsis neonatorum.

9. Compare early- and late-onset sepsis.

10. How does the newborn manifest infection compared with an older child? Why is it particularly important to identify newborn sepsis early?

11. Why are tests for drug levels often needed for antibiotics?

12. How can diabetes cause both intrauterine growth restriction and large-for-gestational-age infants?

13. Explain these complications that may occur in the infant of a diabetic mother.
    a. Respiratory distress syndrome
    b. Hypoglycemia
    c. Hypocalcemia
    d. Polycythemia

14. Describe the typical appearance of a macrosomic infant of a diabetic mother (IDM).

15. List signs of neonatal hypoglycemia.

16. Why does the IDM infant with polycythemia require adequate hydration?

17. List infant behaviors that should cause a nurse to suspect prenatal drug exposure.

18. Why are gavage feedings sometimes needed for the drug-exposed infant, even if born at term?

19. Early screening and treatment for PKU are necessary to prevent ________________.

CRITICAL THINKING EXERCISES

1. Imagine that you are the nurse caring for an infant who requires resuscitation at birth. List the things you would want to have readily available. Write out your actions and what you think the actions of other team members will be from the time the infant is brought to the warmer until he or she is breathing adequately.

2. How might the actions in the above scenario change if there were thick meconium in the amniotic fluid?

3. Compare an infant of a diabetic mother with other newborns. What similarities and differences do you note? Can any of these be explained by how well the woman's diabetes was controlled during pregnancy?

4. Observe the reception the mother of an infant exposed to drugs prenatally receives when she visits the nursery. Are the nurses' reactions positive or negative? If they are not positive, what nursing actions might better benefit the mother?

CASE STUDY

Steven is 12 hours old. He was born vaginally with forceps following a 16-hour labor. He has bilateral cephalhematomas. His mother is Rh negative and Steven is Rh positive. His bilirubin level was 7.5, and his Coombs' test was positive on a cord blood sample.

1. Which of the above information indicates a pathologic condition?

2. What other assessments should be performed?

Twenty-four hours after birth, Steven's bilirubin level is 13.5, and his skin is jaundiced.

3. What treatment does Steven require at this time? How does the treatment affect his bilirubin level?

4. Identify the required nursing interventions for Steven once treatment for jaundice has begun.

5. What are the possible side effects of this treatment?

Steven's bilirubin level continues to rise and becomes dangerously high.

6. What complication can occur with dangerously high levels of bilirubin?

7. What treatment should Steven receive at this time to lower his bilirubin levels?

8. What blood type should be used for Steven's treatment and why?

9. How is an exchange transfusion performed?

10. What are the expected results of the transfusion?

11. What are some possible complications of an exchange transfusion?

12. What is the nurse's role in an exchange transfusion?

REVIEW QUESTIONS

Choose the correct answer.

1. Naloxone for neonatal use is supplied in 1 mg/ml vials. The correct volume of naloxone for a neonate weighing 5 pounds 2 ounces is approximately

   a. 0.1 ml.
   b. 0.2 ml.
   c. 0.3 ml.
   d. 0.4 ml.

2. If meconium is present in the amniotic fluid, the infant's mouth and pharynx should be suctioned after the head is born but before the rest of the body. The primary reason for this action is to

   a. limit transfer of infectious substances to the lower airways.
   b. reduce the likelihood that secondary apnea will occur.
   c. prevent persistence of abnormal cardiac shunts.
   d. avoid drawing meconium into the lower airways with the first breath.

3. Infants receiving phototherapy should be fed every 2 to 3 hours to

   a. promote excretion of bilirubin from the bowel.
   b. prevent development of hypothermia.
   c. increase the lifespan of fetal erythrocytes in the blood.
   d. increase renal and liver perfusion.

4. The nurse notes that a 24-hour-old infant is lethargic and his temperature is below normal, a change from an earlier assessment that was normal. Her mother states that she did not breast feed well and that the infant spit up the small amount she had ingested. The nurse's next action should be to

   a. reassure the mother that infants are often sluggish this soon after birth.
   b. feed the infant formula to determine accurately how much intake she is getting.
   c. determine whether there is jaundice over the thoracic and abdominal areas.
   d. assess for signs of sepsis and report assessments to the physician.

5. A mother who has diabetes is concerned because her 36-hour-old baby is "so yellow." She tells the nurse that she thought her baby's problems were over when his blood glucose stabilized even though he was smaller than expected. The best nursing response is that

   a. her baby's liver is also less mature than expected and cannot handle normal red blood cell breakdown.
   b. her baby lived in a lower-than-normal oxygen environment during pregnancy and must eliminate more red blood cells.
   c. the baby's high blood glucose levels immediately after birth caused a slight dehydration that increases jaundice.
   d. early feedings slowed elimination of meconium that would have also eliminated excess bilirubin.

6. The nurse notes that a 12-hour-old infant is jittery, but his blood glucose level is normal. The infant seems hungry but only takes 1/4 ounce of formula with difficulty. The nurse's next action should be to
   a. recheck the glucose level 30 minutes after the feeding.
   b. apply a bag to collect the next sample of urine.
   c. limit infant contact with the mother for the next 12 hours.
   d. swaddle the infant tightly and try to feed more formula.

7. Choose the caregiver teaching that is most appropriate for the infant who was exposed to cocaine prenatally.
   a. Breast feeding is especially important to the infant's recovery from prenatal drug exposure.
   b. Align the infant's face with yours to allow prolonged eye contact that better facilitates bonding.
   c. Do not burp your baby until at least 1 ounce of formula has been taken.
   d. Swaddle your baby with arms and legs flexed to reduce startling.

31

Women's Health Care

MATCHING KEY TERMS

Match the term with the correct definition.

1. _______ climacteric
2. _______ condyloma
3. _______ dysmenorrhea
4. _______ dyspareunia
5. _______ dysplasia
6. _______ menarche
7. _______ menorrhagia
8. _______ metrorrhagia

a. Wartlike growth on genitalia
b. Painful menstruation
c. Onset of menstruation
d. Bleeding from uterus at time other than menstruation
e. Abnormal development of tissue
f. Excessive bleeding at the time of menstruation
g. Painful coitus in women
h. Menopause

KEY CONCEPTS

1. What are the three major preventable problems in women?

2. When should breast self-examination be done?

3. What are the current recommendations for screening mammography?

4. What is the recommendation for vulvar self-examination?

5. What preparation should a woman make for a pelvic examination with Pap test?

6. Describe the signs, symptoms, and treatment for each benign breast disorder.
   a. Fibroadenoma

   b. Fibrocystic breast changes

   c. Ductal ectasia

   d. Intraductal papilloma

7. Describe major management methods for breast cancer.

8. Define each type of amenorrhea and state common causes for each.
   a. Primary

   b. Secondary

9. List common causes of abnormal uterine bleeding.

10. What is the nurse's role when caring for women who have abnormal uterine bleeding?

11. What treatment is typical for each type of menstrual cycle pain?
    a. Mittelschmerz

    b. Primary dysmenorrheal

    c. Endometriosis

12. What nursing measures are appropriate when a woman has PMS?

13. Explain the purpose for each technique that may be used in medical termination of pregnancy and state any side or adverse effects, if applicable.

	Purpose	Side/Adverse Effects
Mifepristone		
Dilation and aspiration with curettage		
Laminaria		
Prostaglandin E_2		

14. Why should a woman promptly report unexpected uterine bleeding after menopause?

15. What is the purpose of giving estrogen with progestin to relieve the symptoms of menopause?

16. List risks of estrogen-progesterone replacement therapy.

17. What signs occur when a woman has osteoporosis?

18. What screening tests may be used to identify female reproductive tract cancers early?

19. Complete the following table on sexually transmissible diseases as you read your text.

	Signs and Symptoms	Treatment	Teaching
Candidiasis			
Trichomoniasis			
Bacterial vaginosis			
Chlamydia			
Gonorrhea			
Syphilis			
Herpes genitalis			
Condylomata acuminata			
Acquired immunodeficiency syndrome			

20. How does pelvic inflammatory disease occur? What are its results?

CRITICAL THINKING EXERCISES

1. Talk with a woman who has had breast cancer about her feelings upon learning the diagnosis and during the wait between diagnosis and treatment.

2. When caring for people who have experienced age-related fractures, such as a hip fracture, note how many of them are older and female. Do you note any other adverse effects of osteoporosis?

REVIEW QUESTIONS

Choose the correct answer.

1. Breast self-examination should be performed using the
   a. palm of the left hand to palpate the right breast in a wedge pattern.
   b. horizontal pattern to palpate across both breasts at one pass.
   c. middle three fingertips of the left hand to palpate the right breast.
   d. thumb of the opposite hand to palpate each breast in a circular pattern.

2. Your friend calls to tell you that she noticed a small amount of nipple retraction in her right nipple when she was showering. As a nurse, you should advise her to
   a. perform a complete breast self-examination to determine if any lumps are present.
   b. wait until 1 week after her next menstrual period and then do a breast self-examination.
   c. note if there is any change in the amount of nipple retraction for 2 weeks.
   d. see her primary health care provider for a professional examination.

3. A woman will have screening for fecal occult blood. Choose the correct instructions.
   a. Do not take nonsteroidal anti-inflammatory drugs for 48 hours before collecting the sample.
   b. Eat two servings of red meat each day for 3 days before obtaining the specimen.
   c. Collect a small sample of stool from the first stool expelled each morning for 3 days.
   d. Refrigerate the samples until they can be returned to the laboratory for testing.

4. Preoperative nursing care for the woman anticipating a modified radical mastectomy for breast cancer includes preparation for
   a. restricted arm movement on the operative side for 2 weeks after surgery.
   b. a small dressing applied to the operative site.
   c. drainage tubes that will remove fluid that accumulates under the operative area.
   d. a hospital stay of 3 to 4 days.

5. To relieve her menstrual cramps, a woman should be taught to take ibuprofen
   a. within 8 hours of the onset of menstruation.
   b. before onset of menstruation and cramps.
   c. every 4 hours during the 2 days preceding menstruation.
   d. on an empty stomach before the pain becomes severe.

6. Your friend is having hot flashes as she enters menopause. She is interested in hormone replacement to improve these symptoms but is fearful of breast cancer. As a nurse, you should tell her that
   a. her physician or nurse-practitioner can evaluate her actual risk and help her make a better decision.
   b. the risk of breast cancer is very small for women who are under the age of 60 when menstrual periods stop.
   c. taking the estrogen with progestin will reduce the risk for estrogen-induced breast cancer.
   d. the benefits of estrogen replacement therapy far outweigh any risks associated with it.

7. When teaching the woman to take alendronate (Fosamax), the nurse should tell her to
   a. take the tablet with a full glass of milk to prevent gastric pain.
   b. take the medication at night just before bedtime to promote absorption.
   c. reduce intake of calcium supplements after being on the drug for 1 month.
   d. remain upright for at least 30 minutes after taking the drug each morning.

8. The woman who has age-associated urinary incontinence should be taught to
   a. avoid alcohol and caffeinated drinks.
   b. reduce fluid intake before special events.
   c. limit ingestion of foods that acidify urine.
   d. urinate at least every 2 hours while awake.

9. To reduce the risk for toxic shock syndrome, women should be taught to
   a. avoid changing tampons until they are thoroughly saturated.
   b. use a diaphragm with spermicidal jelly during the menstrual period.
   c. wash hands thoroughly before inserting a tampon or diaphragm into the vagina.
   d. limit the use of superabsorbent tampons to the times when flow is heavy.

32

Communicating With Children and Families

HELPFUL HINT

Review sections on language and cognitive development in Chapters 4 through 8 in your textbook.

MATCHING KEY TERMS

Match the term with the correct definition.

1. ______ empathy
2. ______ empowerment
3. ______ active listening
4. ______ professional boundaries
5. ______ sensory information
6. ______ self-esteem
7. ______ win-win solution

a. Information gained from sight, taste, touch, smell, and hearing
b. Personal value that individuals place on themselves
c. Seeing a situation from another person's perspective while remaining objective
d. Limits that separate professional from personal relationships; observed in work settings
e. Attending to another person to gain an understanding of the actual as well as implied message
f. Actions taken to enable another person to participate fully in decision making
g. Resolution of a conflict that parties can support

COMPONENTS OF EFFECTIVE COMMUNICATION

Answer as either true (T) or false (F).

8. ______ Communication involves more than expressing words from one person to another.
9. ______ Touch communicates more meaning to a younger child than it does to an older child.
10. ______ The child or family members may feel intimidated when the nurse stands over them while talking.
11. ______ A nurse watching a television program with the child is an example of communicating attentiveness to the child.
12. ______ Eye contact is a communication connector.
13. ______ Infants are too young to sense emotions from a speaker's tone of voice.
14. ______ Talking with a child with your hands on your hips is an example of a closed body posture.
15. ______ An appropriate time to teach a 4-year-old about surgery is immediately after the parents have gone home.

FAMILY-CENTERED COMMUNICATION

16. What does family-centered care emphasize?

    ____

    ____

17. List five key components of open communication in a family-centered care environment.
    a.
    b.
    c.
    d.
    e.

18. The nurse's ability to __________________________ is critical in establishing good rapport with families.

19. Identify seven strategies to manage conflict.
    a.
    b.
    c.
    d.
    e.
    f.
    g.

20. Why is it important for nurses to be knowledgeable about culture?

THERAPEUTIC RELATIONSHIPS: DEVELOPING AND MAINTAINING TRUST

21. List three behaviors that are warning signs of nurse overinvolvement.
    a.
    b.
    c.

NURSING CARE: COMMUNICATING WITH CHILDREN AND FAMILIES

Answer as either true (T) or false (F).

22. ______ The optimal time to prepare a toddler for a painful procedure is just before the procedure is done.
23. ______ Explanations should include what the child will experience through the senses.
24. ______ It is better not to tell a child how long a painful or invasive procedure will take.
25. ______ Once a procedure is completed, it should not be discussed with the child.

Rewrite each of the following statements so that they are more appropriate for a nurse talking to a 6-year-old child.

26. "It's time for your dressing change." ____
____
27. "I am going to get you on the floor now." ____
____
28. "I am going to give you a shot." ____
____
29. "Let's get your vitals taken." ____
____

COMMUNICATING WITH CHILDREN WHO HAVE SPECIAL NEEDS

30. Suggest three strategies the nurse could use to communicate with a child who has a severe visual impairment.
    a.
    b.
    c.

31. Suggest three strategies for communicating with a child who is deaf.
    a.

    b.

    c.

32. Suggest three strategies for communicating with a child who has a profound neurologic impairment.
    a.

    b.

    c.

SUGGESTED LEARNING ACTIVITIES

1. Review Table 32-4, "Considerations in Choosing Language" in your textbook. Think about the words you use when talking to children. How often have you used potentially ambiguous, hard, or unfamiliar language? Make a conscious effort to use clear, softer, and more familiar language. Once you have had the opportunity to try this "new" language, consider its effects. What were the children's reactions to each style of communication?

STUDENT LEARNING APPLICATION

Enhance your learning by discussing your answers with other students.

A mother brings her 4-year-old son, Juan, to the pediatrician's office for a well-child examination. The physician completes the examination and reminds her that Juan is due for immunizations during this visit. The nurse walks into the examining room holding a syringe in her hand. She looks at Juan and says, "This shot is so you won't get diphtheria, pertussis, or tetanus. I am going to put the needle in your leg (points to thigh area). You can cry or yell, but I need you to keep your leg still. It is going to hurt." She gives the injection and says, "Here is a Band-Aid to put on the sore spot. That wasn't too bad, was it?" The nurse leaves before Juan has a chance to respond.

1. What effective communication techniques were used by this nurse?

2. What communication pitfalls do you recognize in this nurse-child interaction?

3. What suggestions can you offer to make the nurse's communication more effective?

Martina is a 3-year-old with a diagnosis of liver failure. Martina is deaf. Her mother, who is present, primarily speaks Spanish but can understand some English. When Jan, the nursing student, enters Martina's room, the child cries and wants to be held by her mother. Jan approaches Martina to take vital signs, but the child cries even louder.

4. What does Martina's behavior communicate to you?

5. What should Jan do about measuring vital signs at this time?

6. How can Jan establish a rapport with the mother? with Martina?

7. What measures should Jan take to communicate with Martina's mother? with Martina?

REVIEW QUESTIONS

Choose the best answer.

1. A 5-year-old is scheduled for a CT scan of her head. What is the best time for her mother to initiate a discussion about the procedure?
   a. Immediately before the procedure begins
   b. Two hours before the procedure
   c. The day before the procedure
   d. A few days before the procedure

2. Which of the following nurse actions indicates that the nurse understands the components of effective communication?
   a. The nurse stands right next to the chair where the child is seated.
   b. The nurse asks an adolescent if she can give her a hug.
   c. The nurse speaks to a child who is aphonic in a loud, clear voice.
   d. The nurse talks with her arms folded across her chest.

3. An adolescent tells the nurse, "I don't like this hospital room." Which of the following is an active listening response to this child's statement?
   a. "Don't you know this is the best room in the house?"
   b. "Let me see whether there are other rooms available."
   c. "What's wrong with this room?"
   d. "So, you would prefer a different room?"

4. The developmentally appropriate strategy for the nurse to use when doing preoperative teaching with a 10-year-old is to:
   a. keep explanations under 5 minutes.
   b. organize information sequentially.
   c. use puppets to explain the surgery.
   d. start preoperative teaching 3 hours before the surgery.

5. A child with a hearing impairment needs to have an arm cast. What can the nurse do to facilitate communication with the child throughout the cast application process?
   a. Face the child when speaking.
   b. Speak at a slower pace than usual.
   c. Talk clearly and directly into the child's ear.
   d. Keep gestures to a minimum.

6. Which of the following examples describes how a nurse can display an open body posture?
   a. Speaking to a child with head bowed
   b. Frequently shifting weight from one leg to the other while speaking
   c. Leaning away from the child while talking
   d. Talking while hands are moving freely

7. A child has just been diagnosed with diabetes. The child's father tells the nurse, "My wife will be back in the morning. Before she left, she told me that she has a lot of questions about what to do." What is the most appropriate response for the nurse to make at this time?
   a. "You will be meeting with the clinical specialist tomorrow. Ask her tomorrow."
   b. "Did the clinical specialist give you any papers to read? If not, I'll get a pamphlet for you."
   c. "Your wife might want to write down her questions so she won't forget anything when she comes back tomorrow."
   d. "Why don't you tell me what information you got from the clinical specialist today?"

33

Physical Assessment of Children

HELPFUL HINT

Review the physical assessment of the infant and child in a nursing health assessment textbook.

MATCHING KEY TERMS

Match the term with the correct definition.

1. ______ auscultation
2. ______ circumduction
3. ______ crepitation
4. ______ development
5. ______ fasciculation
6. ______ fremitus
7. ______ growth
8. ______ history
9. ______ inspection
10. ______ obtund
11. ______ palpation
12. ______ percussion
13. ______ systematic assessment

a. Vibration perceptible on palpation or auscultation
b. Organized method of collecting data
c. Use of touch to determine temperature, moisture, and organ placement
d. Circular movement of a limb or an eye
e. Aggregate of subjective data that describe past and present health status
f. Tapping of the body to determine density, location, and size of organs
g. Elicitation and evaluation of sounds produced by body
h. Observation to identify physical findings
i. Dry, crackling sound or sensation
j. Small, local, involuntary muscle contraction visible under the skin
k. To render dull or blunt
l. Change that occurs over time in functional, psychosocial, and cognitive behavior
m. Measurable physical and physiologic changes that occur over time

GENERAL APPROACHES TO PHYSICAL ASSESSMENT

Answer as either true (T) or false (F).

14. ______ It is appropriate to auscultate the heart, lungs, and abdomen while an infant is sleeping.
15. ______ Stranger anxiety makes the physical examination of an older infant more difficult.
16. ______ Parents should not be present during a young child's physical examination.
17. ______ In all age groups, invasive procedures should be saved until the end of the examination.

18. ______ Adolescents should be allowed to participate in deciding who will be present during the physical examination.

19. ______ For adolescents, the physical examination proceeds from head to toe.

TECHNIQUES FOR PHYSICAL EXAMINATION

Fill in the blanks.

20. Using an ophthalmoscope is an example of ________ inspection.

21. In palpating the lymph nodes for general assessment, the nurse uses the ____________________.

22. In palpating the lymph nodes specifically for heat, the nurse uses the ____________________.

23. When percussing the liver, the nurse would expect to hear ________ sounds.

24. The ____________________ of the stethoscope is most effective in auscultating low-pitched sounds.

Match each type of history with its description.

25. ______ Complete history

26. ______ Episodic history

27. ______ Well-interim history

a. Information about a specific problem is added to an existing database.

b. Information about a child from conception to present.

c. Information gathered from last well visit to current visit.

Answer as either true (T) or false (F).

28. ______ Axillary temperatures are preferable to rectal temperatures because they are less invasive.

29. ______ The apical impulse is palpated to determine the position of the heart.

30. ______ All irregular heart rhythms in children require immediate attention.

31. ______ The respiratory rate in infants can be counted by observing the movement of the abdomen.

32. ______ A blood pressure cuff that covers three-quarters of the distance between the child's antecubital fossa and shoulder will give a falsely low reading.

33. Give two ways of measuring the length of an infant.

____

____

34. Why is the head circumference measured at every visit until the child is 3 years old?

____

____

Fill in the blanks.

35. All scales must be ____________________ before use.

36. Chest circumference is measured at the ____________________.

37. Midarm circumference is a measure of _______________ and _______________.
38. An adolescent who is 62 inches tall and weighs 120.5 pounds has a body mass index (BMI) of _______.
39. To complete a growth chart on a child's height, the nurse should do the following:
    a. Use a chart appropriate for the child's ________ and ______________________.
    b. Find the child's age on the _______________ axis.
    c. Find the child's height on the _______________ axis.
    d. Mark where the two lines _______________.
    e. Note the _______________.
40. Depigmentation of the skin is called __________________.
41. On a child, the nurse assesses skin turgor on the ___________ or ______________.
42. Unusual hair loss is called ___________; excessive hair growth is called_______________.
43. When a child has head lice, nits are found on the ______________________.
44. Capillary refill should be within ______________________seconds.
45. When assessing a child's face, the nurse examines cranial nerves ___________ and _______________.
46. Frequent wiping of the nose indicates that the child probably has ______________.
47. The philtrum is the ____.
48. How does the nurse examine cranial nerve XII?

    ____

49. By eliciting the gag reflex, the nurse assesses cranial nerve _______.

Match each test with its description.

50. ______ Allen
51. ______ sweep
52. ______ Ishihara
53. ______ Weber
54. ______ Snellen
55. ______ shisper

a. Tests ability to hear via bone conduction
b. Tests visual acuity in a 30-month-old child
c. Tests hearing acuity in an 8-year-old child
d. Tests color vision
e. Tests for hearing loss
f. Tests visual acuity in a 12-year-old child

Answer as either true (T) or false (F).

56. ______ Breathing is more diaphragmatic in a school-age child than in a toddler.
57. ______ Prior to auscultation of breath sounds, have a toddler sit upright on the parent's lap.
58. ______ Normal breath sounds are called adventitious.
59. ______ The apical pulse is also called the point of maximal impulse (PMI).
60. ______ Auscultation of the heart is best done by listening with the bell of the stethoscope only.

61. ______ A pause between the closing of the pulmonic and aortic valves is a normal finding in children.

62. ______ Functional heart murmurs require immediate intervention.

63. When should adolescent females start performing monthly breast self-examinations?

____

64. When assessing the abdomen, why does auscultation follow inspection?

____

65. Describe how to test for rebound tenderness.

____

____

66. How can the nurse decrease adolescent anxiety during a genital examination?

____

67. Why are adolescent males taught to do monthly testicular examinations?

____

Match each term with its description.

68. ______ lordosis
69. ______ Ortolani maneuver
70. ______ genu varum
71. ______ scoliosis
72. ______ kyphosis

a. Performed until the child is 1 year old
b. Common in young children
c. Related to poor posture
d. Bowleg
e. Lateral nonpainful curvature of the spine

Answer as either true (T) or false (F).

73. ______ To evaluate neurologic functioning in a child younger than 5 years of age, use the DDST II.

74. ______ The nurse should test all of the cranial nerves at the beginning of the physical examination.

75. ______ *Obtunded* is a term used to describe one of the altered levels of consciousness.

76. ______ As part of the neurologic examination, it is important to assess a toddler's orientation to person, place, and time.

77. ______ Depression may alter a child's ability to solve problems.

78. ______ Tests designed to assess cerebellar function vary with the child's age.

79. ______ Responses to eliciting the Babinski reflex depend on the child's ability to walk.

80. ______ Neurologic "soft" signs are normal variants and require no further assessment.

STUDENT LEARNING ACTIVITY

1. Perform a complete history and physical assessment on an infant, a child, and an adolescent. Describe your findings clearly and coherently in writing.

STUDENT LEARNING APPLICATIONS

Enhance your learning by discussing your answers with other students.

During a physical assessment on an infant, child, or adolescent, many variables can alter either the process or the findings. Describe how you would handle a physical assessment in each of the following situations.

1. A toddler's parents are not present during the examination.

2. A school-age child's level of cognitive functioning is far below average.

3. An adolescent is experiencing moderately severe abdominal pain.

4. A 9-month-old infant is exhibiting a high degree of stranger anxiety.

5. A preschooler believes that undergoing the physical examination is punishment for being bad.

REVIEW QUESTIONS

Choose the best answer.

1. A 1-year-old child is at the pediatrician's office for a well-interim visit. When interviewing the parents, the nurse should:
   a. obtain a complete history from conception to the present.
   b. record information about the child's chief complaint.
   c. obtain a family history.
   d. gather data about what has occurred since the last visit.

2. Before auscultating a toddler's lungs, the nurse should:
   a. examine the child's ears and throat.
   b. ask the parent(s) to leave the room.
   c. allow the child to examine the stethoscope.
   d. do none of the above.

3. The nurse begins auscultation of the abdomen in the:
   a. RUQ.
   b. RLQ.
   c. LUQ.
   d. LLQ.

4. Which of the following is an abnormal finding?
   a. Posterior fontanel is flat and soft in an 8-month-old infant.
   b. A 7-month-old sits using hands for support.
   c. Breathing is abdominal in a 3-month-old child.
   d. A 5-year-old's pupils dilate when focusing on a distant object.

5. Which of the following is a normal finding in a school-age child?
   a. Bone conduction is greater than air conduction.
   b. Cerumen is found in the external auditory meatus.
   c. Discharge is present in the ear canal.
   d. The tympanic membrane is stationary.

6. An assessment technique of the chest and lungs normally reserved for the advanced nursing practitioner is:
   a. inspection.
   b. auscultation.
   c. palpation.
   d. percussion.

7. The point of maximal impulse (PMI) is located at the fifth intercostal space in the midclavicular line after about age:
   a. 2 months.
   b. 18 months.
   c. 4 years.
   d. 7 years.

8. An example of a "soft" neurologic sign is:
   a. a short attention span.
   b. left handedness.
   c. nonmirroring movement of the extremities.
   d. none of the above.

9. Which of the following sounds occurs when parts of the lungs lose their lubricating fluid?
   a. High-pitched wheezing
   b. Pleural friction rub
   c. Rales
   d. Sonorous rhonchi

10. Which of the following reflexes is elicited by suddenly and briskly dorsiflexing the child's foot and applying moderate pressure?
   a. Achilles
   b. Babinski
   c. Clonus
   d. Patellar

34 Emergency Care of the Child

HELPFUL HINT

Review anatomy and physiology of the cardiac and respiratory systems.

MATCHING KEY TERMS

Match the term with the correct definition.

1. ______ cardiopulmonary resuscitation
2. ______ dental emergency
3. ______ envenomation
4. ______ hypothermia
5. ______ ingestion
6. ______ submersion injury
7. ______ trauma
8. ______ triage

a. Injury from an external cause
b. Protocol performed when an individual's respiratory and cardiovascular systems require support to maintain vital functions
c. Cooling of body temperature to subnormal levels
d. Injury or infection of a tooth in which prompt medical attention is critical for the survival of the tooth or to alleviate pain
e. Swallowing of a potentially toxic substance
f. Sorting process used to decide the urgency of an individual's illness or injury and to allocate appropriate resources effectively
g. Injuries resulting from a near-drowning incident
h. Injection of venom by an animal

GENERAL GUIDELINES FOR EMERGENCY NURSING CARE

9. List five interventions that can facilitate a more positive and comfortable emergency experience for a child and family.
   a.
   b.
   c.
   d.
   e.

10. When family members hear that their teenager sustained serious injuries in an automobile accident, they become very emotional in the waiting room. Identify three guidelines that the nurse could use to handle this situation.
    a.

    b.

    c.

Match each medication with its use in pediatric emergency care.

11. ______ Activated charcoal
12. ______ Atropine sulfate
13. ______ Bretylium tosylate
14. ______ Dextrose
15. ______ Epinephrine
16. ______ Nalaxone
17. ______ Sodium bicarbonate

a. Reverses the effects of some narcotics
b. Treats symptomatic bradycardia
c. Treats bradycardia or asystolic arrest
d. Treats ventricular tachycardia
e. Treats severe acidosis
f. Reduces drug absorption in toxic ingestions
g. Treats hypoglycemia

GROWTH AND DEVELOPMENT ISSUES IN EMERGENCY CARE

Match each age group with the appropriate nursing interventions.

18. ______ Infant
19. ______ Toddler
20. ______ Preschooler
21. ______ School-age
22. ______ Adolescent

a. Ascertain child's level of understanding and allow time for questions.
b. Allow the child to have familiar objects to help him feel safe.
c. Use a soothing voice and touch, rock, or cuddle the child.
d. Explain procedures carefully and allow choices.
e. Distract the child with bright objects or noises.

The Family of a Child in Emergency Care

23. ________ and ________ are the two most common emotions experienced by parents of children cared for in emergencies.

Emergency Assessment of Infants and Children

24. Describe the role of the triage nurse.

    ____

25. Name three essential factors in an initial pediatric triage assessment.
    a.

    b.

    c.

26. List the components of primary assessment.

A: ____________________

B: ____________________

C: ____________________

D: ____________________

E: ____________________

Answer as either true (T) or false (F).

27. ______ A respiratory rate over 60 breaths per minute is considered abnormal for a child of any age.

28. ______ Tachycardia and decreased peripheral perfusion are early signs of cardiovascular compromise in a child.

29. ______ Infants and young children have a higher percentage of fluid located in the intracellular compartment.

30. ______ For the first several months of life, the presence of nasal secretions can cause respiratory compromise in infants.

31. ______ Abdominal breathing is abnormal for infants and young children.

32. What are the four components of a secondary assessment?

a.

b.

c.

d.

33. Give the suggested order for measuring vital signs in children.

____

____

34. Identify the elements of an AMPLE history.

A: ____________________

M: ____________________

P: ____________________

L: ____________________

E: ____________________

35. Which laboratory tests are considered standard protocol in an emergency setting?

____

36. Why is determining the child's weight essential in emergency care?

____

Cardiopulmonary Resuscitation of the Child

37. What are the two most common causes of cardiopulmonary arrest in children?
    a.

    b.

38. Ventilations should be given at a rate of ____________________, or approximately one breath every ______ seconds.

39. What is the emergency intervention for an obstructed airway in a conscious child?

____

40. What is the emergency intervention for an obstructed airway in an unconscious child?

____

41. What is the rationale for NOT performing blind finger sweeps for infants and children?

____

42. What is the emergency intervention for removal of a foreign object from an infant?

____

43. Before and during cardiac compressions, the nurse feels for a pulse in the infant at the ________________; for a child over 1 year of age, at the ________________.

44. According to the American Heart Association, chest compressions are performed at a rate of ________________.

45. The drug of choice for management of cardiac arrest is ________________.

THE CHILD IN SHOCK

Indicate whether each statement refers to hypovolemic (H), cardiogenic (C), or distributive (D) shock.

46. ______ This is the most common type of shock seen in children.

47. ______ This occurs when myocardial function is unable to produce cardiac output that meets the metabolic demands of the body.

48. ______ This occurs when microbial toxins are in the bloodstream.

49. ______ Early signs include warm extremities and purpuric skin lesions.

50. ______ Diuretics are prescribed because of increased intravascular volume.

51. ______ Periorbital edema, crackles, and diaphoresis are clinical manifestations.

52. ______ Initial treatment involves administration of colloids.

Answer as either true (T) or false (F).

53. ______ Hypotension is an early sign of shock in children.
54. ______ Septic shock is the most common cause of hypovolemic shock.
55. ______ Early signs of cardiogenic shock include hypothermia followed by hyperthermia.
56. ______ Vasoconstrictors are used in cardiogenic shock to increase cardiac output.

PEDIATRIC TRAUMA

Answer as either true (T) or false (F).

57. ______ Injury is the leading cause of death for children.
58. ______ Injuries from blunt trauma are often less obvious, yet more serious, than injuries from penetrating trauma.
59. ______ Unrestrained individuals involved in an automobile accident are more likely to be injured than are restrained individuals.
60. ______ The greatest number of pedestrian injuries occurs in children aged 5 to 9 years.
61. ______ An example of a penetrating injury is a gunshot wound.
62. State the goal of the primary survey.
63. Identify the four elements of a primary survey.
    a.

    b.

    c.

    d.

64. What is included in a secondary survey?

    ____

65. For each of the following types of injury, write two questions that the nurse should ask when obtaining a history of the injury.

    Motor vehicle accident: ______________________

    Fall: ______________________

    Penetrating injury: ______________________

66. List five indicators or physical findings that should raise suspicion of child maltreatment.
    a.

    b.

    c.

    d.

    e.

67. What is the most critical aspect of nursing care of the pediatric trauma patient?

    ____

INGESTIONS AND POISONINGS

68. Most poisonings occur as a result of ______________________________.

69. List the five methods used to treat toxic exposure or ingestion.
    a.

    b.

    c.

    d.

    e.

Answer as either true (T) or false (F).

70. ______ Respiratory acidosis is an early manifestation of aspirin toxicity.

71. ______ Hydrocarbon ingestion is associated with chemical pneumonitis.

72. ______ Milk or water is recommended to dilute ingested acids.

73. ______ Activated charcoal has become the recommended treatment for acute poisoning in the pediatric population.

74. ______ Gastric lavage is used to empty the stomach of the toxic substance in the first 1 to 2 hours after an ingestion.

75. ______ The dosage of activated charcoal is usually administered 3 to 4 g/kg.

76. ______ The antidote for acetaminophen ingestion is mucomyst.
77. ______ Emesis should be induced following ingestion of corrosive substances.
78. ______ A serum lead level that is greater than 10 μg/dl is considered harmful.
79. List three questions that should be asked when a child has ingested a poisonous substance.
    a.
    b.
    c.

ANIMAL, HUMAN, AND SNAKE BITES

80. List four local signs and symptoms of a snake bite.
    a.
    b.
    c.
    d.
81. Describe the nursing care of an injury from a dog bite.

    ____

SUBMERSION INJURIES

82. The injury to organ systems that occurs in drowning is the result of ____________.
83. Explain the relationship between submersion in cold water and the diving reflex.

    ____

84. Assessment of the child with a submersion injury focuses on which body system?

    ____

85. The research demonstrates that the need for ____________ is a highly ranked need identified by families of critically ill children.

HEAT-RELATED EMERGENCIES

86. What is the first priority in the management of all pediatric heat-related illnesses?

    ____

87. Describe the treatment for heat exhaustion.

____

88. What are the clinical manifestations of heat stroke?

____

DENTAL EMERGENCIES

Answer as either true (T) or false (F).

89. ______ If a tooth is loose in the socket, it can be removed.

90. ______ An avulsed tooth can be placed in saline or milk for transport to emergency care.

SUGGESTED LEARNING ACTIVITIES

1. Arrange to observe in an emergency department that handles pediatric clients. Ask the nurses about the kinds of pediatric problems that are seen most often.

STUDENT LEARNING APPLICATION

Enhance your learning by discussing your answers with other students.

You are observing in the emergency department when the paramedics bring in 6-year-old Lindsay, who was struck by an automobile when she darted into the street from between two parked cars. The nurse is performing a primary survey on Lindsay when the child goes into cardiac arrest. A neighbor who saw the accident brings Lindsay's mother to the hospital. She arrives at the emergency department while the trauma team is giving Lindsay cardiopulmonary resuscitation. When the mother is told about Lindsay's condition, she begins crying loudly and repeating, "Please don't let her die." The nurse says, "Don't worry now. We won't."

1. What is the correct sequence for CPR for Lindsay?

2. What medications do you expect the nurse to prepare in this emergency situation?

3. What assessments should be included in Lindsay's primary survey?

4. What questions should be directed to the neighbor who witnessed the situation?

5. What do you think about the nurse's response to Lindsay's mother? Offer an alternative response.

6. What can be done for the mother during this emergency situation?

REVIEW QUESTIONS

Choose the best answer.

1. A 2-year-old boy is brought to the emergency department after swallowing over-the-counter antihistamine tablets about 30 minutes earlier. He is now irritable and lethargic. What is the best approach for gastric emptying in this situation?
   a. Dilute the toxic substance with water or milk.
   b. Administer an antidote such as nalaxone.
   c. Perform gastric lavage.
   d. Administer syrup of ipecac.

2. Which medication is used to treat severe acidosis associated with cardiac arrest?
   a. Epinephrine
   b. Calcium chloride
   c. Sodium bicarbonate
   d. Atropine sulfate

3. Which nursing action might help the toddler to feel more secure in the emergency department?
   a. Perform the most distressing procedures first.
   b. Distract the child by counting numbers.
   c. Give the child a reward for cooperative behavior.
   d. Allow the child to hold his favorite toy.

4. Which of the following is assessed first in an initial triage assessment?
   a. Respiratory rate and effort
   b. Skin color and temperature
   c. Response to environment
   d. Heart rate and rhythm

5. When a child's breathing makes a high-pitched sound on inspiration, what term should the nurse use to identify this breath sound?
   a. Snoring
   b. Stridor
   c. Wheezing
   d. Crackles

6. What is one reason that a small child is at a greater risk for airway problems than is an adult?
   a. The child's thicker, inflexible trachea can more easily obstruct the airway.
   b. Children less than 3 years of age are obligate nose breathers.
   c. The child's airway is narrower and more easily obstructed by small amounts of mucus.
   d. The child's smaller tongue creates more space for foreign body obstruction.

7. Which of the following vitals signs indicates that a 5-year-old child requires immediate attention?
   a. Systolic blood pressure of 80 mm Hg
   b. Bulging, pulsatile posterior fontanel
   c. Heart rate of 94 beats per minute
   d. Respiratory rate of 68 breaths per minute

8. Which finding in a 1-year-old child with hypovolemic shock should be reported immediately?
   a. Flat, anterior fontanel
   b. Palpable peripheral pulses
   c. Moist mucous membranes
   d. Less responsive to painful stimuli

9. What is the most common form of distributive shock?
   a. Septic
   b. Hypovolemic
   c. Cardiogenic
   d. Anaphylactic

10. The primary focus of assessment of cardiovascular status in a child with multiple trauma is to identify:
    a. hypovolemia.
    b. septic shock.
    c. cardiac arrest.
    d. electrolyte imbalance.

11. Which of the following is an indicator of hypovolemic shock in a 2-month-old infant?
    a. Bulging anterior fontanel
    b. Capillary refill of less than 2 seconds
    c. Parental report of two wet diapers in past 24 hours
    d. Extremities warm to the touch

12. When drowning occurs, injury to organ systems is the result of:
    a. hypoxia.
    b. respiratory acidosis.
    c. hypokalemia.
    d. hypoglycemia.

13. After a 10-year-old child falls on his face, his mother notices that the upper central incisors are loose. What should she do?
    a. Remove the loose teeth and put them in a container of milk.
    b. Call the dentist and schedule an appointment within the week.
    c. Leave the teeth alone and call the dentist for an immediate appointment.
    d. Ask the child to wiggle the teeth loose while driving to the nearest emergency department.

14. Which vital sign is measured first in children?
    a. Temperature
    b. Pulse
    c. Respiratory rate
    d. Blood pressure

15. Which of the following is the first compensatory mechanism for decreased cardiac output in children?
    a. Tachycardia
    b. Hypotension
    c. Cyanosis
    d. Diminished breath sounds

35

The Ill Child in the Hospital and Other Care Settings

HELPFUL HINT

In your textbook, review Chapters 4 through 8 on growth and development; Chapter 32, "Communicating with Children and Families"; Chapter 36, "The Child With a Chronic Condition or Terminal Illness"; and Chapter 39, "Pain Management for Children."

MATCHING KEY TERMS

Match the term with the correct definition.

1. ______ denial
2. ______ egocentric
3. ______ regression
4. ______ separation anxiety
5. ______ situational crisis
6. ______ therapeutic play

a. An unanticipated event that poses a threat to an individual's well-being
b. Guided play that promotes the child's psychosocial or psychological well-being
c. Distress and apprehension caused by being removed from parents, home, or familiar surroundings
d. Preoccupation with one's own interests and needs
e. Defense mechanism in which unpleasant realities are kept out of conscious awareness
f. Defense mechanism in which conflict or frustration is resolved by returning to a behavior that was successful in earlier years

SETTINGS OF CARE

7. List four settings where the pediatric nurse can provide health or illness care to children.
   a.

   b.

   c.

   d.

Answer as either true (T) or false (F).

8. ______ One role of the pediatric nurse in a hospital setting is that of tour guide.
9. ______ A child who is dehydrated may be admitted to the hospital for a 24-hour observation.
10. ______ Because of limited time, preparing a child for a procedure in an emergency setting is not an important nursing action.
11. ______ Teaching the child and family is less of a concern in an outpatient facility than it is in an acute care setting.
12. ______ In a rehabilitative setting, nurses must balance nurturing the child with setting limits as the child learns to be more self-sufficient.
13. ______ The nurse working in a school-based clinic needs to be sensitive to parental concerns regarding sexuality issues.
14. ______ In a community clinic, the nurse integrates health promotion into acute care.
15. ______ In home care, the nurse serves as case manager and care coordinator.

STRESSORS ASSOCIATED WITH ILLNESS AND HOSPITALIZATION

16. Identify four factors that influence a child's reaction to illness.
    a.

    b.

    c.

    d.

17. Separation anxiety is most significant in the ____________ and ____________ age groups.
18. Describe behaviors associated with the three stages of separation anxiety.

    Protest: ____

    Denial: ____

    Detachment: ____
19. How is a toddler's acting out behavior in the hospital an indicator of a healthy parent-child attachment?

    ____

    ____
20. How can nurses minimize disruption in a toddler's usual routines during hospitalization?

    ____

    ____

21. How can hospitalization intensify a preschooler's fear of injury?

____

____

22. Describe actions to promote a sense of control during hospitalization for the school-age child.

____

____

23. How might the need to be like everyone else affect adolescents who have diabetes mellitus?

____

____

24. Give two examples of regressive behavior the nurse might observe in a child who is hospitalized.
    a.

    b.

FACTORS AFFECTING A CHILD'S RESPONSE TO ILLNESS AND HOSPITALIZATION

25. Identify three factors that affect how a child copes with illness or hospitalization.
    a.

    b.

    c.

26. Give two strategies that might facilitate a child's ability to cope with illness and hospitalization.
    a.

    b.

27. Identify two potential psychological benefits of hospitalization.
    a.

    b.

PLAYROOMS IN HEALTH CARE SETTINGS

28. How is therapeutic play different from normal play? ______________________

____

29. What is emotional outlet play? ______________________________

____

30. How can the nurse keep the hospital playroom a "safe place" for the child?

____

____

31. Give an example of how a child's cooperation with a treatment plan can be enhanced through play.

____

ADMITTING THE CHILD TO A HOSPITAL SETTING

32. How can the nurse set a positive tone for the child and family on admission?

____

____

33. A focused assessment should include the following five areas:

____

____

____

____

____

THE ILL CHILD'S FAMILY

34. How does the parental role change as a result of hospitalization?

____

____

35. Identify three common reactions that a child might have to a sibling being hospitalized.
 a.

 b.

 c.

DEVELOPMENTAL APPROACHES TO THE HOSPITALIZED CHILD

Match each intervention with the appropriate age group. (Age groups may be used more than once.)

36. ______ Be particularly careful to follow home routines and rituals.
37. ______ Provide a special area for activities with this age group.
38. ______ Provide safe outlets for acting out aggression, such as painting and using play dough.
39. ______ Reassure child that he/she did not cause the illness.
40. ______ Assist the child in contacting friends.
41. ______ Limit the number of caregivers assigned to the child.
42. ______ Provide opportunities for nonnutritive sucking and oral stimulation.

a. Neonates
b. Infants
c. Toddlers
d. Preschoolers
e. School-age children
f. Adolescents

SUGGESTED LEARNING ACTIVITIES

1. Arrange for clinical observations in a school or community clinic, pediatrician's office, home care setting, or some other nonacute care setting. Compare the role of the pediatric nurse in these settings with that of the pediatric nurse in the hospital.

2. Develop a plan for a toddler experiencing separation anxiety during hospitalization.

STUDENT LEARNING APPLICATIONS

Enhance your learning by discussing your answers with other students.

David is a 3-year-old child who had an emergency appendectomy. This is the first day after his surgery. David has not been hospitalized previously. His mother stayed with him last night, and his father is planning to visit this evening after work. The family lives about 60 miles from the hospital. David has a 7-year-old sister, Sara, who is in second grade. The grandmother is taking care of Sara after school today.

1. What stressors do you think the family is experiencing at this time?

2. When you get report on David, you learn that he clings to his mother every time a hospital staff member comes into his room. How can you help David cope with his fears?

3. David's mother tells you that she will be going home tonight with her husband because she needs to make arrangements for Sara's care. What advice would you offer her about leaving David?

4. When you ask David whether he wants to have his blood pressure taken, he says "No." What would you do now?

5. David has cried inconsolably for 2 hours since his parents left. When you go to check on him, you find that he has wet his pajamas. What is your interpretation of these behaviors? How would you explain them to David's mother when she calls to check on him?

REVIEW QUESTIONS

Choose the best answer.

1. Which child is most likely to have difficulty with separation during hospitalization?
   a. A 3-month-old
   b. An 18-month-old
   c. A 3-year-old
   d. A 5-year-old

2. Which type of behavior would be expected when a child is in the despair stage of separation anxiety?
   a. Agitated
   b. Playful
   c. Withdrawn
   d. Anxious

3. A young child cries, kicks, and clings to his mother when she tries to leave. What is the nurse's best comment to the mother about this behavior?
   a. "This child is experiencing ineffective coping."
   b. "Parents should not leave their children when they are hospitalized."
   c. "Wait until the child falls asleep to leave."
   d. "This behavior actually shows a healthy attachment between parent and child."

4. Which of the following would not be developmentally appropriate for a hospitalized adolescent?
   a. Allow the adolescent to wear her own clothing.
   b. Provide privacy when giving treatments.
   c. Suggest that her parents bring in her favorite foods.
   d. Discourage visits from school friends.

5. Which of the following nursing interventions might help the hospitalized toddler feel a sense of security and control?
   a. Follow the child's usual bedtime routine.
   b. Place the child in a crib with a cover over it.
   c. Tell the child what needs to be done and do not offer choices.
   d. Suggest to the parents that they buy the child a new toy.

6. What is the best nursing response to a father who is concerned because his 4-year-old daughter has been using the bathroom independently for over a year now but has had a few "accidents" since she has been hospitalized?
   a. Suggest that he take his daughter to the bathroom more often.
   b. Assure him that this behavior will disappear immediately after discharge.
   c. Explain that children often exhibit regressive behaviors because of the stress of hospitalization.
   d. Set up a reward system to motivate the child to use the bathroom.

7. A 7-year-old child, who is going to have a lumbar puncture later today, tells the nurse, "I'm really nervous about this test." What is the best way to minimize the child's anxiety before the procedure?
   a. Review the lumbar puncture procedure with him.
   b. Give him a relaxation tape to practice.
   c. Read a book to him about being in the hospital.
   d. Distract him by playing his favorite board game.

8. Ten-year-old Meg told the school nurse that she is worried about her twin sister, Mary, who is in the hospital. Which of the following might increase Meg's stress about her sister?
   a. Meg's grandparents are helping to care for her at home.
   b. Meg's parents have explained Mary's illness to her.
   c. Meg wonders if she will get sick, too.
   d. Meg plans to visit her sister today after school.

9. Emotional outlet play would be appropriate in which of the following situations?
   a. A child who does not feel well enough to play
   b. A child who is having a hip spica cast applied in the morning
   c. A child who needs to cough and deep breathe postoperatively
   d. A child who has been physically abused

10. Why might a 4-year-old child think that she caused her younger sibling's illness, which necessitated hospitalization?
   a. Preschool-age children understand disease transmission.
   b. The child feels insecure since the birth of the sibling.
   c. The feeling of closeness to her sibling makes her feel responsible for the illness.
   d. Children are magical thinkers at this age.

36

The Child With a Chronic Condition or Terminal Illness

HELPFUL HINT

Review Elizabeth Kübler-Ross' work on death and dying.

MATCHING KEY TERMS

Match the term with the correct definition.

1. ______ anticipatory grief
2. ______ chronic condition
3. ______ chronic sorrow
4. ______ hospice care
5. ______ illness trajectory
6. ______ normalization
7. ______ palliative care

a. The course of an illness, including its impact on those involved
b. Responses used to counteract an illness or abnormal behavior in order to maintain appropriate and valued social roles
c. A system of comprehensive care that provides support and assistance to clients and families affected by terminal illness
d. Recurrent feelings of grief, loss, and fear related to the child's illness and the loss of the ideal, healthy child
e. The processes of mourning, coping, interacting, planning, and psychosocial reorganization that occur as part of the response to the impending death of a loved one
f. Medical treatment or procedures that promote comfort and quality of life, rather than aiming to cure the underlying disease
g. A condition or an illness that is long term and either without cure or with residual effects that limit activities of daily living

8. How does a chronic condition differ from an acute illness?

____

____

9. In what ways has the experience of childhood chronic illness changed?

____

____

10. What is meant by the term *children with special health care needs*?

____

____

THE FAMILY OF THE CHILD WITH SPECIAL HEALTH CARE NEEDS

11. What does the term *situational crisis* mean?

 ____

 ____

12. The predominant trait exhibited by resilient families is ________________.

13. List four additional traits of the resilient family system.
 a.

 b.

 c.

 d.

Answer as either true (T) or false (F).

14. ______ In resilient families, the child's condition-related needs become the focus around which family activities revolve.

15. ______ For resilient families, coping is an active process that involves learning about their child's condition and available resources.

THE GRIEVING PROCESS

16. The nurse caring for a child with a chronic illness must keep in mind that the most important aspect of a chronic illness is that it affects ________________

 ____.

17. Identify the five stages of the grieving process delineated by Kübler-Ross.
 a.

 b.

 c.

 d.

 e.

Answer as either true (T) or false (F).

18. ______ Children move through the five stages of the grieving process sequentially.
19. ______ Children with a chronic condition tend to use denial more frequently than do adults.

THE CHILD WITH SPECIAL HEALTH CARE NEEDS

20. Children's responses to chronic illness are influenced by their ________________ and their ____________________________.
21. Nurses caring for children with chronic conditions must understand issues concerning ____________________ and ________________ in relation to each stage of growth and development.

Answer as either true (T) or false (F).

22. ______ Temporary regression may be observed in children of all ages.
23. ______ Rearing a child with a chronic illness necessitates that parents learn a different set of child-rearing techniques.

THE CHILD WITH A CHRONIC ILLNESS

24. The goal for a child with a chronic illness is to:

    ____
25. Goals for the family system include:

    ____
26. What is the first factor the nurse must consider when planning care for a child with a chronic illness? ____________________________
27. ____________ is the most important factor in establishing a good relationship with a child and family.
28. List three significant needs of parents of children with a chronic condition.
    a.

    b.

    c.

Answer as either true (T) or false (F).

29. ______ Honesty and trust must be maintained at all times when caring for a child with a chronic condition.
30. ______ Siblings of a chronically ill child may also experience developmental regression.
31. ______ Siblings should not participate in the ill child's physical care.

NURSING CARE: THE CHILD WITH A CHRONIC CONDITION IN THE COMMUNITY SETTING

32. Identify one nursing diagnosis for the child with a chronic condition.

    ____

33. What is the rationale for providing opportunities for autonomy when caring for a child with a chronic condition?

    ____

34. Write an expected outcome for a child who has a disturbed body image resulting from alopecia caused by chemotherapy.

    ____

THE TERMINALLY ILL OR DYING CHILD

Match each age group with the corresponding concept of death.

35. ______ Infants/toddlers
36. ______ Preschoolers
37. ______ School-age children
38. ______ Adolescents

a. Death is temporary and reversible.
b. Death is a sad and irreversible event.
c. Death is viewed as the loss of a caretaker.
d. Death is inevitable and irreversible.

Answer as either true (T) or false (F).

39. ______ One of the primary concerns of dying children is the fear of being alone.
40. ______ It is unusual for parents to talk about the experience of the child's illness and death.
41. ______ An important aspect of supporting the sibling of a child who has died is to acknowledge that the loss is significant.

CARING FOR THE DYING CHILD

42. Identify three self-care measures that can assist nurses caring for terminally ill children.

    a.

    b.

    c.

43. What is the most common issue surrounding a child's impending death?

    ____

    ____

Answer as either true (T) or false (F).

44. ______ Pain control is the primary concern for dying children, family, and nursing staff.

45. ______ Hospice care for terminally ill children is increasing.

46. ______ The nurse should provide privacy for the dying child and family.

47. ______ Adequate oral intake is crucial to the dying child's comfort.

48. ______ The absence of either verbal communication or physical touch is detrimental to the dying child.

49. ______ The young child is usually not aware of the presence of parents during the dying process.

50. ______ Respiratory changes are always the earliest indicators of imminent death.

51. ______ Hypercapnia has a sedative effect.

52. ______ The nurse's response to caring for a dying child correlates to a certain degree with the Kübler-Ross stages of grieving.

SUGGESTED LEARNING ACTIVITIES

1. Investigate the availability of pediatric hospice care in your area.

2. Arrange to make a home visit to the family of a child with a chronic illness. How does home care compare with hospital care?

STUDENT LEARNING APPLICATION

Enhance your learning by discussing your answers with other students.

1. What are your fears or concerns about caring for a child who is dying? Talk with other students about your thoughts. Are your fears or concerns similar to or different from those of the other students?

2. Talk to a nurse who has worked with dying children and their families. What has been the most rewarding aspect of this work? The most difficult? Share what you learned with other students.

REVIEW QUESTIONS

Choose the best answer.

1. The most significant concern of the parents of a dying child is the child's:
   a. pain.
   b. hydration.
   c. safety.
   d. privacy.

2. A 4-year-old child understands death as:
   a. the loss of a caretaker.
   b. a temporary separation.
   c. sad and permanent.
   d. something that happens to everyone.

3. Although an individual may fluctuate between stages of the grieving process, the first stage is usually:
   a. denial.
   b. resentment.
   c. bargaining.
   d. depression.

4. Chronic illness with frequent hospitalizations can affect the psychosocial development of a school-age child by:
   a. leading to feelings of inferiority.
   b. preventing a sense of initiative.
   c. interfering with parental attachment.
   d. blocking the development of identity.

5. What is the best response to an adolescent who asks whether he should talk to his dying brother?
   a. "You might want to hold his hand instead because he cannot hear you."
   b. "Although he may not answer you, your brother can still hear what you are saying."
   c. "He can't hear you but he can feel your presence nearby."
   d. "Talk about happy things because you don't want to upset him."

6. Which of the following represents the predominant trait of resilient families?
   a. Disengaging the family from the community
   b. Maintaining rigid family roles
   c. Engaging in efforts to keep the family intact
   d. Focusing on the child's condition-related needs

7. Which of the following interventions is appropriate when caring for a chronically ill toddler?
   a. Prepare for procedures days in advance.
   b. Arrange for friends to visit in the hospital.
   c. Limit parental participation in the child's care.
   d. Keep security objects nearby.

8. What is the nurse's first consideration when planning care for the child with a chronic illness?
   a. Child's condition
   b. Child's development
   c. Family's coping mechanisms
   d. Family's understanding of prognosis

37

Principles and Procedures for Nursing Care of Children

HELPFUL HINT

Review Chapter 32, "Communicating with Children and Families," and Chapter 35, "The Ill Child in the Hospital and Other Care Settings."

MATCHING KEY TERMS

Match the term with the correct definition.

1. ______ informed consent
2. ______ apical pulse rate
3. ______ enteral
4. ______ antipyretic
5. ______ auscultate
6. ______ lavage

a. To listen to body sounds
b. By way of the digestive system
c. Requirement that both the child and the parent/guardian completely understand the proposed procedures or treatments
d. Agent that reduces or relieves fever
e. Process of washing out or irrigating an organ
f. Heart rate determined by placing stethoscope over the point of maximum intensity (PMI) and counting for 1 minute

PREPARING CHILDREN FOR PROCEDURES

7. List five assessments the nurse should make in preparing a child and family for an invasive procedure.
   a.

   b.

   c.

   d.

   e.

Answer as either true (T) or false (F).

8. ______ Children need to be prepared before any procedure is performed.
9. ______ Parents need to be prepared before a procedure is performed on their child.
10. ______ It is preferable to perform painful or invasive procedures in the treatment room.
11. ______ The nurse should praise children only when they have been cooperative during a procedure.
12. ______ Parents should be asked to step out of the room before an invasive procedure is started.
13. ______ Informed consent is obtained from the parent before any surgical or diagnostic invasive procedures.
14. ______ Children over 7 years of age can give informed consent for procedures.

TRANSPORTING INFANTS AND CHILDREN

15. Name four factors that must be considered when choosing the method of transportation for a hospitalized child.
    a.

    b.

    c.

    d.

USING RESTRAINTS

Answer as either true (T) or false (F).

16. ______ Restraints are applied only as a last resort and not for the staff's convenience.
17. ______ The physician's order for restraints should indicate why the restraints are necessary and how long they should be in place.
18. ______ When restraints are applied, the distal extremity is assessed for temperature, pulses, and capillary refill.
19. ______ Restraints should be removed every 4 hours for range of motion and repositioning.

INFECTION CONTROL

20. List the four body components to which Standard Precautions apply.
    a.

    b.

c.

d.

BATHING INFANTS AND CHILDREN

21. The temperature of water used to bathe a child should not exceed ______________.
22. If a thermometer is not accessible, the nurse can determine whether water temperature is comfortable by ____.
23. When bathing an infant in the tub, the nurse makes sure that the water level does not exceed ____ inches.
24. What is the rationale for avoiding talcum powder after a child's bath?

____

ORAL HYGIENE

Answer as either true (T) or false (F).

25. ______ Young children require supervision with brushing teeth.
26. ______ A quarter-sized amount of toothpaste should be placed on the toothbrush each time the child brushes his teeth.
27. ______ Cleaning teeth is avoided when the child is at risk for gingival bleeding.

FEEDING

28. What is the rationale for not propping a bottle when feeding an infant?

____

29. Name three strategies that might make hospital meals more desirable for young children.
    a.

    b.

    c.

VITAL SIGNS

30. What are the indications for measuring axillary temperatures in children?

____

31. What factors might cause an inaccurate measurement of oral temperature?

____

Answer as either true (T) or false (F).

32. ______ Mercury thermometers are recommended for use only in the acute care setting.

33. ______ A mildly elevated axillary temperature should be confirmed by measuring the child's rectal temperature.

34. Give three reasons for a nurse to measure a child's apical pulse.
    a.
    b.
    c.

35. How long should the nurse count a heart rate when measuring an apical pulse?_____

36. The nurse measuring respirations on a 6-month-old would auscultate breath sounds for ______ seconds.

37. The nurse measuring blood pressure hears a systolic pressure at 88 and continues to hear it down to a measurement of zero. This blood pressure should be recorded as______.

FEVER-REDUCING MEASURES

38. The rationale for not using aspirin as an antipyretic for children is that ____.

39. The drugs (generic names) used to treat fever in children are ________________ and____________________.

40. Long-term use of acetaminophen can cause damage to which organ? _____________

SPECIMEN COLLECTION

41. Regardless of the type of specimen to be obtained, the nurse should use _______________ Precautions.

42. The nurse should not attempt to do a throat culture when ______________________ is suspected.

43. Catheterization at home is usually performed as a _____________ procedure.

44. The most common site for bone marrow aspiration in the child is the ____________________.

GAVAGE AND GASTROSTOMY

45. When and how often should the nurse check placement of a nasogastric tube?
    ____

46. Name three methods for determining placement of a nasogastric tube.
    a.

    b.

    c.

Answer as either true (T) or false (F).

47. ______ The most reliable method for determining nasogastric tube placement is auscultation of air entering the stomach.
48. ______ Tube placement and residual volumes should be checked every 24 hours when continuous enteral feedings are infusing.
49. ______ The only definitive method of determining the correct position of a feeding tube is radiographic confirmation.
50. ______ When a bolus feeding is completed, the child is placed on the left side for 30 minutes.

ENEMAS

51. When giving an enema to a 7-year-old child, the nurse should use a volume of _______ and insert the tube into the rectum no farther than ________.

CARE OF OSTOMIES

Answer as either true (T) or false (F).

52. ______ The consistency of stool through an ostomy is determined by the anatomic location of the stoma.
53. ______ The nursing care of a child with an ostomy differs very little from that of an adult.

OXYGEN THERAPY

54. How does oxygen therapy in children differ from therapy in adults?

    ____

ASSESSING OXYGENATION

55. The nurse measures a child's pulse oximetry to be 98%. What does this finding indicate? ______________________________
56. What action should the nurse take if this child's pulse oximetry drops to 89%?

    ____

CHEST PHYSIOTHERAPY

57. Define *percussion.*

58. Define *postural drainage.*

59. When should chest physiotherapy be performed in relation to meals?

____

TRACHEOSTOMY CARE

60. What are the five elements of routine tracheostomy care?
 a.

 b.

 c.

 d.

 e.

61. How often should the nurse perform tracheostomy care? ______________________
62. Catheter insertion and suctioning time should be limited to _______.
63. The suction catheter is inserted with the suction ______.

SURGICAL PROCEDURES

64. At what point preoperatively should clear liquids be stopped?

____

65. What nursing interventions are appropriate to prevent atelectasis postoperatively?

____

66. Identify five stressors that may be experienced by a child undergoing surgery.
 a.

 b.

 c.

d.

e.

SUGGESTED LEARNING ACTIVITIES

1. Follow a child through a surgical experience. Take note of preoperative procedures and teaching, as well as postanesthesia care. When the child returns to the unit, provide immediate postoperative care. How is this nursing care similar to or different from preoperative and postoperative care of an adult?

STUDENT LEARNING APPLICATION

Enhance your learning by discussing your answers with other students.

Betsy is a 3-year-old child who is going to have a bilateral ureteral reimplantation to correct vesicoureteral reflux. She is scheduled for surgery in the morning. She and her parents have just arrived at her assigned room, and you are assigned to admit Betsy to the unit. Betsy's admission orders include routine urinalysis and complete blood count.

1. How are you going to measure Betsy's vital signs?

2. Betsy is not toilet-trained yet. How would you collect a urine specimen from her?

3. Her mother tells you that she wants to stay with Betsy when you take blood for the CBC. What is your response? Where are you planning to do this procedure?

4. How would you explain the procedure for venipuncture to Betsy?

5. Betsy's father wants to know when she has to stop eating before surgery. What would you tell him?

6. What do you want to know from Betsy and her parents before you do any preoperative teaching?

REVIEW QUESTIONS

Choose the correct answer.

1. A parent wants to wait outside until a procedure is completed on his child. Which of the following would be the nurse's best response?
   a. "It would be better for your child if you were by his side."
   b. "That is fine. I will stay with your child during the procedure."
   c. "It is hospital policy for parents to step out of the room during procedures."
   d. "This test will only take a few minutes. Why don't you stay?"

2. Which of the following temperatures indicates fever?
   a. 100.6° F rectally
   b. 99.5° F rectally
   c. 98.9° F orally
   d. 97.9° F axillary

3. What advice should the nurse offer a parent about reducing a child's fever?
   a. Give the child an alcohol bath.
   b. Sponge bathe the child in tepid water.
   c. Administer baby aspirin.
   d. Dress the child in heavy-weight clothing.

4. Which of the following indicates the nurse is correctly measuring vital signs on an infant?
   a. Measuring oral temperature for 5 minutes
   b. Counting apical pulse for 60 seconds
   c. Recording respiratory rate from the cardiorespiratory monitor
   d. Recording blood pressure as P/46

5. A 9-year-old child asks the nurse where the doctor is going to put the needle for his bone marrow test. The nurse describes the location as the:
   a. lower middle part of his back.
   b. middle part of his chest.
   c. right or left side of his hip.
   d. top bone in his leg.

6. When an extremity is restrained, it is essential for the nurse to assess the affected area for:
   a. clubbing.
   b. pallor.
   c. spasm.
   d. crepitus.

7. Nasogastric tube placement should be checked:
   a. prior to initiating a bolus feeding.
   b. when the feeding is completed.
   c. every 12 hours during continuous feedings.
   d. when residual volumes are excessive.

8. The nurse should discontinue a bolus gavage feeding if which of the following occurs?
   a. Fatigue
   b. Crying
   c. Phlebitis
   d. Vomiting

9. Which of the following statements about ostomies is correct?
   a. The lower the stoma along the intestinal tract, the more liquid is the stool.
   b. Urinary stomas do not begin to drain until the second postoperative day.
   c. A minimal amount of drainage from colostomies is normal up to 4 days after surgery.
   d. Children usually do not require appliances on their stomas.

10. What should the nurse teach parents about chest physiotherapy?
    a. Give treatments before meals.
    b. Schedule treatments about 30 minutes after meals.
    c. Treatments should last about 45 minutes to 1 hour.
    d. Children must be placed in all of the postural drainage positions with each treatment.

11. A 2-year-old is scheduled for surgery tomorrow. The parents have been told to arrive at the short procedure unit at 8:00 A.M. The nurse should expect preoperative feeding instructions to include:
    a. clear liquids until midnight tonight, then nothing by mouth.
    b. stopping solid food at 5:00 A.M., then clear liquids until 7:00 A.M.
    c. fluids including milk and orange juice until arrival at the hospital.
    d. clear liquids until 6:00 A.M., then nothing to eat or drink.

38 Medicating Infants and Children

HELPFUL HINT

Review pharmacodynamics and pharmacokinetics in a pharmacology or nursing fundamentals textbook.

MATCHING KEY TERMS

Match the term with the correct definition.

1. _____ EMLA
2. _____ metered-dose inhaler
3. _____ pharmacodynamics
4. _____ pharmacokinetics
5. _____ central venous access device
6. _____ peripherally inserted central line

a. Central line inserted via antecubital vein into the superior vena cava
b. Hand-held device that delivers "puffs" of medication for inhalation
c. Cream used to numb skin at a depth of 0.5 mm
d. Behavior of medications at the cellular level
e. Venous access device placed in the superior vena cava or jugular vein
f. Time and movement relationships of medications

PHARMACOKINETICS IN CHILDREN

7. Name four factors that influence absorption of medications administered orally.
   a.

   b.

   c.

   d.

Answer as either true (T) or false (F).

8. _____ Infants have a larger body surface area–to–weight ratio than adults.
9. _____ Compared with an adult, a child requires a lower dose per kilogram of a water-soluble medication to achieve its desired effect.
10. _____ The immaturity of the blood-brain barrier in a child results in a decreased distribution of medications to the brain.

11. What factors affect drug excretion in the infant?

____

12. Why would a peak and trough serum level be measured?

____

13. The level at which the serum concentration is lowest is referred to as the medication ____________.

PSYCHOLOGIC AND DEVELOPMENTAL DIFFERENCES

14. Name three ways parents can assist the nurse with administering medications to children.
    a.

    b.

    c.

15. Describe two strategies to elicit cooperation from children of the following age groups when administering medications.

    Toddler:
    a.

    b.

    Preschooler:
    a.

    b.

    School-age child:
    a.

    b.

CALCULATING DOSAGES

Answer as either true (T) or false (F).

16. ______ Standard doses exist for pediatric medications.
17. ______ Pediatric doses are usually calculated based on the child's weight in pounds.
18. ______ The most reliable method for determining pediatric medication dosages is to use the body surface area formula.

ADMINISTRATION PROCEDURES

19. List three procedures that should be followed to avoid medication errors when giving medications to children.
    a.

    b.

    c.

20. Why is the oral route one of the least reliable methods of medication administration?

    ____

    ____

21. What should a nurse do if a child cannot swallow tablets or capsules?

    ____

    ____

22. Why should the nurse mix a powdered medication with a "nonessential" food?

    ____

    ____

MEDICATION ADMINISTRATION

Answer as either true (T) or (F) false.

23. ______ Honey can be mixed with medications and given to infants.
24. ______ A sustained-release tablet can be crushed if the child cannot swallow it.
25. ______ Liquid medication should be placed in the child's mouth along the side of the cheek.
26. ______ Oral medications should be administered with the child in an upright position.
27. How can the nurse hold a 3-year-old child who does not want to take oral medication?

    ____

    ____

28. What nursing action should be taken if the child vomits a medication 15 minutes after it was given?

    ____

29. What procedures should be followed when administering medications via a feeding tube?

    ____

    ____

ADMINISTERING INJECTIONS

30. What are the guidelines for giving an explanation to a child before administering an injection?

____

31. What can the nurse do to make injections less painful?

____

ADMINISTERING INTRAMUSCULAR INJECTIONS

Match each injection site with its indication for use.

32. ______ Vastus lateralis
33. ______ Ventrogluteal
34. ______ Dorsogluteal
35. ______ Deltoid

a. Not used for young children because muscle cannot hold the volume of medication
b. Usually used for children younger than 3 years
c. Safe for children older than 18 months
d. Not used until child has been walking for at least 1 year

Answer as either true (T) or false (F).

36. ______ The nurse should document the site used for an injection.
37. ______ The air bubble technique should be used when preparing pediatric injections.
38. ______ Toddlers can receive up to 1.5 ml of a drug safely in the ventrogluteal site.
39. ______ Viscous medication is less painful when injected through a smaller-gauge needle.

ADMINISTERING SUBCUTANEOUS INJECTIONS

40. A subcutaneous injection should not be used if ______________ is impaired.
41. Name four areas of the body that are preferred subcutaneous injection sites.
    a.

    b.

    c.

    d.

Answer as either true (T) or false (F).

42. ______ Subcutaneous injection sites need to be rotated to prevent the development of abscesses.
43. ______ The angle of needle insertion for a subcutaneous injection is usually 90 degrees.
44. ______ Volumes for subcutaneous injections can be as high as 3 ml.

INTRADERMAL INJECTIONS

45. The intradermal route is most often used for ____________________

46. What sites are used for intradermal injections?

____

47. Describe the procedure for administering an intradermal injection.

____

RECTAL ADMINISTRATION

Answer as either true (T) or false (F).

48. ______ Rectal administration of medications is as safe and reliable as other routes.

49. ______ The child should be placed in a prone position for administration of a rectal suppository.

50. ______ The nurse should direct the child to take a deep breath as medication is inserted into the rectum.

OPHTHALMIC AND OTIC ADMINISTRATION

Answer as either true (T) or false (F).

51. ______ Instillation of ophthalmic drops is a sterile procedure.

52. ______ Otic solutions should be warmed to room temperature before being administered.

53. ______ To administer ear drops to a 5-year-old child, pull the pinna of the ear down and back.

INHALATION THERAPY

54. A ____________ used with a metered-dose inhaler increases the effectiveness of the medication.

55. If a child inhales too quickly when using a metered-dose inhaler with a spacer, she will hear a ____________.

56. How long should a child hold her breath after an inhaling a "puff" of medication from a metered-dose inhaler? ____________________

INTRAVENOUS THERAPY

57. What factors should be considered when selecting a site for an intravenous line?

____

58. List a nonpharmacologic technique for helping a child cope with the discomfort of intravenous catheter insertion. ____________________

59. What are the guidelines for using EMLA cream prior to inserting an intravenous catheter?

____

____

60. Why should a volumetric infusion pump be used when administering IV fluids?

____

61. How frequently should an IV site be assessed? ____________________

62. What assessments should be made? ____________________

63. The formula for calculating maintenance fluid needs is: ____________________

____

____

64. Calculate the maintenance fluid requirements for children of the following weights.

35 kg: ________________

16 kg: ________________

65. What is meant by *IV push medications*?

66. Where does the nurse insert the syringe containing the medication when administering medication via the IV retrograde route?

67. Why is it important to flush the IV tubing after administering an IV piggyback medication?

____

68. How frequently should an intermittent infusion port or heparin lock be flushed?____

69. In what types of situations are central venous access devices used?

____

70. What is an implanted venous access device?

71. The major complications of peripherally inserted central catheters (PICC line) are ____

____

ADMINISTRATION OF BLOOD OR BLOOD PRODUCTS

Answer as either true (T) or false (F).

72. ______ Blood should be infused with a dextrose solution on a piggyback setup.

73. ______ Packed red blood cells are administered to infants and children to prevent circulatory hypervolemia.

74. ______ Blood products should be used within 30 minutes of arrival from the blood bank.

75. ______ An important nursing action is to take the child's vital signs before initiating a blood transfusion.

76. ______ The infusion is discontinued immediately if a transfusion reaction is suspected.

CHILD AND FAMILY EDUCATION

77. List six points that need to be addressed when teaching parents about administering medications to a child at home.
    a.

    b.

    c.

    d.

    e.

    f.

SUGGESTED LEARNING ACTIVITIES

1. Review a child's medication Kardex. Calculate dosages for prescribed medications. Determine whether the prescribed dosage is safe for the child. Observe medication administration. What techniques were helpful to the child? To the nurse?

STUDENT LEARNING APPLICATION

Enhance your learning by discussing your answers with other students.

Kelly is a 9-year-old girl with cystic fibrosis. Kelly is in the hospital for an exacerbation. Her cough has worsened, she has lost weight, and she is mildly dehydrated. She weighs 55 pounds. Kelly's admission orders include IV fluids and medications.

1. Kelly needs to have an IV line placed for fluids and medications. What could you do to minimize her discomfort before and during the venipuncture?

2. There is an order to give Kelly D5 .225 NSS at 65 cc/hr. Calculate her maintenance fluid requirements. How does this order compare with your calculation?

3. There is an order to give tobramycin 40 mg IVPB every 8 hours. The dosage range for children is 6–7.5 mg/kg/day divided every 8 hours. Is Kelly's dose within that range?

4. Two days later, Kelly's maintenance IV line is converted to a heparin lock. How does the care of a heparin lock differ from that of a continuous IV?

5. Kelly's IV line has infiltrated, and a PICC line is discussed. What is a PICC line? What are the advantages of having a PICC line instead of a heparin lock?

6. Kelly needs to take Pancrease capsules before meals and snacks. Her mother tells you Kelly cannot swallow pills. What additional information would you want her to know about giving medications to Kelly?

7. When you approach Kelly to administer her oral medications, she turns her head away and puts her hand over her mouth. What would you do to get Kelly to take her medications? What would you do if Kelly's mother were present?

REVIEW QUESTIONS

Choose the best answer.

1. Physiologic differences in the gastrointestinal system between children and adults affect which component of drug action?
   a. Absorption
   b. Distribution
   c. Metabolism
   d. Excretion

2. Drug toxicity may occur more rapidly in the infant for which of the following reasons?
   a. Larger surface area requires a larger dosage.
   b. Fewer enzymes are available to bind with the drug.
   c. Renal immaturity may delay drug excretion.
   d. The blood-brain barrier becomes less selective with maturity.

3. The pediatric maintenance dosage for Dilantin is 4 to 8 mg/kg/day in three equal doses. A safe morning dose for a child weighing 15 kg is:
   a. 30 mg.
   b. 60 mg.
   c. 90 mg.
   d. any of these dosages would be safe.

4. Which of the following foods is the best choice for mixing with a medication to be administered to an infant?
   a. Honey
   b. Cherry syrup
   c. Similac with iron
   d. Pudding

5. Which of the following sites should the nurse use to administer an intramuscular injection to a 17-month-old child?
   a. Deltoid
   b. Dorsogluteal
   c. Vastus lateralis
   d. Ventrogluteal

6. When administering insulin subcutaneously, the nurse should:
   a. use a 1- to $1\frac{1}{2}$-inch needle.
   b. rotate injection sites.
   c. administer a very small volume such as 0.1 ml.
   d. inject the needle at a 30-degree angle.

7. Which of the following actions is appropriate for the administration of a rectal suppository?
   a. Position the child on his abdomen.
   b. Insert the suppository 1 to 2 inches.
   c. Direct the child to take a deep breath.
   d. Ask the child to get up and walk around after insertion.

8. Which of the following statements about the administration of IV piggyback medications is correct?
   a. The undiluted medication is pushed directly into the IV catheter through the port closest to the patient.
   b. The medication is injected into the port nearest the child and flushed through the tubing slowly.
   c. The IV catheter is used intermittently when medication is infused over a 1- to 2-hour period.
   d. The medication is diluted in at least 20 ml of IV fluid and infused over at least 15 minutes.

39

Pain Management for Children

HELPFUL HINT

Review pain management in a medical-surgical nursing textbook.

MATCHING KEY TERMS

Match the term with the correct definition.

1. ______ AHRQ
2. ______ conscious sedation
3. ______ epidural
4. ______ nocioceptive
5. ______ pain
6. ______ pain threshold
7. ______ patient-controlled analgesia (PCA)
8. ______ transcutaneous electrical nerve stimulation (TENS)

a. Self-administration of an analgesic by a client instructed in how to do so
b. Impulse giving rise to the sensation of pain
c. Agency for Healthcare Research and Quality
d. Method of producing electroanalgesia through electrodes applied to the skin
e. Unpleasant sensory and emotional experience associated with actual or potential tissue damage
f. Situated within the spinal canal, on or outside the dura mater
g. Level of intensity at which pain becomes appreciable or perceptible
h. "Light sedation" during which child retains airway and other protective reflexes and can respond to verbal stimuli

DEFINITIONS AND THEORIES OF PAIN

9. According to McCaffrey and Paero, *pain* is

____

10. The International Association for the Study of Pain defines *pain* as

____

Answer as either true (T) or false (F).

11. ______ The gate control theory supports the use of physiologic and psychologic interventions in pain management.
12. ______ Rubbing a sprained ankle makes the pain worse.
13. ______ A child with arthritis typically experiences acute pain.
14. ______ Acute pain experienced by hospitalized children is often procedural pain.
15. ______ Chronic pain usually affects a child's ability to lead a normal life.

RESEARCH ON PAIN IN CHILDREN

16. A three-step ladder for treating cancer pain was developed by _______________.
17. Guidelines for managing pain in sickle cell disease were developed by ___________.
18. __________added new standards that integrate pain assessment and management into their accreditation standards.

MYTHS ABOUT PAIN AND PAIN MANAGEMENT IN CHILDREN

Answer as either true (T) or false (F).

19. _____ Myelinization is not necessary for pain perception.
20. _____ Emotional factors contribute to the pain experience.
21. _____ Children are at greater risk for respiratory depression from narcotics than are adults.
22. _____ Premature infants lack the neurologic structures required for pain perception.

ASSESSMENT OF PAIN IN CHILDREN

23. To assess pain in infants, the nurse looks for _____________________________ and _______________________ responses.
24. As infants get older, their responses to pain change from generalized to __________ responses.
25. It is important for the nurse to distinguish between pain and _____________ in infants.
26. Toddlers may react to pain with generalized _______________________.
27. Preschoolers may think that pain is a ____________________.
28. Give two reasons why a school-age child might overreact to pain.

    ____

    ____

29. How does adolescent egocentrism affect how adolescents communicate about pain?

    ____

    ____

30. Why is it imperative to use pain assessment tools with children?

    ____

    ____

31. Pain self-report tools are usually appropriate for children older than_____years.
32. Which pain assessment tools use a photographic scale as well as a numerical scale?

    ____

    ____

NONPHARMACOLOGIC AND PHARMACOLOGIC PAIN INTERVENTIONS

33. What are the benefits of regulated breathing techniques?

    ____

34. Explain how children who are using distraction are not pain free.

    ____

35. Guided imagery involves ______________ and ______________.

36. What is biofeedback?

    ____

37. What are the benefits of progressive muscle relaxation in older children?

    ____

38. What is hypnosis?

    ____

39. A TENS unit interferes with the ________________________________

40. For children receiving PCA therapy, ________________ should be readily available.

41. Why is aspirin not recommended for children?

    ____

Answer as either true (T) or false (F).

42. _____ EMLA cream is effective within 10 minutes of application.
43. _____ Nonsteroidal antiinflammatory drugs (NSAIDs) reduce pain and inflammation.
44. _____ Acetaminophen does not inhibit prostaglandin.
45. _____ Opioid analgesics can cause sedation and respiratory depression.
46. _____ Meperidine (Demerol) is more effective than morphine in children.
47. _____ Midazolam (Versed) is used for conscious sedation.
48. _____ Epidural analgesia has fewer side effects than opioid analgesics.

SUGGESTED LEARNING ACTIVITIES

1. Interview a pediatric nurse about his or her experiences with managing pain in children. Discover how the nurse assesses pain in children who have chronic pain. Ask the nurse to explain how he or she designs a plan for managing chronic pain in children.

2. Interview the parent of an infant or a toddler. Learn how the parent knows that the child is in pain.

STUDENT LEARNING APPLICATIONS

Enhance your learning by discussing your answers with other students.

Jose, an 8-year-old boy who weighs 30 kg, is experiencing acute pain. The physician orders 3 mg of morphine sulfate IV every 4 hours for pain. Jose receives 3 mg at 9 A.M. At 9:30 A.M., he rates his pain as 0 on a 0-to-5 rating scale. At noon, he complains of "bad pain" and rates his pain as 5 on the same scale.

1. What do think about Jose's order for pain medication? What changes may be required?

2. What other questions would you ask Jose about his pain?

3. What questions would you ask Jose about what else might be helpful in managing his pain?

4. How would you present your findings to Jose's physician?

REVIEW QUESTIONS

Choose the best answer.

1. The side effects of opioid analgesics include:
   a. constipation.
   b. nausea.
   c. sedation.
   d. all of the above.

2. A hospitalized 12-year-old child is playing Nintendo and rates her pain as 1 on a 0 to 5 rating scale. This activity is an example of:
   a. imagery.
   b. distraction.
   c. play therapy.
   d. self-hypnosis.

3. A child's perception of pain is influenced by the:
   a. parental response to the child's pain.
   b. child's ethnic background.
   c. child's developmental stage.
   d. all of the above.

4. Postoperative pain is an example of:
   a. acute pain.
   b. conscious pain.
   c. chronic pain.
   d. objective pain.

5. Which of the following drugs is classified as an NSAID?
   a. acetaminophen
   b. codeine
   c. ibuprofen
   d. midazolam

6. Which of the following statements about children and pain and its management is true?
   a. Children can easily become addicted to opioid analgesics.
   b. Children who are playing are not in pain.
   c. Past pain experiences affect how a child experiences pain.
   d. Children are more likely than adults to experience respiratory depression from narcotics.

7. Respiratory depression is a side effect of:
   a. acetaminophen.
   b. fentanyl.
   c. ketorolac.
   d. naloxone.

8. The drug Narcan:
   a. causes respiratory depression at high doses.
   b. is used to reverse the adverse effects of chlorpromazine.
   c. is a topical anesthetic.
   d. may result in cardiac arrest if given too rapidly.

40

The Child With an Infectious Disease

HELPFUL HINT

Review the concept of immunity in an anatomy and physiology textbook. Review specific immunizations in a pharmacology textbook.

MATCHING KEY TERMS

Match the term with the correct definition.

1. ______ exanthem
2. ______ host
3. ______ immunity
4. ______ infection
5. ______ pathogen
6. ______ prodrome
7. ______ toxin
8. ______ vector

a. Invasion of the body by another organism
b. Microorganism that produces disease
c. Eruption or rash on the skin
d. Carrier that transfers an infective agent from one host to another
e. Initial stage of a disease
f. Poison produced by pathogenic microorganisms
g. Resistance of the body to the effects of harmful organisms
h. Organism from which a parasite obtains its nourishment

REVIEW OF DISEASE TRANSMISSION

Match each mode of infection transmission with its example.

9. ______ Airborne route
10. ______ Fecal-oral transmission
11. ______ Direct contact transmission
12. ______ Vector-borne
13. ______ Direct inoculation

a. Infection contracted through the use of contaminated needles
b. Transmission of disease through sexual activity
c. Illness resulting from a deer tick bite
d. Infection caused by pathogens shed through sneezing or coughing
e. Illness caused by ingestion of contaminated food

INFECTION AND HOST DEFENSES

14. The first lines of defense in an intact immune are the __________ and _________.

IMMUNITY

Match each vaccine with its description.

15. ______ Live or attenuated
16. ______ Killed or inactivated
17. ______ Toxoid
18. ______ Human immune globulin
19. ______ Antitoxin

a. Bacterial toxins that have been inactivated by either chemicals or heat
b. Vaccine derived from the serum of immunized animals
c. Vaccine contains a pathogen that has had its virulence diminished
d. Can be disease specific and offers temporary passive immunity
e. Contains pathogens inactivated by either chemicals or heat

NURSING CARE: THE CHILD WITH AN INFECTION IN THE COMMUNITY SETTING

20. What information should be included in a nursing assessment of a child with an infection?

____

____

21. What information should the nurse teach a family about using antipyretic medications when a child is febrile?

____

22. What signs and symptoms should be reported to the primary medical caregiver when a child is febrile?

____

VIRAL INFECTIONS

Match each virus with its description.

23. ______ Cytomegalovirus (CMV)
24. ______ Epstein-Barr virus
25. ______ Fifth disease
26. ______ Mumps
27. ______ Poliomyelitis
28. ______ Rabies
29. ______ Roseola infantum
30. ______ Rubella
31. ______ Rubeola
32. ______ Varicella-zoster
33. ______ Variola

a. Infection may proceed to flaccid paralysis.
b. Rash appears after fever subsides.
c. Acute signs of fever, pharyngitis, lymphadenopathy, and hepatosplenomegaly continue for 2 to 4 weeks, followed by gradual recovery.
d. Virus remains latent in a sensory nerve ending, and the dorsal root ganglion and may be reactivated at a later time.
e. Its vaccine can be given after exposure to the virus.
f. This is a common cause of congenital infections in infants.
g. Koplik spots in the buccal mucosa appear 2 days before the red, maculopapular rash.
h. Its classic sign is parotid glandular swelling.
i. This is a mild systemic disease with a fiery red edematous facial rash followed by a maculopapular rash on the trunk and extremities.
j. Infection during the first trimester of pregnancy has serious consequences for the fetus.
k. Though eradicated worldwide, it has the potential for being used as a bioterrorism weapon

34. What is the American Academy of Pediatrics recommendation regarding poliovirus vaccine?

____

____

BACTERIAL, RICKETTSIAL, BORRELIA, HELMINTH, AND FUNGAL INFECTIONS

Answer as either true (T) or false (F).

35. ______ Pertussis is a highly contagious disease associated with a high infant mortality rate.
36. ______ Scarlet fever is caused by group A beta-hemolytic streptococci.
37. ______ In both Lyme disease and Rocky Mountain spotted fever, the vector is a tick.
38. ______ When a child is diagnosed with a helminthic infection, treatment is usually provided for the entire family.
39. ______ Frequent handwashing can prevent the spread of parasitic infections.
40. ______ Manifestations of fungal infections appear quickly after the child contracts the organism.
41. ______ A bull's-eye rash may be a manifestation of diphtheria.
42. ______ An opportunistic fungal infection is limited to the skin, hair, and nails.

SEXUALLY TRANSMITTED DISEASES (STDS)

Match each disease with its treatment.

43. ______ Gonorrhea
44. ______ Syphilis
45. ______ Chlamydia
46. ______ Trichomoniasis
47. ______ Human papilloma virus
48. ______ Herpes simplex virus II

a. Metronidazole
b. Erythromycin
c. Ceftriaxone
d. Acyclovir
e. Penicillin
f. Surgery

SUGGESTED LEARNING ACTIVITIES

1. Obtain information from the local health department on STDs. Plan a presentation to adolescents on preventing STDs with the information you gathered.

STUDENT LEARNING APPLICATION

Seven-year-old Jodie has been admitted to the hospital for oxygen therapy and IV antibiotics for the treatment of pneumonia. Ten days ago, her best friend came down with chickenpox. Jodie has never had chickenpox and has not yet received the varicella vaccine. Two days after admission, Jodie develops a macular rash on her trunk and scalp, and her fever returns.

1. Will Jodie require isolation?

2. Will she be given acyclovir? Why or why not?

3. Will she be given varicella zoster immune globulin? Why or why not?

When entering Jodie's room to take vital signs, the nurse finds her crying. She refuses to eat her lunch, saying she wants to go to the playroom.

4. How should the nurse handle this situation?

Jodie is uncomfortable from the itching caused by the skin lesions. You find her scratching her arms and trunk.

5. What interventions would you implement to relieve the itching and prevent scratching?

REVIEW QUESTIONS

Choose the best answer.

1. Congenital rubella may result in:
   a. encephalitis.
   b. cardiac anomalies.
   c. hydronephrosis.
   d. neural tube defects.

2. Splenic rupture is a complication of:
   a. CMV infection.
   b. Epstein-Barr virus.
   c. erythema infectiosum.
   d. varicella-zoster.

3. Which intervention would not be appropriate when caring for a child with pertussis?
   a. Monitoring intake and output
   b. Administering a cough suppressant
   c. Providing child with periods of uninterrupted rest
   d. Administering erythromycin

4. A "white strawberry tongue" is a clinical manifestation of which infectious disease?
   a. Poliomyelitis
   b. Roseola
   c. Rubeola
   d. Scarlet fever

5. Using an insect repellent when in the woods can help prevent:
   a. CMV infection.
   b. helminth infections.
   c. Rocky Mountain spotted fever.
   d. scarlet fever.

6. An adolescent comes to the clinic because she has dysuria, urinary frequency, and a mucopurulent discharge. These signs are manifestations of which STD?
   a. Herpes simplex II virus
   b. Syphilis
   c. Chlamydia
   d. Human papilloma virus

7. Which of the following describes the rash associated with Lyme disease?
   a. Erythematous maculopapular rash surrounded by a whitish ring
   b. Fine, red papular rash that appears within 24 hours of tick bite
   c. Petechial rash that begins on extremities and spreads to the rest of the body
   d. Erythematous macula or papule with a clearing in the center

8. Immunization against which illness no longer involves administration of a live virus?
   a. Measles
   b. Polio
   c. Pertussis
   d. Tetanus

41

The Child With an Immunologic Alteration

HELPFUL HINT

Review the immune system in an anatomy and physiology textbook.

MATCHING KEY TERMS

Match the term with the correct definition.

1. ______ active immunity
2. ______ allergy
3. ______ antibody
4. ______ antigen
5. ______ autoimmune disease
6. ______ complement
7. ______ immune system
8. ______ immunodeficiency
9. ______ leukocytes
10. ______ lymphocytes
11. ______ nonspecific immune functions
12. ______ passive immunity
13. ______ specific immune functions

a. Blood cells that mainly function to protect the body against foreign substances
b. Production of autoantibodies against cells of the body by the immune system
c. Protection occurring when serum containing an antibody is given to someone without the antibody
d. Protection that follows exposure to an antigen
e. Defect in the immune system that places a person at high risk for infection
f. Hypersensitivity reaction
g. Primary white blood cells of the immune system
h. Body's internal defense against foreign substances
i. Substance identified by the immune system as foreign
j. Protein produced by the immune system that binds to specific antigens and eliminates them from the body
k. Accessory system to a humoral response composed of proteins that facilitate enzyme action and antigen death
l. Humoral and cell-mediated responses that are activated in a highly discriminatory manner
m. Protective barriers that are activated in the presence of an antigen but are not specific to that antigen

REVIEW OF THE IMMUNE SYSTEM

Match the cells with their functions.

14. ______ Neutrophils
15. ______ Eosinophils
16. ______ Basophils
17. ______ Monocytes
18. ______ B lymphocytes
19. ______ T lymphocytes
20. ______ Helper T cells
21. ______ Suppressor T cells
22. ______ Cytotoxic T cells

a. Phagocytize target cells
b. Responsible for cellular immunity
c. First leukocytes to respond to tissue damage
d. Ingest and introduce antigens into the circulation
e. Inhibit the actions of helper T cells and B cells
f. Neutralize histamine
g. Responsible for humoral immunity
h. Secrete lymphokines that stimulate B cells to manufacture antibodies
i. Secrete histamine, heparin, and serotonin in inflammatory and hypersensitivity reactions

THE CHILD WITH AN IMMUNODEFICIENCY

23. How do immunodeficiency disorders result?

____

24. List the clinical findings associated with immunodeficiency.

____

HUMAN IMMUNODEFICIENCY VIRUS (HIV) INFECTION

25. Name three ways HIV infection can be transmitted from mother to child.
    a.

    b.

    c.

26. The rate of HIV transmission from mother to child decreases when both receive ____________________.

27. What is the goal of antiretroviral therapy for a child with HIV infection?

____

28. On what is the dosage of antiretroviral combination drug therapy for adolescents based?____

29. ________________________ is the antibiotic used for the prophylactic treatment of *Pneumocystis carinii* pneumonia.

30. Which medications are typically given for the following levels of pain?
    a. mild

    b. moderate

    c. severe

CORTICOSTEROID THERAPY

31. How do corticosteroids cause immunosuppression?

    ____

    ____

32. Why is it dangerous to abruptly stop giving corticosteroid medication?

    ____

33. Corticosteroid excess is diagnosed by administering a bolus of ______________.
34. If long-term use of corticosteroids is required, they are usually prescribed to be taken

    ____

35. In a child receiving corticosteroids, what can be done to minimize the risk for GI bleeding? To deal with increased appetite?

IMMUNE COMPLEX AND AUTOIMMUNE DISORDERS

36. Give two examples of immune complex disorders.

    ____

    ____

37. What are autoantibodies?

SYSTEMIC LUPUS ERYTHEMATOSUS (SLE)

Answer as either true (T) or false (F).

38. ______ SLE has periods of remission and exacerbation.
39. ______ SLE affects more males than females.
40. ______ In SLE, antinuclear antibodies are present.
41. ______ In SLE, systemic corticosteroids are used to control the inflammatory process.
42. ______ The clinical manifestations of SLE depend on which body systems are affected.
43. ______ Antimalarial drugs are used to treat joint problems in SLE.

ALLERGIC REACTIONS AND ANAPHYLAXIS

44. What is an allergy?

____

Match each allergic reaction with its example.

45. ______ Immediate hypersensitivity
46. ______ Cytotoxic hypersensitivity
47. ______ Arthus hypersensitivity
48. ______ Delayed cell-mediated hypersensitivity

a. Transfusion reaction
b. Asthma
c. Poison ivy
d. Poststreptococcal glomerulonephritis

49. List the most serious features of anaphylaxis.

____

50. ____________________ is the first line drug of choice in treating anaphylaxis.

51. What are the differences between allergy skin tests and the radioallergosorbent test (RAST)?

____

____

SUGGESTED LEARNING ACTIVITY

Many communities have support groups for people with SLE. Contact one in your community and arrange to attend a meeting. Report on the meeting to your class.

STUDENT LEARNING APPLICATIONS

Caring for a child with HIV infection or AIDS can be very challenging from both the physical and psychosocial perspectives. It is important for health care professionals to be aware of their own feelings about the disease. Think about the following questions and then discuss them with a family member, friend, or another student.

1. Which aspects of caring for a child with HIV or AIDS would you personally find most difficult?

   Providing physical care

   Worrying about contracting HIV infection from the child

   Dealing with the child's family

Knowing that the child has a life-threatening illness

Meeting the child's psychosocial needs

2. If the child contracted HIV prenatally, how would you feel about the child's mother? Could you remain nonjudgmental and supportive?

3. Which of the following HIV-positive adolescents would be most difficult for you to care for? Least difficult? Why?

   14-Year-old Annie, who uses illegal IV drugs

   16-Year-old Beth, who is a teenage prostitute

   17-Year-old David, who is homosexual

REVIEW QUESTIONS

Choose the best answer.

1. When the immune system fails to differentiate the body's cells from foreign cells, which of the following occurs?
   a. Active immunity
   b. Autoimmune response
   c. Cell-mediated response
   d. Humoral response

2. IgA:
   a. crosses the placenta.
   b. provides antibacterial protection.
   c. passes to the neonate in breast milk.
   d. influences B cell differentiation.

3. The test used to assess the immune status of an HIV-positive child is:
   a. CD4+ count.
   b. ELISA.
   c. HIV culture.
   d. p24 antigen.

4. In teaching a family about corticosteroids, which of the following statements should the nurse *not* include?
   a. "Take the medication with food or milk."
   b. "Do not stop the medication abruptly."
   c. "Signs of infection may be masked."
   d. "Changes in appearance are permanent."

5. Signs of SLE include:
   a. erythema marginatum, carditis, and chorea.
   b. discoid rash, photosensitivity, and positive antinuclear antibody (ANA) assay.
   c. fever, erythematous rash, and strawberry tongue.
   d. laryngospasm, edema, and hypotension.

6. The immunoglobulin involved in allergic reactions is:

   a. IgA.
   b. IgD.
   c. IgE.
   d. IgG.

7. Most children with HIV are infected:

   a. through blood and blood products.
   b. perinatally.
   c. through sexual abuse.
   d. through failure to use Standard Precautions.

8. The school nurse is teaching two sixth-graders about their bee sting allergies. Which of the following statements indicate that the children require further teaching?

   a. "I'll wear my khakis instead of jeans on the class trip to the zoo."
   b. "If a bee comes near me, I'll run away as fast as I can."
   c. "If I have to use my Epi-Pen, I can give it in my leg without pulling my khakis down."
   d. "I'll keep the windows closed when riding in the car."

42

The Child With a Fluid and Electrolyte Alteration

HELPFUL HINT

Review the concepts of fluid and electrolyte balance in a biochemistry textbook.

MATCHING KEY TERMS

Match the term with the correct definition.

1. ______ acidosis
2. ______ alkalosis
3. ______ anuria
4. ______ ECF (extracellular fluid)
5. ______ hypernatremic (hypertonic) dehydration
6. ______ hyponatremic (hypotonic) dehydration
7. ______ ICF (intracellular fluid)
8. ______ interstitial fluid
9. ______ intravascular fluid
10. ______ isonatremic (isotonic) dehydration
11. ______ oliguria

a. Serum pH <7.35
b. Serum sodium >150 mEq/L
c. Serum pH >7.45
d. Fluid found within the cells
e. Absence of urine formation
f. Condition that occurs when sodium concentration falls below that of normal body fluids
g. Fluid found outside the cell
h. Fluid surrounding the cells, including lymph fluid
i. Fluid within the blood vessels
j. Diminished amounts of urine output
k. Condition that occurs when sodium concentration is identical to that of body fluids

REVIEW OF FLUID AND ELECTROLYTE IMBALANCES IN CHILDREN

Answer as either true (T) or false (F).

12. ______ Sensible water loss is water that is lost via the respiratory tract and skin.
13. ______ Infants' higher metabolic rates make them more prone to fluid loss than older children.
14. ______ Infants' immature renal function increases their ability to concentrate urine.
15. ______ The proportionate water content for a premature infant is about 60%.
16. ______ Burns, fever, gastroenteritis, and respiratory infections can all result in fluid volume deficit.

Fill in the blanks.

17. Children are more likely to lose ______________ fluid when they have a fever.
18. Body fluids are composed of ____________ and ______________.
19. The primary electrolyte in the ECF is ______________; the primary electrolytes in the ICF are __________________ and __________________.
20. The normal serum pH ranges from ____________ to ____________.
21. What three mechanisms operate to keep the serum pH within the normal range?
    a.

    b.

    c.

22. Two buffers that help maintain normal serum pH are ______________________________ and ______________________________.
23. If the serum pH drops below normal, the rate and depth of respirations will ____________.
24. The kidneys help maintain normal serum pH by regulating ____________________ and ____________________ in the blood.

Match each disorder with its clinical manifestations.

25. _____ Hyponatremia
26. _____ Hypernatremia
27. _____ Hypokalemia
28. _____ Hyperkalemia
29. _____ Hypocalcemia
30. _____ Hypercalcemia

a. Muscle weakness, leg cramps, and ileus
b. Abdominal cramping, tachycardia, and cold, clammy skin
c. Tetany, positive Chvostek's sign, and hypotension
d. Itching, weakness, and bradycardia
e. Flaccid paralysis and cardiac and respiratory arrest
f. Thirst, peripheral edema, and seizures

Match each condition with its causes.

31. _____ Metabolic acidosis
32. _____ Metabolic alkalosis
33. _____ Respiratory acidosis
34. _____ Respiratory alkalosis

a. Ketosis, tissue hypoxia, and bicarbonate loss
b. Hyperventilation, sepsis, and compensation for metabolic acidosis
c. Airway obstruction and respiratory failure
d. Volume depletion and increased alkali intake

DEHYDRATION

Answer as either true (T) or false (F).

35. _____ Isotonic dehydration occurs when water and electrolytes are lost in the same proportion as they occur in the body.
36. _____ In dehydration, fluid loss occurs first in the intracellular fluid.

37. ______ An infant who has lost 7% of his body weight has moderate dehydration.
38. ______ Initial therapy in severe dehydration is aimed at preventing shock.
39. ______ When a child is severely dehydrated, electrolytes such as potassium are replaced by administering them by slow IV push.
40. ______ If a child who is anuric receives potassium, hypokalemia is likely to result.
41. ______ Diluted Gatorade is an acceptable oral rehydrating solution for a toddler.

DIARRHEA

42. Define *diarrhea*.

____

43. Diarrhea caused by infection is usually called ________________.
44. List four other causes of diarrhea.
    a.

    b.

    c.

    d.

45. Why are sports drinks and colas inappropriate fluid choices for a child with diarrhea?

____

46. Explain why an infant with diarrhea should continue to receive breast milk or full-strength formula.

____

47. What common foods are generally well tolerated during diarrhea?

____

48. How can skin breakdown be prevented in infants with diarrhea?

____

VOMITING

Answer as either true (T) or false (F).

49. ______ Vomiting can result from allergic reactions.
50. ______ Emesis with a fecal odor may indicate lower intestinal obstruction.
51. ______ Projectile vomiting is usually due to overfeeding.
52. ______ Oral rehydrating solutions cannot be used when a child has vomited.

SUGGESTED LEARNING ACTIVITIES

1. Design an information sheet describing dehydration for new parents. Be sure to include the following information about dehydration: what causes it, what to look for, what to do if it occurs, when to call the physician, and other important information. Make your information sheet attractive, accurate, and concise.

2. Compare the ingredients in Pedialyte with those in Gatorade. How are they alike? How are they different?

STUDENT LEARNING APPLICATIONS

Enhance your learning by discussing your answers with other students.

Two-month-old Nathan is admitted to the hospital with severe dehydration.

1. As Nathan's nurse, what would you expect to find when assessing the following?
   - Skin turgor
   - Urine output
   - Anterior fontanel
   - Mucous membranes
   - Pulse
   - Blood pressure
   - Sensorium
   - Skin color

2. Because Nathan is not drinking, the physician orders IV fluids. Nathan presently weighs 9 pounds 4 ounces. What are his 24-hour fluid maintenance requirements?

3. Nathan has not voided for at least 4 hours. The physician has included potassium chloride in the IV order. What problem does this pose? How would you handle it?

4. How will you recognize when Nathan is improving?

REVIEW QUESTIONS

Choose the best answer.

1. An otherwise healthy infant is admitted to the hospital with dehydration and diarrhea. She is hyperirritable and agitated, and she has flushed skin and dry mucous membranes. The nurse suspects:
   a. hypercalcemia.
   b. hypokalemia.
   c. hyperkalemia.
   d. hypernatremia.

2. An infant who has been vomiting frequently is at risk for:
   a. metabolic acidosis.
   b. metabolic alkalosis.
   c. respiratory acidosis.
   d. respiratory alkalosis.

3. Which of the following statements about the compensatory mechanisms that maintain normal serum pH is true?
   a. If serum pH rises above normal, the respiratory rate and depth increase.
   b. If serum pH rises above normal, the kidneys conserve hydrogen ions.
   c. Bicarbonate is a chemical that buffers the intracellular fluid.
   d. Respiratory compensatory mechanisms work more slowly than renal mechanisms.

4. Which of the following are indicators of dehydration in a 4-year-old child?
   a. Heart rate of 120 beats per minute and sunken fontanel
   b. Specific gravity of 1.010 and oliguria
   c. Weight gain and absence of tears
   d. Thirst and specific gravity of 1.038

5. Infants with dehydration must be monitored for signs of impending shock. Which of the following is a late sign of shock in the infant?
   a. Decreased blood pressure
   b. Elevated heart rate
   c. Change in skin color
   d. Change in sensorium

6. A preschooler with moderate diarrhea who is just admitted to the hospital and who is not NPO wants something to drink. The nurse's best choice is to offer:
   a. an oral rehydrating solution.
   b. Gatorade.
   c. diluted apple juice.
   d. low-fat milk.

7. An infant with diarrhea has tolerated clear liquids but begins having diarrhea again when she returns to her regular formula. Her diet should be changed to:
   a. boiled skim milk.
   b. soy formula.
   c. IV fluids.
   d. Pedialyte.

8. A child weighing 14 kg is receiving maintenance IV fluids. The child should receive how many milliliters per hour?
   a. 14
   b. 24
   c. 50
   d. 100

9. An infant weighed 6.4 kg at the pediatrician's office 2 days ago. He has had diarrhea since then. He now weighs 5.9 kg. His mucous membranes are dry, his fontanel is sunken, and his capillary refill is about 5 seconds. The infant has:

   a. hypotonic dehydration.
   b. moderate dehydration.
   c. hypernatremic dehydration.
   d. severe dehydration.

10. An infant has viral gastroenteritis. To prevent its spread to other family members, the nurse teaches the family:

    a. proper handwashing techniques.
    b. how to administer antidiarrheal medications.
    c. how to administer antibiotics.
    d. how to calculate daily fluid requirements.

43

The Child With a Gastrointestinal Alteration

HELPFUL HINT

Review the anatomy and physiology of the GI tract in an anatomy and physiology textbook.

MATCHING KEY TERMS

Match the term with the correct definition.

1. ______ achalasia
2. ______ atresia
3. ______ azotemia
4. ______ dysphagia
5. ______ encopresis
6. ______ fistula
7. ______ fundoplication
8. ______ hematemesis
9. ______ melena
10. ______ occult bleeding
11. ______ peristalsis
12. ______ projectile vomiting
13. ______ pylorus
14. ______ tenesmus

a. Presence of urea in the blood
b. Distal opening of the stomach
c. Black, tarry stools, indicating bleeding
d. Abnormal passage between two organs
e. Progressive wavelike motions that propel fluid and food through gastrointestinal (GI) tract
f. Failure of smooth muscle fibers of the GI tract to relax
g. Incontinence of feces
h. Surgical wrapping of the stomach fundus around distal esophagus to prevent gastric reflux
i. Vomiting that is projected with force up to 4 feet
j. Abnormal closure or absence of a body passage
k. Vomiting of blood, either red or "coffee grounds"
l. Inability to swallow or difficulty in swallowing
m. Bleeding that is detectable only by microscopic or chemical means
n. Ineffective, painful, or continuous urge to defecate

REVIEW OF THE GASTROINTESTINAL SYSTEM

15. What are the primary functions of the upper GI system?

____

16. What are the primary functions of the lower GI system?

____

17. What are the functions of the liver?

____

18. Prenatally, how are nutrients brought to, and waste products removed from, the fetus?

____

DISORDERS OF PRENATAL DEVELOPMENT

Answer as either true (T) or false (F).

19. ______ The diagnosis of cleft lip and palate can be determined through inspection.
20. ______ Infants with cleft lip are at risk for problems with parent-infant attachment.
21. ______ Cleft palate repair precedes cleft lip repair.
22. ______ To keep a cleft palate repair incision site clean, the nurse gives water after all feedings.
23. ______ Children with cleft palates require frequent hearing tests.

Fill in the blanks.

24. ______________ is a significant prenatal clue in the diagnosis of tracheoesophageal fistula (TEF).
25. An infant with TEF is at constant risk for ______________.
26. What are the "3 Cs" that suggest TEF?

    ____

    ____

    ____

27. How does an infant with TEF receive nutrition prior to surgery?

    ____

28. Describe how to care for an esophagostomy.

    ____

Match each disorder with its description.

29. ______ Hiatal hernia
30. ______ Congenital diaphragmatic hernia
31. ______ Imperforate anus
32. ______ Gastroschisis
33. ______ Omphalocele
34. ______ Umbilical hernia

a. Condition in which viscera are outside of the abdominal cavity and not covered with a sac
b. Incomplete development of the anus
c. Protrusion of a portion of the stomach through the esophageal hiatus of the diaphragm
d. Herniation of the gut into the umbilical cord
e. Herniation of abdominal contents into the thoracic cavity through the diaphragm
f. Condition in which gut pushes outward at the umbilicus during straining or crying

MOTILITY DISORDERS

35. Describe the home dietary management of gastroesophageal reflux (GER) in a 5-month old infant.

____

36. List the drugs used to treat GER that have the following actions.
    a. Decrease acid secretions

    b. Accelerate gastric emptying

    c. Provide barrier protection

37. Describe how chronic constipation can lead to encopresis.

____

38. __________ and __________ are thought to be common causes of irritable bowel syndrome (IBS).

39. Clinical manifestations of IBS include:

____

INFLAMMATORY AND INFECTIOUS DISEASES

Answer as either true (T) or false (F).

40. ______ Stress ulcers are considered primary ulcers.
41. ______ Dietary management of ulcers includes a bland diet with added milk.
42. ______ *H. pylori* is a bacterium associated with duodenal ulcers.
43. ______ *Giardia* is the most common pathogen causing gastroenteritis in daycare settings.
44. ______ There is no pharmacologic treatment for rotavirus.
45. ______ In gastroenteritis, dehydration and electrolyte imbalances must be corrected promptly.
46. ______ Headache, irritability, nuchal rigidity, and seizures are manifestations of *Salmonella*.
47. ______ The cardinal symptom of appendicitis is pain that eventually localizes at McBurney's point.
48. ______ Sudden cessation of pain in a child with appendicitis is indicative of spontaneous remission.
49. Describe the differences between Crohn's disease and ulcerative colitis.

____

____

____

50. Which four categories of drugs are used to treat inflammatory bowel disease?
    a.

    b.

    c.

    d.

OBSTRUCTIVE DISORDERS

51. Describe the vomiting that occurs with pyloric stenosis.
52. The classic signs of intussusception include ____________________________.
53. How is hydrostatic reduction of an intussusception attempted?

    ____

54. ____________ is caused by a malrotation of the bowel.
55. What is the cardinal sign of Hirschsprung disease in the newborn?

    ____

56. A life-threatening complication of Hirschsprung disease is ________________.

MALABSORPTION DISORDERS

Answer as either true (T) or false (F).

57. ______ Isomil is an appropriate formula for an infant with lactose intolerance.
58. ______ Celiac disease results from the inability to digest celiac.
59. ______ Corn and rice products must be avoided in celiac disease.
60. ______ Corticosteroids are used to decrease mucosal inflammation in celiac crisis.

HEPATIC DISORDERS

For each type of hepatitis, list its mode(s) of transmission.

61. Hepatitis A virus (HAV) ____________________________________
62. Hepatitis B virus (HBV) ____________________________________
63. Hepatitis C virus (HCV) ____________________________________
64. Hepatitis delta virus (HDV) ____________________________________
65. Hepatitis E virus (HEV) ____________________________________
66. What are the clinical manifestations of fulminating hepatitis?

    ____

67. ______________ usually progresses in a cephalocaudal direction.
68. Vaccinations for hepatitis _____ and hepatitis _____ are currently available.

Answer as either true (T) or false (F).

69. ______ The Kasai procedure corrects biliary atresia.
70. ______ In biliary atresia, water-soluble vitamins are not absorbed.
71. ______ Pruritus can be alleviated with colloidal oatmeal baths.
72. ______ Manifestations of portal hypertension include ascites, GI bleeding, and severe edema.
73. In children, cirrhosis generally results from ____________________________ and ____________________.
74. The three major complications of cirrhosis are

    ____

    ____

    ____

75. ____ is the definitive therapy for cirrhosis.

SUGGESTED LEARNING ACTIVITIES

1. Role play with another student. In this scenario, one of you is the nurse and the other is the parent of a newborn with a cleft lip and palate. The "parent" refuses to hold or even look at the infant. How would the "nurse" promote parent-infant attachment in this situation? You may want to include another student as an observer/"coach."

2. Observe one of the diagnostic procedures discussed in this chapter, such as fiberoptic endoscopy, abdominal flat plate radiography, or colonoscopy. Based on your observations and readings, design a teaching plan for this procedure for an 8-year-old child.

STUDENT LEARNING APPLICATIONS

Enhance your learning by discussing your answers with other students.

Melissa, age 16 years, has just been diagnosed with Crohn's disease.

1. From what you know about adolescent development, what would you guess Melissa's chief concerns are about this diagnosis?

2. As her nurse, how would you determine whether your guesses are accurate?

3. How might this disease affect Melissa's physical and psychosocial development?

4. Melissa tells you, "Well, I guess this means that I won't be going to college." How would you respond to this statement?

REVIEW QUESTIONS

Choose the best answer.

1. At his 1-year-old checkup, you note that Jason has thin arms and legs and abdominal distention. His mother reports that he has been irritable, has lost his appetite, and has foul-smelling stools. He has fallen behind on the growth chart. Jason probably has:
   a. Crohn's disease.
   b. Hirschsprung's disease.
   c. IBS.
   d. celiac disease.

2. Which of the following is not an appropriate intervention following surgery for Hirschsprung disease?
   a. Assess surgical site for swelling, redness, and drainage.
   b. Monitor rectal temperature every 4 hours for evidence of fever.
   c. Reunite parents with child as soon as possible.
   d. Keep child NPO until bowel sounds return.

3. A 5-year-old, admitted to rule out appendicitis, tells the nurse, "It doesn't hurt anymore." The nurse suspects that the:
   a. child is afraid of surgery.
   b. appendix has ruptured.
   c. child wants to please the nurse.
   d. child cannot communicate about pain accurately.

4. A 6-year-old is admitted to the hospital with severe abdominal pain, bloody diarrhea, high fever, headache, and nuchal rigidity. The child probably has:
   a. an intussusception.
   b. cirrhosis.
   c. a perforated appendix.
   d. a *Shigella* infection.

5. For the child with encopresis, mineral oil is often prescribed to:
   a. facilitate absorption of fat-soluble vitamins.
   b. eliminate pain associated with bowel movements.
   c. evacuate fecal impactions.
   d. initiate the normal gastrocolic reflex.

6. An adolescent has just been diagnosed with an ulcer. Which of these statements indicates that she requires clarification about her therapeutic regimen?
   a. "I won't take my ulcer medication and milk of magnesia close together."
   b. "I'll switch to orange soda from cola."
   c. "I'll take two Motrin when the pain comes back."
   d. "I'll see if breathing exercises can help me relax more."

7. When performing a newborn assessment, the nurse observes that the infant is cyanotic and has nasal flaring and retractions. Also, no breath sounds can be auscultated on the left side, and he palpates an apical pulse on the right side of the sternum. The nurse immediately notifies the physician because he suspects:
   a. a tracheoesophageal fistula.
   b. a cleft palate.
   c. pyloric stenosis.
   d. a diaphragmatic hernia.

8. Careful handwashing before and after client contact can prevent the spread of:
   a. hepatitis A virus.
   b. hepatitis B virus.
   c. ulcerative colitis.
   d. all of the above.

9. A child with lactose intolerance may be able to drink milk if it is taken with:
   a. Colace.
   b. LactAid.
   c. lactulose.
   d. Lomotil.

10. In teaching parents about the use of elbow restraints following surgical repair of a cleft lip, which statement should the nurse *not* include?
    a. "Restraints may be removed for sleep."
    b. "Remove restraints for 10 or 15 minutes every 2 hours."
    c. "Apply restraints loosely but tight enough to prevent elbow bending."
    d. "Continue to use the restraints for 8 days."

11. A newborn with a tracheoesophageal fistula is waiting for transfer to a neonatal intensive care unit. The nurse's priority intervention is:
    a. arranging for transportation.
    b. preventing aspiration.
    c. providing psychosocial support for the parents.
    d. providing small, frequent feedings.

12. Which of the following tests is not typically ordered when GER is suspected?
    a. Fiberoptic endoscopy
    b. Barium enema
    c. pH studies
    d. Scintigraphy

13. Which of the following dietary modifications is appropriate for GER?
    a. An infant is given small, frequent feedings.
    b. A toddler eats solid foods before drinking liquids.
    c. A school-age child avoids colas and chocolate.
    d. All of the above are appropriate.

44

The Child With a Genitourinary Alteration

HELPFUL HINT

Review the anatomy and physiology of the renal system in an anatomy and physiology textbook.

MATCHING KEY TERMS

Match the term with the correct definition.

1. ______ arteriovenous fistula
2. ______ arteriovenous graft
3. ______ dysuria
4. ______ edema
5. ______ frequency
6. ______ hypercalciuria
7. ______ hyperlipidemia
8. ______ hypoalbuminemia
9. ______ proteinuria
10. ______ urgency

a. Sudden urge to urinate
b. Excessive calcium in the urine
c. Presence of protein in the urine
d. Tube inserted between an artery and a vein for hemodialysis
e. Presence of abnormally large amounts of fluid in intercellular spaces of the body
f. Connection between an artery and a vein
g. Low levels of albumin in the blood
h. High levels of serum cholesterol and triglycerides
i. Pain when urinating
j. Urination at short time intervals

REVIEW OF THE GENITOURINARY SYSTEM

11. The newborn's bladder is located in the ______________ cavity.
12. Children's shorter urethras predispose them to ________________________.
13. The ____________________ is the kidney's functional unit.
14. A child's bladder capacity is approximately equal to _____ ml/kg of body weight.
15. Normal urine pH ranges from ________ to _________.

ENURESIS

Answer as either true (T) or false (F).

16. ______ Children typically achieve nighttime bladder control before daytime bladder control.
17. ______ Diurnal enuresis may be helped by biofeedback.
18. ______ Dysuria may result from excessive calcium loss in the urine.

19. ______ Imipramine, an antidepressant, may be prescribed for nocturnal enuresis.
20. ______ Secondary enuresis may be the result of stress.

URINARY TRACT INFECTIONS (UTIS)

Match each disorder with its description.

21. ______ Cystitis
22. ______ Pyelonephritis
23. ______ Hydronephrosis
24. ______ Vesicoureteral reflux

a. Structural defect that allows urine to backflow into the ureters
b. Inflammation of the bladder
c. Kidney infection
d. Dilation of the renal pelvis

25. The diagnostic study for a UTI is ____________.
26. Bladder catheterization and ____________________________ are two invasive ways of collecting a urine specimen that will accurately detect bacteria in the urine.
27. A voiding cystourethrogram is ordered to detect ________________.
28. Pyelonephritis is treated with ______________________ antibiotics.
29. Hypertension in childhood might result from renal scarring due to __________.
30. List five ways of preventing UTIs in young children.

a.

b.

c.

d.

e.

CRYPTORCHIDISM

Answer as either true (T) or false (F).

31. ______ Preterm infants have a higher incidence of cryptorchidism.
32. ______ Most infants with cryptorchidism require surgery.
33. ______ Orchiopexy is the surgical correction for cryptorchidism.
34. ______ Children with cryptorchidism are at increased risk for testicular cancer.

HYPOSPADIAS AND EPISPADIAS

Fill in the blanks.

35. Infants with hypospadias should not be ____________________ before surgical correction.
36. Dorsal placement of the urethral opening in males is called ____________________; ventral placement is called ____________________.
37. __________ is a downward curvature of the penile shaft.
38. After surgery, urinary diversions, such as indwelling catheters or ____________________, are used to allow the meatus to heal.

MISCELLANEOUS DISORDERS AND ANOMALIES OF THE GENITOURINARY TRACT

Match each disorder with its description.

39. ______ Hydrocele
40. ______ Phimosis
41. ______ Testicular torsion
42. ______ Bladder exstrophy
43. ______ True pseudohermaphroditism

a. Inability to retract the prepuce after about age 3 years
b. Presence of both ovarian and testicular tissues with abnormal genital structures
c. Painless swelling of the scrotum
d. Urinary bladder located outside of the body at birth
e. Painful swelling of the scrotum

ACUTE POSTSTREPTOCOCCAL GLOMERULONEPHRITIS

44. List the clinical manifestations of acute poststreptococcal glomerulonephritis.

____

____

45. Describe the role that antigen-antibody complexes play in acute poststreptococcal glomerulonephritis.

____

____

46. In severe renal insufficiency, BUN, and creatinine ____________________.
47. ______________ indicates that acute poststreptococcal glomerulonephritis is starting to resolve.

NEPHROTIC SYNDROME

48. List the clinical manifestations of nephrotic syndrome.

____

____

49. Which drug is used initially to achieve remission in nephrotic syndrome?

50. When is a child with nephrotic syndrome considered to be in remission?

____

ACUTE RENAL FAILURE

Match each disorder with the types of acute renal failure they cause. (Answers may be used more than once.)

51. ______ Glomerulonephritis
52. ______ Pyelonephritis
53. ______ Dehydration
54. ______ Hemolytic uremic syndrome
55. ______ Hemorrhagic shock
56. ______ Neurogenic bladder
57. ______ Kidney stones

a. Prerenal
b. Intrarenal
c. Postrenal

Answer as either true (T) or false (F).

58. ______ Hemolytic uremic syndrome is the most frequent cause of acute renal failure in children.
59. ______ Kayexalate is administered to manage hypokalemia.
60. ______ Hyponatremia results from water overload in acute renal failure.
61. ______ In acute renal failure, children develop metabolic alkalosis.

CHRONIC RENAL FAILURE AND END-STAGE RENAL DISEASE (ESRD)

62. Dialysis removes ____________________ and ____________________ from the blood and regulates ____________________ and ____________________.
63. Vascular access for hemodialysis is achieved through a double-lumen central line or a(n) ____
64. In peritoneal dialysis, the dialysis fluid is placed in the __________________ cavity.
65. Manifestations of ESRD include

    ____

66. Children with ESRD require either dialysis or ____________.
67. ____________________ is the most common complication of kidney transplantation.
68. Children with kidney transplants are at high risk for infection because of

    ____

SUGGESTED LEARNING ACTIVITIES

1. Visit a dialysis center and interview one of the nurses. Report to your class on the most challenging aspects of the nurse's work.

2. Contact a medical supply company. Find out the cost of the equipment and supplies needed for peritoneal dialysis. Calculate the approximate cost per month. Find out whether the costs are covered entirely by medical insurance. Report to your class.

STUDENT LEARNING APPLICATIONS

Enhance your learning by discussing your answers with other students.

Five-year-old Jack is brought to the pediatrician by his parents, who have noticed that Jack has "puffiness" around his eyes and ankles and that his "belly is getting bigger." They also report that "he's just not himself" and that he has no appetite. You find that his vital signs are within normal limits for his age and sex. You note pitting edema of his lower extremities and abdomen. Urine tests are negative for occult blood and +4 for protein.

1. Based on these findings, what would you expect Jack's diagnosis to be?

After a brief hospitalization, Jack is discharged to home. He will be treated with prednisone, penicillin, and a no-added-salt diet.

2. What will you teach the family about the actions and side effects of prednisone and how to administer it?

3. Jack's mother does not understand the need for penicillin "because the doctor said he doesn't have an infection." How will you explain this?

4. What will you teach the family about the reason for the no-added-salt diet?

Jack goes into remission after 2 weeks. The physician recommends that Jack be given a pneumococcal vaccination. His father does not understand this recommendation, saying, "All of Jack's shots are up to date."

5. How will you address this?

REVIEW QUESTIONS

Choose the best answer.

1. A 7-year-old with cystitis will require:
   a. a renal ultrasound.
   b. oral antibiotics.
   c. a suprapubic aspiration.
   d. all of the above.

2. A 9-year-old is admitted to the hospital with acute glomerulonephritis. In taking the child's history, the nurse is not surprised to find that the child has had:
   a. back pain for a few days.
   b. dysuria since the previous night.
   c. a history of hypertension.
   d. a sore throat last week.

3. A child with nephrotic syndrome who is steroid dependent:
   a. will have an antibiotic added to the steroid.
   b. initially responds well to prednisone but relapses while on a tapering schedule.
   c. requires a kidney biopsy to determine the exact cause of the disease.
   d. will eventually require dialysis.

4. A child with grade I vesicoureteral reflux is treated with:
   a. antibiotics.
   b. diuretics.
   c. muscle relaxants.
   d. surgery.

5. Recurrent urinary tract infections are clinical manifestations of:
   a. enuresis.
   b. hypospadias.
   c. glomerulonephritis.
   d. vesicoureteral reflux.

6. Acute renal failure is suspected when a child presents with:
   a. dysuria and fever.
   b. oliguria and elevated BUN.
   c. edema and proteinuria.
   d. fatigue and hypertension.

7. A pale, listless 5-year-old is brought to the emergency department. The child has many bruises, decreased urine output, and bloody diarrhea. The nurse plans emergency care based on his suspicion of:
   a. child abuse.
   b. nephrotic syndrome.
   c. glomerulonephritis.
   d. hemolytic uremic syndrome.

8. The most common cause of chronic renal failure in children is:
   a. congenital renal abnormalities.
   b. insulin-dependent diabetes.
   c. ESRD.
   d. nephrotoxic antibiotic use.

9. Corticosteroids are used in the treatment of:
   a. glomerulonephritis.
   b. nephrotic syndrome.
   c. phimosis.
   d. vesicoureteral reflux.

10. In a child with ESRD, recombinant erythropoietin is used to treat:
    a. rejection of a transplanted kidney.
    b. renal osteodystrophy.
    c. hypertension.
    d. anemia.

45

The Child With a Respiratory Alteration

HELPFUL HINT

Review the anatomy and physiology of the respiratory system in an anatomy and physiology textbook.

MATCHING KEY TERMS

Match the term with the correct definition.

1. ______ atelectasis
2. ______ crackles
3. ______ dysphagia
4. ______ dyspnea
5. ______ grunting
6. ______ hypercapnia
7. ______ hypocapnia
8. ______ hypoxemia
9. ______ hypoxia
10. ______ nasal flaring
11. ______ nasal polyps
12. ______ orthopnea
13. ______ retractions
14. ______ rhonchi
15. ______ stridor
16. ______ tachypnea
17. ______ wheezing

a. Abnormal movement of the chest wall during inspiration
b. Sound, similar to a grunting noise, that can be heard with or without a stethoscope
c. Shrill, harsh sound heard during inspiration, expiration, or both
d. Increased respiratory rate
e. Widening of the nares that indicates air hunger
f. Increased levels of carbon dioxide in the blood
g. Difficulty breathing except in an upright position
h. Collapsed or airless part of the lung
i. High-pitched musical whistles heard with or without a stethoscope
j. Breath sounds caused by passage of air through thick secretions that do not clear with coughing
k. Difficulty breathing
l. Decreased levels of carbon dioxide in the blood
m. Rales
n. Decreased oxygenation of cells and tissues
o. Decreased levels of oxygen in the blood
p. Difficulty swallowing
q. Semitransparent herniations of respiratory epithelium

REVIEW OF THE RESPIRATORY SYSTEM

Answer as either true (T) or false (F).

18. ______ Lack of surfactant places an infant at greater risk for respiratory distress syndrome.
19. ______ Retractions are commonly seen in older children and adults with respiratory distress.

20. ______ The tonsils help filter circulating lymph fluid.
21. ______ Arterial blood gases are used mainly to assess acid-base balance.
22. ______ A sweat test is used to diagnose allergies.
23. ______ Pulse oximetry is used to measure oxygen saturation in the blood.

ALLERGIC RHINITIS

24. The onset of allergic rhinitis rarely occurs before age ______________.
25. Classic manifestations of allergic rhinitis include

____

____

26. ______________________ involves injecting the child with progressively larger doses of the allergen.

SINUSITIS

27. Acute sinusitis often follows a(n) ____________.
28. Chronic sinusitis is associated with allergic rhinitis and ____________.
29. Pain associated with sinusitis may be relieved by administering __________________ and applying ______________________.

OTITIS MEDIA

Answer as either true (T) or false (F).

30. ______ Risk factors for otitis media include using a pacifier, attending a daycare center, and bottle feeding.
31. ______ Ear drainage indicates otitis media with effusion.
32. ______ Tympanostomy tubes usually fall out spontaneously.

PHARYNGITIS AND TONSILLITIS

Match each term with its description.

33. ______ Pharyngitis
34. ______ Tonsillitis
35. ______ Adenoiditis

a. Inflammation of the palatine tonsils
b. Inflammation of the pharyngeal tonsils
c. Inflammation of the throat and surrounding lymph tissue

LARYNGOMALACIA

36. The hallmark of laryngomalacia is ________________ stridor that ____________ when the infant is supine.

CROUP

Match each type of croup with its description.

37. ______ Acute spasmodic croup
38. ______ Laryngotracheobronchitis
39. ______ Epiglottitis
40. ______ Tracheitis

a. Occurs more often in anxious, excitable children
b. Life-threatening medical emergency
c. Most common form of croup
d. Usually follows an upper respiratory infection

Answer as either true (T) or false (F).

41. ______ Children with stridor at rest should be taken to an emergency department.
42. ______ The HiB vaccine has reduced the incidence of tracheitis.
43. ______ Children who receive racemic epinephrine in the emergency department should be observed for at least 3 hours after treatment.
44. ______ Sedatives are used to keep a child with croup calm.

EPIGLOTTITIS

45. Manifestations of epiglottitis include

____

____

46. When epiglottitis is suspected, never use a ______________________ to inspect the child's throat.

BRONCHITIS

47. Bronchitis is usually caused by a ________________.
48. Treatment includes ____________, ____________, and ____________.

BRONCHIOLITIS

49. Respiratory syncytial virus (RSV) is the causative agent in bronchiolitis in more than ______% of the cases.
50. Why is RSV so easily communicable?

____

51. What effects can ribavirin (Virazole) have on health care providers and visitors?

____

____

52. List two products that may be used monthly as RSV prophylaxis in preterm infants.

a.

b.

PNEUMONIA

53. What can be done to promote pulmonary drainage in a child with pneumonia?

____

____

54. The oxygen saturation of a child with pneumonia, who has no underlying chronic pulmonary disease, should be maintained at >______%.

FOREIGN BODY ASPIRATION

55. List six foods that are commonly aspirated by young children.

 a.

 b.

 c.

 d.

 e.

 f.

56. Manifestations of an obstructed airway in a child who has aspirated are ____________ and __________________.

PULMONARY NONINFECTIOUS IRRITATION

57. Adult respiratory distress syndrome can be precipitated by

____

58. ______________________________ is associated with asthma in children.

59. ____________________ poisoning is a complication of smoke inhalation.

RESPIRATORY DISTRESS SYNDROME (RDS)

Answer as either true (T) or false (F).

60. ______ RDS can result from insufficient amounts of surfactant.

61. ______ The incidence of RDS increases as gestational age increases.

62. ______ Central cyanosis is an early sign of RDS.

63. ______ Fluid replacement is used to both treat and prevent RDS.

APNEA

Match each term with its description.

64. ______ Apnea
65. ______ Periodic breathing
66. ______ Apparent life-threatening event

a. Three or more respiratory pauses lasting longer than 3 seconds with less than 20 seconds of respiration between pauses
b. Cessation of breathing for at least 20 seconds, or for a shorter period if accompanied by bradycardia and cyanosis
c. Sudden episode of apnea with changes in color and muscle tone accompanied by coughing or gagging

67. A nurse witnessing an apneic episode should note
____
____

68. When home apnea monitoring is prescribed, parents need instruction about ____________________ and ____________________.

SUDDEN INFANT DEATH SYNDROME (SIDS)

Answer as either true (T) or false (F).

69. ______ SIDS usually occurs during sleep.
70. ______ SIDS usually occurs after the age of 6 months.
71. ______ Infants should be placed supine or side-lying for sleep.
72. ______ Parents of an infant who has died from SIDS who experience guilt have most likely abused the infant in the past.

ASTHMA

73. In recent years the incidence and mortality rates for asthma have both ____________.
74. Wheezing is typically heard on ________________________.
75. Tachypnea ______________ carbon dioxide levels in the blood.
76. Beta$_2$-adrenergic agonists are used to __________________.
77. Increasingly severe asthma that does not respond to vigorous treatment is called ____________________________.
78. __________________ is an ideal sport for children with asthma.
79. Corticosteroids are used during an acute asthma attack to _____________.
80. Children with asthma monitor their condition at home by using ___________.
81. Mast cell inhibitors are given 30 minutes before _______________.
82. Two breathing exercises to slow the respiratory rate are _____________ and ________________.

BRONCHOPULMONARY DYSPLASIA (BPD)

Answer as either true (T) or false (F).

83. ______ BPD results from lung injury related to receiving supplemental oxygen and mechanical ventilation.
84. ______ Pursing of the lips and nasal flaring are early signs of impending respiratory distress.
85. ______ In BPD, diuretics are used to treat hypertension.
86. ______ Infants with BPD have irreversible developmental delays.

CYSTIC FIBROSIS (CF)

Answer as either true (T) or false (F).

87. ______ CF is an autosomal dominant inherited disorder.
88. ______ CF affects the functioning of the exocrine glands.
89. ______ Children with CF present with malnutrition because of poor diet.
90. ______ Meconium ileus may be the first indicator of CF.
91. ______ Cor pumonale results from increased pulmonary resistance.
92. ______ Aerobic exercise may be as effective as chest physiotherapy in relieving pulmonary obstruction in CF.
93. ______ Enzyme dosage is adjusted according to weight gain.
94. ______ A child with CF requires extra salt and fluids when the weather is hot.

TUBERCULOSIS (TB)

Match each term with its description.

95. ______ TB exposure
96. ______ TB infection
97. ______ TB disease

a. Recent contact with a person who has contagious TB
b. Positive skin test with signs and symptoms of TB
c. Positive skin test with no signs and symptoms

Answer as either true (T) or false (F).

98. ______ Children with TB are rarely contagious.
99. ______ The Mantoux test is the preferred method of screening for TB.
100. ______ Children with TB infection are treated with Bacillus Calmette-Guérin for 9 months.
101. ______ In infants, a negative tuberculin skin test rules out TB infection.

SUGGESTED LEARNING ACTIVITIES

1. Interview a public health nurse about the incidence of TB in your community. Has your community seen an increase in new cases of TB? If yes, to what does the nurse attribute this increase? Share your findings with the class.

2. Investigate an asthma self-help group for children in your community. How does it meet the child's informational and psychosocial needs? Report to your class.

STUDENT LEARNING APPLICATIONS

Enhance your learning by discussing your answers with other students.

Parents bring their 2-month-old daughter, Tina, to the pediatrician. They are very anxious because she has been crying "all the time and won't eat or sleep." They also tell you that she feels "very hot." Tina is diagnosed with acute otitis media, and amoxicillin is prescribed for 14 days.

1. What would you teach the parents about the causes, risk factors, and course of acute otitis media?

2. What would you teach them about the treatment and follow-up?

Tina's parents remain extremely anxious. Their anxiety seems out of proportion to the situation. You are tempted to say, "It's just an ear infection. Lighten up."

3. Why would you *not* say that?

4. Why do you think the parents are so upset?

5. How can you determine whether you are correct?

In talking with Tina's parents, you discover that both of them had siblings who died before their first birthdays.

6. How does this information change your perception of their anxiety?

7. How can you effectively intervene with this family?

REVIEW QUESTIONS

Choose the best answer.

1. A toddler is admitted to the hospital with croup. He is tachypneic with substernal retracting and nasal flaring. He has a harsh, barklike cough. His pulse oximetry reading on room air is 98%. The most accurate nursing diagnosis for him is:
   a. ineffective breathing pattern.
   b. ineffective airway clearance.
   c. impaired gas exchange.
   d. all of the above.

2. In preparing a 6-year-old child for a tonsillectomy, the nurse should not:
   a. direct the teaching at the child's parents.
   b. reassure the child that she will be able to talk following the surgery.
   c. explain that her throat will be sore after surgery.
   d. explain that she will have to drink a lot after surgery.

3. A preschooler arrives in the emergency department. She is very anxious and irritable and refuses to lie down to be examined. She is sitting up, leaning forward on her hands, and drooling saliva. She is warm to the touch and her color is pale. The nurse should:
   a. take the child's vital signs.
   b. notify the physician immediately.
   c. ask the parents to wait outside the examining room.
   d. start an intravenous line.

4. Parents bring their 8-month-old son to the emergency department because "he's breathing so fast that he can't even eat, and he's so hot." Physical examination reveals respiratory rate of 60, nasal flaring, intercostal retracting, and moderate expiratory wheezing. The nurse suspects that the infant has:
   a. acute spasmodic croup.
   b. bronchiolitis.
   c. epiglottitis.
   d. aspirated a foreign body.

5. The nurse is preparing a child for a bronchoscopy. The child most likely has:
   a. apnea.
   b. bronchiolitis.
   c. aspirated a foreign body.
   d. pneumonia.

6. Which of the following drugs increases the central respiratory drive?
   a. Isoniazid
   b. Albuterol
   c. Caffeine
   d. Ribavirin

7. Active bleeding in a child following a tonsillectomy is indicated by:
   a. refusal to drink fluids.
   b. frequent swallowing.
   c. "coffee grounds" emesis.
   d. all of the above.

8. A child experiences bronchoconstriction 5 hours after an acute asthma attack. This is an example of which kind of inflammatory response?
   a. Immediate
   b. Intermediate
   c. Delayed

9. A nurse teaching a family about the use of pancreatic enzymes in the treatment of CF should include which of the following?
   a. "Give the preparation three times a day and before bedtime."
   b. "Dissolve the enzymes in warm whole milk."
   c. "Increase the dosage if the child has loose, fatty stools."
   d. "Chewing the enzymes will increase their efficacy."

10. A child with exercise-induced asthma can prevent an attack by:
    a. covering the nose and mouth with a scarf when exercising outside in the cold.
    b. inhaling a corticosteroid before exercise.
    c. inhaling through the mouth during exercise.
    d. taking prednisone before exercising.

11. A test used in the diagnosis of CF is
    a. RAST.
    b. sweat chloride.
    c. culture for *Pseudomonas.*
    d. Mantoux.

12. Which of the following therapies is least likely to be used for a child with CF who is hospitalized with a respiratory infection?
    a. Chest physiotherapy every 3 hours
    b. Intravenous antibiotics
    c. Cough suppressant medications
    d. Postural drainage

13. An infant is hospitalized following an apparent life-threatening event. The apnea monitor suddenly alarms. The nurse should first:
    a. assess the infant.
    b. question witnesses about the triggering event.
    c. initiate CPR.
    d. reset the monitor.

46

The Child With a Cardiovascular Alteration

HELPFUL HINT

Review the anatomy and physiology of the heart and fetal circulation in an anatomy and physiology textbook.

MATCHING KEY TERMS

Match the term with the correct definition.

1. ______ angioplasty
2. ______ cardiomegaly
3. ______ compensation
4. ______ decompensation
5. ______ dysrhythmia
6. ______ palpitation
7. ______ pulmonary edema
8. ______ pulmonary hypertension
9. ______ pulmonary venous congestion
10. ______ shunt
11. ______ systemic venous congestion
12. ______ valvuloplasty

a. Increased systemic venous pressure leading to excessive fluid in the systemic veins
b. Abnormal blood flow from one part of the circulatory system to another
c. Maintenance of adequate blood flow accomplished by cardiac and circulatory adjustments
d. Procedure to open a valve
e. Increased pulmonary pressure leading to excessive fluid in the pulmonary veins
f. Procedure that dilates vessels
g. Disturbance of rhythm
h. Enlarged heart
i. Collection of excess fluid in alveoli
j. Sensation of rapid or irregular heart beat
k. Inability of the heart to maintain adequate circulation
l. Increased pressure in pulmonary arteries and arterioles

MORE DEFINITIONS

Recall the definitions of the terms in italics in the following statements. Then, apply your knowledge and determine whether each statement is true (T) or false (F).

13. ______ *Afterload* is the amount of force against which ventricles contract.
14. ______ *Central venous pressure* (CVP) is measured in the left ventricle.
15. ______ Drug's *chronotropic* effect has an impact on the heart's rate.
16. ______ Drug's *inotropic* effect has an impact on *myocardial contractility*.

17. ______ *Preload* is measured by determining CVP.
18. ______ *Pulmonary vascular resistance* affects the left ventricle.
19. ______ *Regurgitation* is the result of turbulent blood flow.
20. ______ *Systemic vascular resistance* is the amount of pressure exerted by the systemic vascular bed.

REVIEW OF THE CARDIOVASCULAR SYSTEM

Fill in the blanks.

21. In fetal circulation, gas exchange occurs at the ________________.
22. In fetal circulation, oxygenated blood from the placenta flows from the right atrium into the left atrium through the ________________________.
23. After birth, the fetal shunt between the pulmonary artery and the aorta, which is called the ___________________, closes.
24. After birth, pulmonary vascular resistance __________________ and the systemic arterial pressure ________________________.

CARDIOVASCULAR ASSESSMENT

Answer as either true (T) or false (F).

25. ______ Clubbing of nail beds indicates chronic hypoxia.
26. ______ A gallop is a missing heart sound.
27. ______ The point of maximal impulse at the seventh intercostal space indicates cardiomegaly.
28. ______ Cool extremities in a warm room may indicate decreased cardiac output.
29. ______ Dyspnea is an indicator of congestive heart failure.
30. ______ S2 is auscultated at the heart's apex and correlates with the palpable pulse.
31. ______ Squatting may indicate acyanotic heart disease.
32. ______ Cardiac catheterization can be an interventional as well as diagnostic procedure.

PHYSIOLOGIC CONSEQUENCES OF CONGENITAL HEART DISEASE

33. In infants, early manifestations of CHF include

____

Match each drug or class of drugs with its description.

34. ______ Furosemide
35. ______ Spironolactone
36. ______ Thiazide diuretic
37. ______ Digoxin
38. ______ Vasodilator

a. Acts on distal renal tubules
b. Potassium-sparing diuretic
c. Relaxes smooth muscles; decreases afterload
d. Increases cardiac output; has positive inotropic and negative chronotropic effects
e. Potent loop diuretic

39. In an infant, fluid retention is monitored by ______________________________.

40. Before administering digoxin, the nurse should count ______________________, check ______________________, and observe ______________________.

41. Polycythemia compensates for ______________________________.

42. Treatment of hypercyanotic episodes includes

____

LEFT-TO-RIGHT SHUNTING LESIONS AND OBSTRUCTIVE LESIONS

43. ______________________________ is managed medically with indomethacin.

44. Classic signs of ______________________________ are decreased pulses and blood pressure in the lower extremities.

45. ______________________________ is an abnormal opening between the ventricles, whereas ______________________________ is an abnormal opening between the atria.

46. Endocardial cushion defect is also known as ______________________.

47. Narrowing of the pulmonary artery is called ______________________.

48. Thickening of the aortic valve is known as ______________________.

CYANOTIC LESIONS WITH ALTERED PULMONARY BLOOD FLOW

Match each defect with its description.

49. ______ Transposition of the great arteries
50. ______ Hypoplastic left heart syndrome
51. ______ Pulmonary atresia
52. ______ Tetralogy of Fallot
53. ______ Tricuspid atresia
54. ______ Truncus arteriosus

a. Defect composed of four distinct lesions
b. Condition in which pulmonary artery and aorta are one vessel
c. Failure of the pulmonary valve to develop
d. Absence of tricuspid valve
e. Inadequate development of left side of the heart
f. Reversal of the aorta and pulmonary artery

ACQUIRED HEART DISEASE

Answer as either true (T) or false (F).

55. ______ Gram-positive microorganisms are usually responsible for infective endocarditis.

56. ______ Immune complexes play a role in rheumatic fever.

57. ______ Kawasaki disease is an immune-mediated condition resulting in vasculitis.

58. ______ Antibiotic prophylaxis with penicillin for at least 5 years is part of the management of rheumatic fever without cardiac complications.

59. ______ Vegetation seen on echocardiogram suggests Kawasaki disease.

60. ______ Congenital heart malformations require infective endocarditis prophylaxis.

61. ______ Normal blood pressure for a child is defined as a systolic and/or diastolic blood pressure less than the 90th percentile for age and gender.

62. ______ Children with essential hypertension often have a family history of the disease.
63. ______ Renal disease is a complication of secondary hypertension.
64. ______ Nonpharmacologic therapies for hypertension are usually not effective.

CARDIOMYOPATHIES

65. Which type of cardiomyopathy is a major cause of sudden cardiac death in adolescents?

    ____

66. Which type results from an infection or exposure to a toxin?

67. Drugs used to decrease ventricular hypercontractility and outflow tract obstruction are _______ and _______ blockers.

DYSRHYTHMIAS

68. Vagal maneuvers may be used terminate an episode of __________________________.
69. Bradydysrhythmias are associated with ________________________.
70. In __________________________, there is no cardiac output.
71. Briefly placing an ice bag over an infant's face may stimulate a _____________ response.
72. In asystole, _______________________ is administered to stimulate cardiac activity.

HIGH CHOLESTEROL IN CHILDREN AND ADOLESCENTS

73. Risk factors for coronary artery disease in children and adolescents include:

    ____

    ____

74. In children, borderline levels for LDL cholesterol are ______________ mg/dL, and a high level for LDL is greater than _________ mg/dL.

SUGGESTED LEARNING ACTIVITIES

1. Role-play with two other students. Have one student act as the nurse and another act as a parent who has just been told that his or her child has a cardiac defect and will require surgery. Have the third student observe the interaction. After 10 minutes, discuss the role-play. The "nurse" can describe how it felt to deal with the "parent." The "parent" can describe which of the "nurse's" interventions were effective and which could use improvement. The observer can describe the interchange from an objective viewpoint.

2. Interview the parent of a child who has had cardiac surgery in the past. Try to discover what the health care team did that was helpful for the family during the child's hospitalization. What could have been done better?

3. Observe a cardiac catheterization. Design a teaching plan that describes to a 12-year-old child what to expect.

STUDENT LEARNING APPLICATIONS

Enhance your learning by discussing your answers with other students.

Michael is a healthy 10-year-old African-American undergoing a routine physical. His height and weight are at the 75th percentile. His blood pressure is at the 95th percentile for his age and gender, but a review of his chart reveals that his blood pressure has been slightly below the 90th percentile on previous visits.

1. On the basis of these findings, what questions would you, as his nurse, ask Michael and his parents?

2. How would you further assess his blood pressure?

The physician makes the diagnosis of essential hypertension and decides to initiate nonpharmacologic therapy.

3. How would you assess the family's need for information about the following treatments?
   - Weight control

   - Physical conditioning

   - Dietary modifications

   - Relaxation techniques

4. What key features of these treatments would you stress when you present the information?

5. How would you evaluate the effectiveness of your presentation?

REVIEW QUESTIONS

Choose the best answer.

1. In his physical assessment of an infant with a ventricular septal defect (VSD), the nurse notices dyspnea, hepatosplenomegaly, and periorbital edema. He understands that these are clinical manifestations of:
   a. heart failure.
   b. endocarditis.
   c. fluid overload.
   d. decreased central venous pressure.

2. Percentiles for average blood pressure are based on a child's:
   a. weight and gender.
   b. age and gender.
   c. gender and race.
   d. age and weight.

3. Which of the following nursing interventions is not appropriate when caring for an infant with cardiovascular alterations?
   a. Discouraging breast feeding
   b. Limiting bottle feedings to no longer than 30 minutes
   c. Maintaining a neutral thermal environment
   d. Providing periods of uninterrupted rest

4. Children with hypertension who are receiving loop diuretics are at risk for imbalances of:
   a. calcium.
   b. chloride.
   c. potassium.
   d. sodium.

5. A toddler is hospitalized with CHF and is receiving digoxin and furosemide. She has vomited twice in the past 4 hours. The nurse's best action is to:
   a. increase the child's fluid intake.
   b. omit the next dose of furosemide.
   c. check the child's blood pressure prior to the next dose of digoxin.
   d. get an order to draw a digoxin level.

6. An infant with a left-to-right shunt is admitted to the hospital in CHF. Yesterday, she weighed 3.6 kg. A finding that indicates a worsening of her condition today is:
   a. weight of 3.67 kg.
   b. urine output of 40 ml in the past 8 hours.
   c. rales in the lower lobes.
   d. all of the above.

7. While the nurse is doing a newborn assessment, he finds that the infant's blood pressure in her arms is much higher than in her legs. The nurse suspects that the infant has:

    a. aortic stenosis.
    b. atrioventricular canal.
    c. coarctation of the aorta.
    d. truncus arteriosus.

8. Parents of a toddler with tetralogy of Fallot explain that they do not want him to overexert himself, so they always keep him in his playpen or crib to limit his mobility. Based on this information, the most appropriate nursing diagnosis is:

    a. activity intolerance.
    b. risk for altered parenting.
    c. caregiver role strain.
    d. risk for altered growth and development.

9. While the nurse is taking routine vital signs, she notices that the infant is having a hypercyanotic episode. What should the nurse do first?

    a. Continue getting vital signs for a baseline comparison.
    b. Place the infant in a knee chest position.
    c. Get a pulse oximetry reading.
    d. Give morphine sulfate.

10. Parents of children with congenital heart problems often experience loss of control when the child is hospitalized. The nurse who understands this will:

    a. encourage parents to participate in their child's care.
    b. explain procedures prior to performing them.
    c. answer questions honestly.
    d. do all of the above.

11. The father of a child with a congenital heart defect asks the nurse why his daughter has to take penicillin before she gets her teeth cleaned by the dentist. The nurse explains that this is necessary to prevent:

    a. infective endocarditis.
    b. congestive heart failure.
    c. rheumatic fever.
    d. infected gums.

12. Which of the following are indicators of infective endocarditis?

    a. Positive blood cultures
    b. Vegetation seen on Holter monitoring
    c. Decreased erythrocyte sedimentation rate
    d. All of the above

47

The Child With a Hematologic Alteration

HELPFUL HINT

Review the anatomy and physiology of the hematologic system in an anatomy and physiology textbook.

MATCHING KEY TERMS

Match the term with the correct definition.

1. ______ autoimmune disorder
2. ______ chelation
3. ______ erythropoiesis
4. ______ extramedullary
5. ______ granulocytes
6. ______ hematopoiesis
7. ______ hemolysis
8. ______ hemosiderosis
9. ______ pancytopenia
10. ______ reticulocytes
11. ______ reticuloendothelial system

a. Outside of the bone marrow
b. Collection of cells capable of phagocytosis
c. Reduction in all types of blood cells
d. Breakdown of red blood cells (RBCs)
e. Increase in tissue iron stores
f. Production of RBCs
g. Immature RBCs
h. Production of blood cells
i. Disorder in which the body launches an immunologic response against itself
j. Neutrophils, eosinophils, or basophils
k. Binding of a metallic ion with a structure that results in inactivation of the ion

REVIEW OF THE HEMATOLOGIC SYSTEM

12. Explain the function of:
    a. RBCs:

    b. White blood cells (WBCs):

    c. Platelets:

13. Define each term:
    a. Anemia:

    b. Polycythemia:

    c. Lymphopenia:

    d. Megakaryocytes:

IRON DEFICIENCY ANEMIA (IDA)

14. How does the introduction of cow's milk into the diet before 1 year of age affect the development of IDA?

____

15. Why are infants with IDA lethargic?

____

16. Give two reasons why adolescents are prone to IDA.
    a.

    b.

17. What foods can interfere with iron absorption?

SICKLE CELL DISEASE (SCD)

18. Under what three conditions do RBCs change to a sickle shape?
    a.

    b.

    c.

19. Sickled RBCs cause microvascular occlusion. What does this lead to?

____

Match each complication of sickle cell disease with its clinical manifestation.

20. ______ Vaso-occlusive crisis
21. ______ Acute chest syndrome
22. ______ Dactylitis
23. ______ Stroke
24. ______ Acute splenic sequestration
25. ______ Aplastic crises
26. ______ Priapism

a. Altered level of consciousness
b. Painful, persistent erection of penis
c. Pallor, lethargy, and fainting
d. Swelling of hands and feet
e. Signs of hypovolemic shock
f. Fever, cough, and chest pain
g. Pain depending on organ or tissues affected

BETA-THALASSEMIA

27. Beta-thalassemia is inherited in a(n) ______________________________ pattern.
28. The major complication of the treatment of beta-thalassemia is ________________.
29. In beta-thalassemia, chelation removes ______________________ from the body.
30. The drug used to manage hemosiderosis is ____________________________.

HEMOPHILIA

31. Describe the parents of a girl with hemophilia.

    ____

32. In hemophilia A, the missing blood clotting component is ____________________; in hemophilia B, the missing component is ____________________________.
33. What are the manifestations of bleeding into the joints? ______________________

    ____

34. Hemophilia is a genetic disorder carried on the ______ chromosome.

VON WILLEBRAND'S DISEASE (VWD)

Answer as either true (T) or false (F).

35. ______ vWD is an acquired bleeding disorder.
36. ______ Prolonged and excessive bleeding and menorrhagia are signs of vWD.
37. ______ The von Willebrand protein carries coagulation factor IX.
38. ______ vWD is sometimes treated with desmopressin acetate (DDAVP).

IMMUNE THROMBOCYTOPENIC PURPURA (ITP)

Answer as either true (T) or false (F).

39. ______ ITP is the result of the destruction and decreased production of the platelets.
40. ______ ITP is an autoimmune disorder.
41. ______ Petechiae and bruising are clinical manifestations of ITP.
42. ______ Splenectomy is the treatment of choice for acute ITP.
43. ______ ITP can be either an acute or a chronic disorder.

DISSEMINATED INTRAVASCULAR COAGULATION (DIC)

Answer as either true (T) or false (F).

44. ______ Excessive bleeding and excessive clotting occur at the same time in DIC.

45. ______ In DIC, bleeding occurs because of the depletion of platelets and clotting factors.

46. ______ Excessive bruising and oozing from venipuncture sites are late signs of DIC.

APLASTIC ANEMIA

47. In aplastic anemia, the bone marrow stops producing ____________________, ________________________, and ____________________________.

48. Clinical manifestations of aplastic anemia include ____________________________

____

49. Medications used to treat aplastic anemia include steroids, cyclosporin, anti-thymocyte/anti-lymphocyte globulin, and ____________________________.

SUGGESTED LEARNING ACTIVITIES

With one or several other students in a discussion group, review the genetic implications of inherited hematologic disorders by discussing the following questions.

1. Sickle cell disease is an autosomal recessive disorder.
   a. When both parents have the trait, what are the chances that:
      - a child will have neither the trait nor the disease?
      - a child will have the disease?
      - a child will have the trait?

   b. When one parent has the disease and the other has the trait, what are the chances that:
      - a child will have neither the trait nor the disease?
      - a child will have the disease?
      - a child will have the trait?

   c. When neither parent has the disease but one has the trait, what are the chances that:
      - a child will have neither the trait nor the disease?
      - a child will have the disease?

- a child will have the trait?

2. Hemophilia is an inherited X-linked recessive disorder.
   a. When the mother is a carrier and the father does not have hemophilia, what are the chances that:
      - a daughter will have the disease?
      - a daughter will be a carrier?
      - a son will have the disease?
      - a son will be a carrier?

   b. When the mother is a carrier and the father has hemophilia, what are the chances that:
      - a daughter will have the disease?
      - a daughter will be a carrier?
      - a son will have the disease?
      - a son will be a carrier?

STUDENT LEARNING APPLICATIONS

Enhance your learning by discussing your answers with other students.

Joellen is a 12-year-old girl who was admitted to the hospital in a vaso-occlusive sickle cell crisis. Her pain is localized in her right arm and shoulder, and she rates it as 3.5 on a 0 to 5 scale. Her vital signs are slightly elevated, with her oral temperature at 38.2° C. She weighs 40 kg.

1. Joellen is receiving morphine sulfate for pain. As her nurse, what nonpharmacologic measures for pain management might you also use for Joellen?

The physician orders IV fluids for Joellen to run at 2X maintenance.

2. What are Joellen's basic fluid maintenance requirements for a 24-hour period? What should her hourly IV rate be in order to provide 2X maintenance fluids?

3. You want to assess Joellen's knowledge about prevention of sickle cell crises. How would you do this?

4. While caring for Joellen, you notice that she has a productive cough. She also starts to complain about pain in her chest. How would you address this new problem?

REVIEW QUESTIONS

Choose the best answer.

1. An example of an autoimmune disorder is:
   a. HDN.
   b. DIC.
   c. ITP.
   d. vWD.

2. If a preschooler with mild hemophilia is experiencing joint pain, the nurse should:
   a. administer children's aspirin.
   b. apply cold compresses.
   c. do passive range-of-motion exercises.
   d. give the child a warm bath in the tub.

3. Which of these statements about chelation therapy is true?
   a. It is used to rid the body of excess sulfate.
   b. It is used to treat one of the complications of factor VIII therapy.
   c. It is used to manage hemosiderosis.
   d. It often results in increased bleeding.

4. An example of a disorder inherited in autosomal dominant pattern is:
   a. hemophilia A.
   b. beta-thalassemia.
   c. vWD.
   d. ABO-Rh incompatibility.

5. Which of these statements by an adolescent with iron deficiency anemia indicates that she needs more teaching about her iron supplement?
   a. "I'll take my pill with orange juice."
   b. "I'll keep the pills out of reach of my younger brother and sister."
   c. "I'll double the dose during my periods."
   d. "It's normal for my bowel movements to be black while I'm taking iron."

6. Four-year-old Sara is admitted to the hospital with sickle cell disease. Her vital signs are temperature of 37.2° C, heart rate 124, respiratory rate 38, and blood pressure 70/40. She is pale and listless and has splenomegaly. She is experiencing:
   a. aplastic crisis.
   b. acute chest syndrome.
   c. a cerebrovascular accident (CVA).
   d. acute sequestration crisis.

7. A 6-year-old hospital patient complains of a headache. This could be a sign of a serious complication if the child has:

   a. aplastic anemia.
   b. hemophilia.
   c. sickle cell disease.
   d. any of the above.

8. A toddler with hemophilia is at risk for:

   a. altered growth related to poor appetite.
   b. developmental delay related to activity restrictions.
   c. infection related to decreased WBCs.
   d. all of the above.

48

The Child With Cancer

HELPFUL HINT

A pharmacology textbook will provide a more extensive discussion of chemotherapy.

MATCHING KEY TERMS

Match the term with the correct definition.

1. ______ benign cells
2. ______ blast cells
3. ______ clean margins
4. ______ extramedullary
5. ______ immunosuppression
6. ______ intrathecal
7. ______ malignant cells
8. ______ neutropenia
9. ______ protocal
10. ______ thrombocytopenia

a. Immature lymphocytes
b. Plan of research-based care outlining drug therapy and follow-up interventions
c. Within the spinal column
d. Decrease in number of white blood cells that results in reduced ability to fight infection
e. Reduction in platelet count
f. Slow-growing cells forming a tumor with distinct borders
g. Outside the bone marrow
h. Evidence of normal, disease-free tissue in the outermost layer of cells of a surgical sample
i. Abnormal cells that have invasive and unregulated growth
j. Weakening of the body's normal immune response

REVIEW OF CANCER

11. Any tumor that arises from new, abnormal growth is called a ___________.
12. The two ways that cancer cells spread are ___________ and ___________.
13. Why is staging done for tumors?

____

Answer as either true (T) or false (F).

14. ______ The cause of most childhood cancers in unknown.
15. ______ The cardinal signs of cancer in children are the same as an adult.
16. ______ Cancer in children is a common occurrence.
17. ______ Cancer is the leading cause of death due to disease in childhood.

18. List the seven overt signs and symptoms of cancer in children:
    a.
    b.
    c.
    d.
    e.
    f.
    g.

19. List the five covert signs and symptoms of cancer in children.
    a.
    b.
    c.
    d.
    e.

20. How is a child positioned for a bone marrow aspiration?

___

THE CHILD WITH CANCER

21. Identify the three primary treatment modalities for children with cancer.
    a.
    b.
    c.

22. Chemotherapy is the use of __________ to kill cancer cells.
23. Identify the three body systems whose cells are most often affected by chemotherapy.

    a.

    b.

    c.

24. Define *nadir.*

    ____

25. ________________ places the child with cancer at risk for the development of opportunistic infections.

Identify each of the following signs and symptoms as a side effect of chemotherapy (C), radiation (R), or both (B).

26. ______ Skin reactions
27. ______ Nausea and vomiting
28. ______ Alopecia
29. ______ Bone marrow suppression
30. ______ Stomatitis
31. ______ Fatigue
32. Which class of antiemetic drugs has been found to be more effective than other antiemetics in treating chemotherapy-induced nausea and vomiting?

    ____

33. What is the purpose of a biopsy?

    ____

34. How would a central venous catheter facilitate chemotherapy administration?

    ____

35. The side effects of radiation therapy are specific to the __________ and __________.
36. The side effects of radiation therapy usually appear _________ days after treatment is initiated.
37. _________________________ is the most common side effect of radiation therapy.
38. Hematopoietic stem cells are able to differentiate into _________________________.
39. What is an autologous bone marrow transplant?

40. What is an allogenic bone marrow transplant?

41. For which childhood cancers has bone marrow transplantation (BMT) become standard ___________ therapy?

42. What is conditioning?

43. The major problem associated with an allogenic transplants is ___________.

44. What are biologic response modifiers?

____

LEUKEMIA

45. Leukemia is caused by the proliferation of _______________.

46. List five clinical manifestations of leukemia.

    a.

    b.

    c.

    d.

    e.

47. The diagnostic test that confirms a diagnosis of leukemia is ___________________.

48. In leukemia, normal bone marrow is replaced by malignant ___________________.

49. The preferred treatment for leukemia is ___________________.

50. When is a child with acute lymphocytic leukemia considered to be in remission?

    ____

51. Why are allopurinol and intravenous fluids with sodium bicarbonate given before chemotherapy?

52. List two sanctuary sites.

    ______________________________ and ______________________________

53. List five nursing diagnoses for the child with leukemia.

    a.

    b.

    c.

    d.

    e.

54. Why are rectal temperatures contraindicated for the child with neutropenia?

    ____

55. A child is at severe risk of infection when his or her absolute neutrophil level is ______________.

56. What should the nurse teach the child with leukemia and family about oral hygiene?

    ____

57. Why are live-virus vaccines contraindicated for the child with leukemia?

    ____

58. What action is indicated if an immunosuppressed child is exposed to someone with chickenpox?

    ____

59. What precautions should be taken for a child who is thrombocytopenic?

    ____

60. What types of foods or fluids should be offered to the child who is nauseated?

    ____

Answer as true (T) or false (F).

61. ______ When a child is nauseated, warm liquids are better tolerated than cold liquids.

62. ______ Offering the child his favorite food will distract a child from his nausea.

63. ______ Hair may grow back in different color and texture after chemotherapy.

64. ______ Skin that is erythematous as a result of radiation can be massaged with any type of lotion.

65. ______ Oral temperatures are contraindicated for the child with mouth ulcers.

BRAIN TUMORS

66. Manifestations of brain tumors vary with ___________ and ___________.
67. What are the two hallmark symptoms of brain tumors in children?

    ____

68. Currently, the imaging modality used to evaluate brain tumors is ______________.
69. Which treatment modalities are used to treat brain tumors in children younger than 3 years?

    ____

70. Why is the Trendelenburg position contraindicated following a craniotomy?

    ____

OTHER CHILDHOOD CANCERS

Answer as either true (T) or false (F).

71. _____ The abdominal mass on a child with Wilms' tumor should be palpated every shift for changes.
72. _____ Treatment for tumor lysis syndrome includes allopurinol and hydration with IV fluids containing sodium bicarbonate.
73. _____ The primary treatment modality for non-Hodgkin's lymphoma is surgery.
74. _____ Neuroblastoma is a solid tumor that is found in infants and children.
75. _____ In the majority of cases, neuroblastoma manifests as a primary abdominal mass.
76. _____ Ewing's sarcoma is the most common primary bone malignancy in children.
77. _____ Treatment of osteogenic sarcoma involves surgery and chemotherapy.
78. _____ Most cases of retinoblastoma are diagnosed before 3 years of age.

CREATE YOUR OWN STUDY GUIDE

Provide the description/pathophysiologic information for each condition or tumor listed in the following table.

	Description/Pathophysiology
Wilms' tumor	
Hodgkin's disease	
Non-Hodgkin's lymphoma	
Brain tumor	
Neuroblastoma	
Osteosarcoma	
Ewing's sarcoma	
Rhabdomyosarcoma	
Retinoblastoma	

CREATE YOUR OWN STUDY GUIDE

Describe the clinical manifestations and treatment for each condition or tumor listed in the following table.

	Clinical Manifestations	Treatment
Wilms' tumor		
Hodgkin's disease		
Non-Hodgkin's lymphoma		
Brain tumor		
Neuroblastoma		
Osteosarcoma		
Ewing's sarcoma		
Rhabdomyosarcoma		
Retinoblastoma		

SUGGESTED LEARNING ACTIVITIES

1. What are the guidelines for administration of chemotherapy at your clinical site?

2. If there is an oncology clinic at your clinical site, talk with the nurses about their responsibilities in the oncology clinic. Do the nurses need more advanced preparation in pediatric oncology?

STUDENT LEARNING APPLICATION

Enhance your learning by discussing your answers with other students.

The parents of 7-year-old Tom are concerned because he has had a low-grade fever for a week. His appetite and energy levels are decreased. They have also noticed bruises on Tom's legs even though he has not been physically active. A complete blood count shows blast cells on the differential. Tom is referred to a pediatric oncologist because leukemia is suspected; he is then admitted to the hospital.

This is Tom's first day in the hospital, and you are caring for him.

1. What diagnostic studies would you expect to be ordered for Tom?

2. Respond to the following questions asked by Tom's father: "What is a bone marrow biopsy? Why does Tom need this test?"

When a bone marrow biopsy confirms acute lymphocytic leukemia (ALL), chemotherapy is initiated.

3. What are the nurse's responsibilities when caring for a child receiving chemotherapy?

4. What nursing assessments will you make while Tom is receiving chemotherapy?

When his parents leave the room to go to the cafeteria for lunch, Tom asks you several questions. How would you respond to his questions below?

5. "Do I have to have a transplant?"

6. "What are my chances?"

7. "How long do I have to get chemo?"

8. "Will I lose my hair?"

REVIEW QUESTIONS

Choose the best answer.

1. Bone marrow transplantation is considered standard therapy for which childhood cancer?
   a. Acute myelocytic leukemia
   b. Wilm's tumor
   c. Osteosarcoma
   d. Hodgkin's disease

2. The most common side effect of radiation therapy is:
   a. vomiting.
   b. bone marrow suppression.
   c. fatigue.
   d. erythema at the site.

3. Which position is contraindicated for a child following surgery to remove a brain tumor?
   a. Supine
   b. Prone
   c. Trendelenberg
   d. Low Fowler's

4. When a child's own bone marrow is used in a bone marrow transplant, it is called a(n):
   a. allogenic transplant.
   b. autologous transplant.
   c. homogenic transplant.
   d. None of these terms is correct.

5. Which of the following is *not* a biologic response modifier?
   a. Monoclonal antibodies
   b. Interleukin
   c. Tumor necrosis factors
   d. Interferon

6. A child has a history of a fever of unknown origin, excessive bruising, and fatigue. This combination of symptoms is suggestive of which childhood cancer?
   a. Leukemia
   b. Neuroblastoma
   c. Lymphoma
   d. Osteosarcoma

7. A diagnosis of leukemia is confirmed by which of the following studies?
   a. Lumbar puncture
   b. Bone scan
   c. Bone marrow biopsy
   d. Complete blood count

8. What precautions should be taken for a child with a platelet count of 18,000?
   a. Eat a low-bacteria diet.
   b. Use a soft-bristled toothbrush.
   c. Get extra rest.
   d. Start an iron supplement.

9. Which of the following would be the best fluid for the child who is nauseated from chemotherapy?
   a. Child's favorite flavored milkshake
   b. Room temperature water
   c. Sips of cold soda
   d. Hot tea with honey

10. What would the nurse tell an adolescent receiving chemotherapy about alopecia?
    a. "Don't worry. Most chemotherapy does not cause hair loss."
    b. "Your hair might grow back in a different color or texture."
    c. "Your hair will come back when you are finished all of your chemotherapy."
    d. "Aren't you lucky. The bald look is in right now."

11. Which of the following would not be included in a plan of care for a child with Wilms' tumor?
    a. Palpate the abdominal mass for any changes.
    b. Teach the child and family about a nephrectomy.
    c. Talk with the family about postoperative chemotherapy.
    d. Assess the urine for microscopic or gross hematuria.

12. The prevention of tumor lysis syndrome would include which of the following?
    a. Hydration and alkalinizing the urine
    b. Administering bicarbonate to make the urine acidic
    c. Assessing urine for hematuria
    d. Administering leukovorin rescue

13. What is the risk for infection if a child's absolute neutrophil count is less than 400 cells/mm^3?
    a. Severe
    b. Moderate
    c. Minimal
    d. Not significant

14. Which of the following is considered a hallmark symptom of brain tumor in children?
    a. Ataxia
    b. Morning vomiting
    c. Visual changes
    d. Seizure

49

The Child With an Integumentary Alteration

HELPFUL HINT

Review skin assessment in Chapter 23, "Physical Assessment of Children." Review Chapter 39, "Pain Management for Children."

MATCHING KEY TERMS

Match the term with the correct definition.

1. ______ debridement
2. ______ desquamation
3. ______ ecchymosis
4. ______ eschar
5. ______ erythema
6. ______ excoriation
7. ______ intertrigo
8. ______ keratosis
9. ______ lichenification
10. ______ pruritis
11. ______ urticaria

a. Thickening and hardening of the skin
b. Scratch or abrasion of the skin
c. Itching
d. Sloughing of the skin in scales or sheets
e. Redness of the skin
f. Overgrowth and thickening of the cornified epithelium
g. Vascular reaction of the skin characterized by pruritic wheals
h. Dark plaque associated with tissue necrosis
i. Discoloration of skin or mucous membranes caused by leakage of blood into subcutaneous tissue
j. Maceration of two closely apposed skin surfaces.
k. Removal of foreign material and devitalized or contaminated tissue from a traumatic or infected lesion to expose healthy tissue

REVIEW OF THE INTEGUMENTARY SYSTEM

12. List the five major functions of the skin.

    a.

    b.

    c.

d.

e.

Answer as either true (T) or false (F).

13. ______ The skin is the body's largest organ.
14. ______ The epidermis is completely replaced every 4 months.
15. ______ Mongolian spots are more commonly seen in infants of color.
16. ______ Vascular birthmarks are extremely uncommon.

INFECTIONS OF THE SKIN

Impetigo

17. The most common bacterial skin infection of childhood is ___________.
18. The organisms responsible for most of the cases of impetigo are ___________ and ___________________.
19. How is impetigo spread to other parts of the body and from person to person?

____

20. Describe the appearance of primary lesions of impetigo.

____

21. What is the treatment for impetigo? __________________________
22. What is a complication of impetigo caused by beta-hemolytic streptococci?

____

23. What should parents be taught about preventing the spread of impetigo?

____

Cellulitis

24. What is cellulitis?
25. Which areas of the body are most commonly affected by cellulitis?

____

26. Name three clinical manifestations of cellulitis.

a.

b.

c.

27. How is cellulitis treated?

28. Identify four nursing interventions for a child with cellulitis on his lower leg.
    a.
    b.
    c.

Candidiasis

29. What is the organism responsible for causing thrush?

30. Describe the clinical manifestations of thrush.

    ____

31. What questions should the nurse ask the mother of an infant with oral candidiasis during ________ an assessment?

32. The medication used to treat oral candidiasis is ________________.

33. How should the prescribed medication be administered to an infant with oral candidiasis?

    ____

    ____

Tinea Infections

34. Identify the body parts affected in the following tinea infections.
    a. Tinea capitis: ______________________________
    b. Tinea corporis: ______________________________
    c. Tinea pedis: ______________________________

35. What medications are used in the treatment of the following tinea infections, and how are they administered?
    a. Tinea capitis: ______________________________
    b. Tinea corporis: ______________________________
    c. Tinea cruris: ______________________________
    d. Tinea pedis: ______________________________

Answer as either true (T) or false (F).

36. ______ Children receiving a prolonged course of griseofulvin therapy should undergo liver function studies.

37. ______ Tinea infections are not contagious to others.

38. ______ Tinea infections heal more quickly if the affected area is kept warm and moist.

Herpes Simplex Virus (HSV) Infection

39. What is herpetic whitlow?

____

40. What medication can lessen the severity of HSV-1? ____________________

41. How would the nurse advise the parents of a child with HSV-1 lesions on the lips who does not want to eat or drink? ____________________________

Lice Infestations

Answer as either true (T) or false (F).

42. ______ Lice can be transmitted only by direct contact with an infested person.

43. ______ Clean hair is a deterrent to head lice.

44. Describe what the nurse is looking for when assessing a child for head lice.

____

45. What is the recommended treatment for killing active lice?

____

46. Give three interventions that should be taken if head lice are found.

a.

b.

c.

Mite Infestation (Scabies)

47. How is scabies transmitted?

48. Name the clinical manifestations of scabies.

____

49. How should a scabicide lotion be applied to the skin?

____

Atopic Dermatitis

50. What causes the intense pruritis associated with atopic dermatitis?

____

51. Describe the appearance of the skin in childhood-onset eczema.

____

52. List three interventions that can relieve itching for a child with atopic dermatitis.
   a.
   b.
   c.

Seborrheic Dermatitis

53. Seborrheic dermatitis is also known as ____________________.
54. Name two clinical manifestations of seborrheic dermatitis.
   a.
   b.
55. Name two interventions used to treat seborrheic dermatitis of the scalp.
   a.
   b.

Contact Dermatitis

56. What is contact dermatitis?

57. Name three interventions that can relieve itching from contact dermatitis.
   a.
   b.
   c.

58. What initial interventions should be taken if a child is exposed to poison ivy?

____

Answer as either true (T) or false (F).

59. ______ Diaper dermatitis is easier to prevent than to treat.

60. ______ The diaper area should be cleaned with water and mild soap after each voiding or bowel movement.

61. ______ Rubber pants should not be used because they hold in moisture and cause skin breakdown.

Acne Vulgaris

62. What parts of the skin are involved in acne vulgaris?

63. Develop an explanation of acne for a young adolescent.

____

64. What should the nurse teach an adolescent about the following medications in order to prevent adverse effects?

a. Tretinoin (Retin-A):

b. Tetracycline:

c. Isotretinoin (Accutane):

65. What guidelines for daily skin care should be followed by the adolescent with acne?

____

____

Insect Bites or Stings

66. What precautions should be taken when a child is allergic to bee stings?

____

67. What intervention should be taken when a child gets a bee sting?

____

68. Why should insect repellents containing diethyloluamide (DEET) not be used on small children?

Miscellaneous Skin Disorders

69. Describe the management of frostbite.

____

70. What should children and parents know about preventing frostbite?

____

71. Describe the best method of removing a tick.

____

Match each skin disorder with its definition.

72. ______ Stevens-Johnson syndrome
73. ______ Molluscum contagiousum
74. ______ Psoriasis
75. ______ Warts

a. Viral infection of the skin and mucous membranes
b. Chronic inflammatory condition caused by rapid proliferation of keratinocytes
c. Skin infection caused by a human papilloma virus
d. Autoimmune disease that may be triggered by infections or medications

BURN INJURIES

Match each description of burn injury with the corresponding level of burn depth. (Answers may be used more than once.)

76. ______ Blisters within minutes of burn injury
77. ______ Peels after 24 to 48 hours
78. ______ Has a mottled, waxy, white dry surface
79. ______ White, cherry red, or black appearance

a. Superficial
b. Partial thickness
c. Full thickness

Match each description of burn injury with the corresponding levels of severity. (Answers may be used more than once.)

80. ______ Partial-thickness burns of greater than 20% of total body surface area (TBSA)
81. ______ Full-thickness burn of less than 2% TBSA, not involving special areas
82. ______ Partial-thickness burns of 10% to 20% TBSA
83. ______ Burns of eyes, ears, face, hands, feet, perineum, or joints

a. Minor
b. Moderate
c. Major

84. What should the nurse teach parents about preventing sunburn in children?

____

____

85. List the three commonly used topical antimicrobial agents for burns.

    a.

    b.

    c.

86. Define *burn shock*.

87. Name four possible complications of an electrical injury.

    a.

    b.

    c.

    d.

SUGGESTED LEARNING ACTIVITIES

1. Develop a one-page instruction sheet for the parents of any of the disorders presented in this chapter.

2. If possible, arrange an observational experience at a pediatric burn center.

3. What are your fears and concerns about caring for a child who has had a major burn injury?

STUDENT LEARNING APPLICATION

Enhance your learning by discussing your answers with other students.

The Child With Head Lice

Six-year-old Kelly was sent to the school nurse because her teacher noticed that she had been scratching her head for the past few days.

1. How should the school nurse check Kelly for head lice?

The examination of Kelly's head revealed nits throughout her hair. When the nurse called Kelly's mother to discuss the matter, her mother comments, "I wash Kelly's hair almost every day. She is a neat child. How could she get lice?"

2. How should the nurse respond to this comment?

3. What are the implications of this problem for the other children in the classroom? For other members of Kelly's family?

4. How should the nurse explain the treatment for head lice to the mother?

5. What measures should be taken in Kelly's classroom?

6. What can children be taught about preventing head lice?

The Child With a Burn Injury

Two-year-old Erica was burned when she pulled on a tablecloth and hot coffee spilled on her chest. On arrival at the emergency department, Erica is alert. Her vital signs are temperature 98.4° F, heart rate 102, respiratory rate 24, and blood pressure 86/54. A 5 × 10-cm area on her upper chest area is red, and four fluid-filled blisters are observed.

1. How would you classify the depth and severity of Erica's injury?

2. What would you expect to be included in Erica's treatment?

Erica's parents are told that she can go home but that they will need to take care of her burned area until it heals.

3. What will you teach them about caring for a burn wound?

4. What concerns do you have about preventing burns in Erica's home?

5. How should you respond to Erica's mother when she asks you, "Will she have a scar?"

REVIEW QUESTIONS

Choose the best answer.

1. A child cut his hand a few days ago. Now the area is swollen and painful, and a red streak extends from it up to the forearm. These are signs of:
   a. impetigo.
   b. cellulitis.
   c. contact dermatitis.
   d. eczema.

2. Which medication is appropriate for the treatment of tinea capitis?
   a. Griseofulvin orally for 6 to 8 weeks
   b. Lotrimin cream to affected areas three times a day until lesions are healed
   c. Tinactin spray twice per day to affected lesions
   d. Penicillin four times a day for 10 days

3. The stinger of a honeybee should be removed by:
   a. squeezing it out of the skin.
   b. using tweezers to lift it out.
   c. scraping it out horizontally.
   d. applying heat to draw out the stinger.

4. What should an adolescent female with severe acne know about Accutane before initiating treatment?
   a. She will need to use sunscreen to reduce photosensitivity.
   b. Accutane can cause menstrual irregularities.
   c. Accutane is teratogenic if taken during pregnancy.
   d. Exposure to sunlight should be avoided while taking Accutane.

5. What should the nurse teach parents about skin care for the child with atopic dermatitis?
   a. After bathing, apply moisturizing cream when the skin has been thoroughly dried.
   b. Avoid clothing made of cotton and polyester because these materials are irritating.
   c. Dress the child warmly at bedtime to prevent itching due to coldness.
   d. Moisturizing creams can be applied whenever the skin looks dry.

6. Which of the following actions is appropriate for the prevention of diaper dermatitis?
   a. Apply medicated powder to perineum after each diaper change.
   b. Wash diaper area with a mild soap and water after each voiding or bowel movement.
   c. Keep the diaper area open to air during rest periods.
   d. Change diapers at least every 4 hours.

7. Assessment of the skin of a child with diaper dermatitis is likely to reveal:
   a. keratosis.
   b. ecchymoses.
   c. lichenification.
   d. pruritis.

8. Assessment of a child with nits would reveal:
   a. very small black bugs jumping throughout the hair.
   b. white specks firmly attached to the hair shaft.
   c. small flakes resembling dandruff that are easily removed from the hair.
   d. clusters of nits at the crown of the head and front hairline.

9. The depth of a burn that appears red to pale ivory, with a moist surface and fluid-filled blisters, is most likely:
   a. superficial.
   b. superficial partial thickness.
   c. deep partial thickness.
   d. full thickness.

10. What is the first priority when initiating treatment on a child with a major burn injury?
    a. Fluid resuscitation
    b. Prevention of sepsis
    c. Airway assessment
    d. Correcting metabolic imbalances

11. What is the most common cause of burn injuries in children under 3 years of age?
    a. Flame
    b. Electrical
    c. Chemical
    d. Scald

12. Burn shock results from:
    a. hypovolemia
    b. sepsis.
    c. toxins.
    d. metabolic acidosis.

50

The Child With a Musculoskeletal Alteration

HELPFUL HINT

Review the anatomy and physiology of the musculoskeletal system in an anatomy and physiology textbook.

MATCHING KEY TERMS

Match the term with the correct definition.

1. ______ avascular necrosis
2. ______ dislocation
3. ______ dysplasia
4. ______ ossification
5. ______ osteoblasts
6. ______ osteoclasts
7. ______ osteotomy
8. ______ paresthesia
9. ______ polydactyly
10. ______ pseudarthrosis
11. ______ reduction
12. ______ subluxation
13. ______ syndactyly
14. ______ valgum
15. ______ varum

a. Failure of the bones to fuse
b. Abnormal bending away from the midline
c. Displacement of a bone from its normal articulation with a joint
d. Extra fingers or toes
e. Tissue damage resulting from inadequate blood supply to the area
f. Surgical cutting of the bone
g. Partial dislocation of a joint
h. Abnormal development of tissue
i. Abnormal bending toward the midline
j. Fusing or webbing of two or more fingers or toes
k. Repositioning of bone fragments into neutral alignment
l. Mesodermal cells whose activity produces bone
m. Sensation of numbness and tingling
n. Bone cells that absorb and remove old bone tissue
o. Process of forming bone from osseous tissue or cartilage

16. Write the opposite of each of the following terms.
    a. Abduction : ____________________
    b. Eversion: ____________________
    c. Internal rotation: ____________________
    d. External fixation: ____________________

Recall the definition of the italicized term in each of the following. Then, identify whether the statement is true (T) or false (F).

17. ______ Artificial limbs are called *orthoses*.
18. ______ *Arthroscopy* is a medical treatment for joint injuries.
19. ______ *Callus* becomes hardened through osteoclastic activity.
20. ______ *Superior mesenteric artery syndrome* resembles intestinal obstruction.
21. ______ In an *autologous blood transfusion*, a person receives blood from a close relative.
22. ______ *Crepitus* results when the ends of a broken bone move against each other.
23. ______ *Ankylosis* is a condition in which a joint is difficult to move.
24. ______ *Plantar flexion* involves bending the foot upward.

REVIEW OF THE MUSCULOSKELETAL SYSTEM

25. Define the three classes of joints.
    a. Synarthrotic:
    b. Amphiarthrotic:
    c. Diarthrotic:
26. Where are the following types of muscles found?
    a. Smooth:
    b. Striated:
    c. Cardiac:

Casts and Traction

27. List the five "P's" of vascular impairment.
    a.
    b.
    c.
    d.
    e.

28. ____________ is the most serious complication associated with skeletal traction.
29. Cervical traction is used to treat ____________.
30. ____________ traction is always continuous.
31. Dunlop traction is used to treat fractures of the _______________.
32. ____________ traction is used for hemarthrosis associated with hemophilia.
33. ____________ traction is used to stabilize fractured femurs.
34. Crutchfield tongs are used to stabilize fractures of the _______________ and _______________ vertebrae.

Limb Defects and Clubfoot

Answer as either true (T) or false (F).

35. ______ Clubfoot is readily apparent by clinical examination at birth.
36. ______ An infant's clubfoot cannot be manipulated into a neutral position.
37. ______ Long-term follow-up for clubfoot is not necessary after corrective surgery.
38. ______ Nonsurgical management of clubfoot requires serial casting.
39. ______ Genu valgum is commonly referred to as "bowlegs."
40. ______ Children requiring casts for limb abnormalities are at risk for altered growth and development.
41. ______ Genu varum is a normal variation in toddlers.
42. ______ A child with webbed fingers has polydactyly.
43. ______ Metatarsus adductus is commonly known as "clubfoot."

Developmental Dysplasia of the Hip

44. What are the manifestations of developmental dysplasia of the hip in the following age groups?
    a. Newborn:

    b. Older infant:

    c. Toddler:

45. The Pavlik harness maintains the hip in which three positions?

    ____

46. Improper positioning of an infant's hip in a Pavlik harness can interrupt the blood supply to the head of the femur, resulting in _______________.

47. List five actual or potential problems encountered when caring for a child in a Pavlik harness.

    a.

    b.

    c.

    d.

    e.

Legg-Calvé-Perthes Disease (LCP)

Answer as either true (T) or false (F).

48. ______ LCP can result in arthritis and skeletal deformities.
49. ______ LCP results in avascular necrosis of the femoral head.
50. ______ Surgical correction increases overall treatment time.
51. ______ In LCP, both hips are usually affected.

Slipped Capital Femoral Epiphysis (SCFE)

52. The typical adolescent with SCFE is ________ average for height and weight.
53. The adolescent with SCFE often presents with ________________ pain.
54. ________________ traction is often used preoperatively to prevent spasms.
55. Surgical correction involves inserting a screw across the ____________ .

Fractures

56. A compound fracture is ____________.
57. Describe compartment syndrome.

    ____

58. A child with a compound fracture is at risk for ____________.
59. Proper healing of a fracture requires correct reduction and ____________.
60. Open reduction requires the surgical insertion of a(n) ____________ device.
61. Fractures in infants usually result from birth trauma or ____________ trauma.
62. The most common sites for fractures in children are ____________.
63. Epiphyseal injuries are fractures that occur between the shaft of a long bone and the ____________.
64. Fat emboli occur most frequently after _______ injuries or fractures of ______ bones.

Soft Tissue Injuries

Match each term with its description.

65. ______ Sprain
66. ______ Strain
67. ______ Contusion
68. ______ Dislocation

a. Articulating surfaces of joint no longer in contact
b. Damage to soft tissue, muscle, or subcutaneous tissue
c. Excessive muscle stretch, resulting in tears and pulls
d. Stretched or torn ligaments

Osgood-Schlatter Disease

69. To what is Osgood-Schlatter disease thought to be related?

____

____

70. List three clinical manifestations of Osgood-Schlatter disease.

____

____

____

____

Osteogenesis Imperfecta

71. Describe osteogenesis imperfecta.

____

72. Identify three clinical manifestations of osteogenesis imperfecta.

   a.

   b.

   c.

Osteomyelitis

Answer as either true (T) or false (F).

73. ______ Osteomyelitis may follow otitis media.
74. ______ Cellulitis can result in osteomyelitis.
75. ______ Osteomyelitis occurs most frequently in infants.
76. ______ Children with osteomyelitis require complete bed rest.
77. ______ Areas of sequestrum are highly susceptible to antibiotics.

Juvenile Arthritis

78. Briefly describe juvenile arthritis.

____

79. What is uveitis?

80. When are SAARDs used?

____

81. Juvenile arthritis is the leading cause of ________________ in children.

Muscular Dystrophies

82. Muscular dystrophies are

____

83. What is the most common type of muscular dystrophy?

84. What is the most common cause of death resulting from muscular dystrophy?

____

Scoliosis, Kyphosis, and Lordosis

Answer as either true (T) or false (F).

85. ______ Paralytic scoliosis is the predominant form of scoliosis.
86. ______ Uneven shoulder height is an indicator of scoliosis.
87. ______ Bracing is used to correct existing curves in scoliosis.
88. ______ Spinal fusion is used to treat severe scoliosis.
89. ______ Superior mesenteric artery syndrome is a complication of bracing for scoliosis.
90. ______ After washing and drying the skin, Keri-lotion should be applied before putting on a tee shirt and brace for scoliosis.
91. ______ Lordosis is a lateral curvature of the spine.
92. ______ Kyphosis is a convex curvature of the spine, usually in the thoracic area.

SUGGESTED LEARNING ACTIVITIES

1. Spend some time with a school nurse doing scoliosis screening. Report on the procedure, the reactions of the students, and the screening results to your class.

2. Arrange to observe in a newborn nursery. Observe the nurses' techniques for assessing skeletal abnormalities.

STUDENT LEARNING APPLICATIONS

Enhance your learning by discussing your answers with other students.

Twelve-year-old Kai is admitted to the hospital with a fractured femur. He is in Russell traction, and he says to you, "I hate this thing! Why are you doing this to me?"

1. How would you explain to Kai about traction and why he needs it?

2. How would you address the "doing this to me" aspect of Kai's question?

3. How would you facilitate trust?

4. How would you enlist Kai's cooperation in maintaining proper alignment and in doing range-of-motion exercises and neurovascular assessments?

REVIEW QUESTIONS

Choose the best answer.

1. Screening for idiopathic scoliosis is done:

   a. prenatally.
   b. in the newborn period.
   c. during the school-age years.
   d. in middle adolescence.

2. A disorder that is obvious in the newborn period is:

   a. clubfoot.
   b. polydactyly.
   c. syndactyly.
   d. all of the above.

3. When developmental dysplasia of the hip is diagnosed:

   a. treatment is begun immediately.
   b. treatment is postponed until the child is able to bear weight.
   c. surgery is scheduled as soon as the child weighs 10 pounds.
   d. bilateral casting is done at 1 month of age.

4. Uncorrected scoliosis can result in:

   a. superior mesenteric artery syndrome.
   b. reduced respiratory function.
   c. fusion of the vertebrae.
   d. none of the above.

5. A child with lordosis may present with:

   a. a concave deformity and obesity.
   b. scoliosis and kyphosis.
   c. a convex deformity and pain in the lower back.
   d. unequal shoulder height and leg length discrepancy.

6. A newborn has been casted for a clubfoot. Parents should be taught about:

   a. assessing for genu varum.
   b. preventing pathologic fractures.
   c. frequent follow-up visits.
   d. preventing deformities in the hands.

7. A child has a closed fracture of the right radius, with slight ecchymosis below the elbow. She always rates her pain as either 9 or 10 on a 10-point scale. Her right hand is cooler than her left, and she cannot extend the fingers of her hand because they "burn." She is probably experiencing:

   a. compartment syndrome.
   b. epiphyseal injuries.
   c. early signs of an infection.
   d. all the above.

8. In taking the history of a child with juvenile arthritis, the nurse would probably discover that the child is taking:

   a. acetaminophen.
   b. aspirin.
   c. morphine.
   d. prednisone.

9. A male adolescent is diagnosed with Osgood-Schlatter disease. In taking a history, the nurse is not surprised to find that he:

   a. is below the 20th percentile for height and weight.
   b. is a medal-winning swimmer.
   c. is on the football team.
   d. has a family history of arthritis.

10. A painful limp, pain in the knee and hip joints, and quadriceps muscle atrophy are clinical manifestations of:

    a. Legg-Calvé-Perthes disease.
    b. Osgood-Schlatter disease.
    c. osteogenesis imperfecta.
    d. Duchenne muscular dystrophy.

11. An appropriate intervention for a child's sprained ankle is:

    a. ibuprofen.
    b. ice packs applied for 20 minutes.
    c. elastic bandage wrap.
    d. all of the above.

12. What is the best way to assess sensory function in a 6-year-old child with a lower leg cast?

    a. Ask "Do you feel this?" when pressing down on the little toe.
    b. Check capillary refill in the middle toe.
    c. Tell the child to wiggle his toes.
    d. Ask "Which toe am I pinching?" when pinching the great toe.

13. A child is hospitalized with musculoskeletal trauma following a severe scooter crash. The nurse would expect to find:

    a. elevated alkaline phosphatase (ALP).
    b. positive rheumatoid factor (RF).
    c. decreased erythrocyte sedimentation rate (ESR).
    d. all of these.

14. A musculoskeletal condition that typically results in death in late adolescence is:

    a. osteogenesis imperfecta.
    b. Legg-Calvé-Perthes disease.
    c. juvenile arthritis.
    d. Duchenne muscular dystrophy.

51

The Child With an Endocrine or Metabolic Alteration

HELPFUL HINT

Refer to an anatomy and physiology textbook for a more extensive discussion of the endocrine system.

MATCHING KEY TERMS

Match the term with the correct definition.

1. ______ hormone
2. ______ gland
3. ______ pituitary
4. ______ euthyroid
5. ______ glucagon
6. ______ hyperglycemia
7. ______ hypoglycemia
8. ______ hypothalamus

a. An endocrine gland attached to the base of the brain that secretes many hormones
b. Chemical substance produced by one gland or tissue and transported by the blood to other tissues, where it causes a specific effect
c. Blood glucose levels below 70 mg/dL
d. Portion of the brain that secretes releasing factors
e. Organ or structure that secretes a substance to be used in some other part of the body
f. Normal thyroid function
g. In a nondiabetic person, fasting blood glucose level greater than or equal to 110 mg/dL
h. Counteracts the action of insulin

REVIEW OF THE ENDOCRINE SYSTEM

Match each hormone with the pituitary lobe that produces it. (Answers may be used more than once.)

9. ______ Oxytocin
10. ______ Adrenocorticotropic hormone (ACTH)
11. ______ Thyroid-stimulating hormone (TSH)
12. ______ Luteinizing hormone (LH)
13. ______ Antidiuretic hormone (ADH)
14. ______ Growth hormone (GH)
15. ______ Prolactin

a. Anterior pituitary lobe
b. Posterior pituitary lobe

DIAGNOSTIC TESTS AND PROCEDURES

16. How are alterations in endocrine functioning usually diagnosed?

____

17. Accurate measurements of _______________ and _______________ are essential when assessing a child for endocrine function.

NEONATAL HYPOGLYCEMIA

18. Hypoglycemia in the neonate is defined as a plasma glucose concentration of less than _______________.
19. The neonates who are most likely to experience hypoglycemia are ___________ infants and infants who are ___________________________.
20. List five signs that indicate a neonate is hypoglycemic.
    a.
    b.
    c.
    d.
    e.
21. What is the intervention for a neonate who is hypoglycemic but asymptomatic?

    ____

    ____
22. What assessments are indicated if a neonate is at increased risk for hypoglycemia?

    ____

    ____
23. What complication can occur when a neonate is receiving IV glucose?

    ____

    ____

HYPOCALCEMIA

24. *Neonatal hypocalcemia* is defined as total serum calcium concentration of less than ___________.
25. Why does neonatal hypocalcemia occur most often in infants of diabetic mothers?

    ____

    ____
26. What is the best time to administer an oral calcium supplement?

PHENYLKETONURIA AND INBORN ERRORS OF METABOLISM

27. What is the genetic transmission pattern of phenylketonuria?

28. Phenylketonuria results in damage to which body system?

29. When should the neonate be screened for phenylketonuria?

30. What is the treatment of phenylketonuria?

Answer as either true (T) or false (F).

31. ______ The child with galactosemia must be on a lifelong low-protein limited–amino acid diet.
32. ______ Maple syrup urine disease causes ketoacidosis 2 to 3 days after birth.
33. ______ Tay-Sachs disease can be treated through dietary modifications.

CONGENITAL ADRENAL HYPERPLASIA

34. In congenital adrenal hyperplasia, the adrenal gland is not able to manufacture ________________________________ but instead produces excess __________.
35. What finding in the newborn infant would raise suspicion of congenital adrenal hyperplasia?

36. The treatment of congenital adrenal hyperplasia involves lifelong _______________.

CONGENITAL AND ACQUIRED HYPOTHYROIDISM

Answer as either true (T) or false (F).

37. ______ Newborn screening for hypothyroidism should be done between 10 and 14 days of age.
38. ______ If untreated, congenital hypothyroidism can result in mental retardation.
39. ______ Treatment of congenital hypothyroidism requires lifelong thyroid hormone replacement.
40. ______ The most common cause of acquired hypothyroidism in children is an autoimmune process.
41. ______ A decreased TSH level is the most sensitive indicator of primary hypothyroidism.

Match each disorder with its characteristic signs and symptoms. (Disorders may be used more than once.)

42. ______ Decreased activity
43. ______ Accelerated linear growth
44. ______ Increased appetite
45. ______ Weight gain
46. ______ Edema of face, hands, and eyes
47. ______ Cold intolerance

a. Hypothyroidism
b. Hyperthyroidism

48. What should parents be taught about administering levothyroxine to their infant?

____

____

HYPERTHYROIDISM (GRAVES DISEASE)

49. List three approaches to the management of hyperthyroidism.

a.

b.

c.

50. The child receiving propylthiouracil must be monitored for which two significant adverse effects?

____

51. Why may treatment for Grave's disease be tapered after a few years?

____

DIABETES INSIPIDUS

52. Diabetes insipidus results when there is a deficiency of ______________________.

53. List the two classic manifestations of diabetes insipidus.

a.

b.

54. Describe the response of a child with diabetes insipidus to being deprived of all fluids for 8 hours.

____

____

55. What medication is used to treat diabetes insipidus?

56. How is this medication administered?

SYNDROME OF INAPPROPRIATE ANTIDIURETIC HORMONE (SIADH)

57. What is the body's response to excessive ADH?

____

58. In SIADH:
    a. urine output is ____________________
    b. urine specific gravity is ____________________
    c. serum sodium levels are ____________________
    d. urine osmolality is ____________________

59. The child with fluid overload is at risk for injury related to ______________ caused by hyponatremia.

PRECOCIOUS PUBERTY

60. Define precocious puberty. ____
61. What is a major consequence of precocious puberty? ____________________
62. The treatment for precocious puberty is ____________________.
63. How does the treatment in question #62 work to inhibit precocious puberty?

____

GROWTH HORMONE (GH) DEFICIENCY

Answer as either true (T) or false (F).

64. ______ A sign that a child may have a growth hormone deficiency is weight less than 5th percentile for age and gender.
65. ______ Delayed puberty is a manifestation of growth hormone deficiency.
66. ______ Stimulation testing is necessary to confirm a diagnosis of growth hormone deficiency.
67. ______ Growth hormone replacement is administered subcutaneously 6 to 7 times per week.

DIABETES MELLITUS

68. The primary source of energy for body cells is ____________________.

69. Glucose is stored in the liver and muscles in the form of _____________.

70. The main function of insulin is ________________________.

71. What is the etiology of type 1 diabetes mellitus? ___________________

Identify the physiologic basis for the following signs and symptoms of type 1 diabetes mellitus.

72. Hyperglycemia:

73. Polyuria:

74. Excessive thirst:

75. Hunger:

76. Weight loss:

77. A fasting serum glucose level exceeding _______ and a random level exceeding _______ is indicative of type 1 diabetes mellitus.

Answer as either true (T) or false (F).

78. ______ The child in the "honeymoon" phase requires increased insulin therapy to prevent hyperglycemia.

79. ______ The goal of insulin therapy is to assist the beta cells with insulin production.

80. ______ Oral hypogylcemic agents are not effective in the management of type 1 diabetes mellitus.

81. ______ Food intake should be balanced with insulin dosage.

82. ______ The family should adhere to a consistent schedule for meal times and amount of food intake.

83. ______ Exercise raises blood sugar levels.

84. ______ Exercise should be scheduled to coincide with insulin peak times.

85. ______ A 15- to 30-g carbohydrate snack can be eaten when the child is planning 1 hour of exercise.

86. Give three examples of a 15-g serving of carbohydrates for the treatment of hypoglycemia.

    a.

    b.

    c.

87. What situations could result in hypoglycemia?

    ____

88. What intervention for hypoglycemia should be taken if the child is unconscious?

    ____

DIABETIC KETOACIDOSIS (DKA)

89. Why is rehydration the initial step in resolving DKA?

    ____

90. In the treatment of DKA, what type of insulin is used and how is it administered?

    ____

SUGGESTED LEARNING ACTIVITIES

1. Arrange an observational experience in an outpatient endocrine clinic. Because many children with endocrine alterations are treated in outpatient settings, this would provide firsthand knowledge of pediatric endocrine alterations.

2. Develop a teaching plan for the parents of a newborn diagnosed with congenital hypothyroidism.

3. Review teaching materials for type 1 diabetes mellitus used at your clinical site. Compare them with teaching materials at another site.

4. Talk with children who have type 1 diabetes mellitus and their families about management and living with this chronic disease.

STUDENT LEARNING APPLICATION

Enhance your learning by discussing your answers with other students.

Lizzy is a 7-year-old child who has been sent to the emergency department from the pediatrician's office for possible DKA. Her parents brought her to the pediatrician because she has had increased urination and abdominal pain. She has lost weight over the past few weeks. The ED nurse observes Lizzy breathing rapidly and deeply and notes that her breath has a fruity odor. Lizzy's blood glucose is 580 mg/dL. Her parents are shocked when they are told that Lizzy is experiencing DKA. Her father says, "We thought she might have a urinary tract infection."

1. Why might her parents have thought that Lizzy had such an infection?

2. What is the basis for Lizzy's symptoms?

3. What interventions would you expect for Lizzy?

4. What would you expect Lizzy's insulin schedule to be?

Lizzy and her parents receive intensive teaching about type 1 diabetes mellitus management. She is placed on a schedule of three insulin injections per day. A few days later, her mother calls the nurse because Lizzy is pale, shaky, and diaphoretic.

5. What do you think is happening to Lizzy?

6. What action would you take?

Lizzy has been active in soccer and softball at her school, and she wants to continue to play.

7. What can Lizzy do to prevent problems during a game or practice?

REVIEW QUESTIONS

Choose the best answer.

1. Which of these statements about congenital hypothyroidism is correct?
   a. Mental retardation caused by hypothyroidism is reversible with treatment.
   b. The most common cause of congenital hypothyroidism is thyroiditis.
   c. The child with congenital hypothyroidism requires lifelong thyroid hormone replacement.
   d. Screening for this disorder is usually done between 3 and 6 months of age.

2. The child with precocious puberty is at risk for:
   a. altered reproductive ability.
   b. delayed development of secondary sex characteristics.
   c. short adult stature.
   d. endocrine tumors.

3. A clinical manifestation of growth hormone deficiency is:
   a. weight less than 5% percentile for age.
   b. hyperglycemia.
   c. precocious puberty
   d. height less than 5% percentile for age and gender.

4. A nursing intervention for a child with SIADH is to:
   a. offer fluids frequently to increase fluid intake.
   b. explain the reason for restricting fluids.
   c. assist the child in selecting low sodium foods.
   d. assess the child for dehydration.

5. When performing a physical assessment on a child with hyperthyroidism, the nurse would be alert for:
   a. coarse hair.
   b. dry, thick skin,
   c. cold intolerance.
   d. tremors.

6. The child experiencing SIADH would be assessed for signs of the electrolyte imbalance called:
   a. hyponatremia.
   b. hypernatremia.
   c. hypocalcemia.
   d. hypokalemia.

7. The etiology of type 1 diabetes mellitus is thought to be:
   a. viral.
   b. genetic.
   c. environmental.
   d. autoimmune.

8. A child received NPH insulin subcutaneously at 8:00 A.M. At what time is this child most likely to become hypoglycemic?
   a. 9:00 to 11:00 A.M.
   b. 12:00 NOON to 2:00 P.M.
   c. 2:00 to 4:00 P.M.
   d. 6:00 to 8:00 P.M.

9. Which of these situations could lead to hypogylcemia?
   a. Insufficient insulin
   b. Decreased exercise
   c. Missed meal
   d. Minor illness

10. An appropriate diabetes task for the preschool child would be to include which of the following?
    a. Perform finger puncture for blood.
    b. Choose injection sites according to a rotation schedule.
    c. Push the plunger on the syringe.
    d. Identify a "code" word to describe hypoglycemia.

11. Sick day rules for the child with type 1 diabetes mellitus include which of the following?
    a. Do not give insulin if the child is nauseated or vomiting.
    b. Test blood glucose levels at least twice a day.
    c. Test urine for ketones with each void.
    d. Offer fluids with calories if the child is not eating.

12. One adrenergic sign of hypoglycemia is:
    a. blurred vision.
    b. clammy skin.
    c. irritability.
    d. increased respiratory rate.

13. If not properly balanced with insulin and diet, exercise can lead to:
    a. hypoglycemia.
    b. hyperglycemia.
    c. ketoacidosis.
    d. hypokalemia.

14. The best action for a child who is experiencing hypoglycemia is to:
    a. drink 4 ounces of fruit juice.
    b. eat a chocolate bar.
    c. drink a can of diet soda.
    d. get some exercise.

52

The Child With a Neurologic Alteration

HELPFUL HINT

Review the physiology of the nervous system in an anatomy and physiology textbook. Also, refer to a pharmacology textbook for a more detailed discussion of anticonvulsant medications.

MATCHING KEY TERMS

Match the term with the correct definition.

1. ______ blood-brain barrier
2. ______ cerebral herniation
3. ______ Cushing's response
4. ______ decerebrate posture
5. ______ decorticate posture
6. ______ Monro-Kellie doctrine
7. ______ myelinization

a. Abnormal flexion of the upper extremities and extension of the lower extremities
b. Formation of the proteolipid coating of nerves
c. Separation between brain tissue and blood
d. Shift of brain tissue sideways or downward, causing severe neurologic dysfunction
e. Abnormal extension of upper extremities with internal rotation of upper arms and wrists
f. Compensatory mechanism of cranial contents that maintains steady volume and pressure
g. Late sign of increased intracranial pressure (ICP)

REVIEW OF THE CENTRAL NERVOUS SYSTEM

8. Identify the week(s) during gestation when the following occur.
   a. Neural tube closes:

   b. First period of rapid brain cell growth:

   c. Second period of rapid brain cell growth:

   d. Myelin sheath begins to form:

9. Name the three main sections of the brain.

   a.

   b.

   c.

10. What is the function of cerebrospinal fluid (CSF)?

Match each term with its description.

11. ______ Dura mater
12. ______ Tentorium
13. ______ Pia mater
14. ______ Axial skeleton
15. ______ Cerebrum
16. ______ Brain stem

a. Fills the upper portion of the skull
b. Outer layer of meninges
c. Contains the pons, medulla, midbrain, thalamus, and third ventricle
d. Tent-like structure separating cerebellum from occipital lobe
e. Innermost layer of meninges
f. Protects structures of the central nervous system

INCREASED INTRACRANIAL PRESSURE

17. How does the brain compensate for increased ICP?

    ____

18. Identify two clinical manifestations of increased ICP for each of the following age groups.

    a. Infants:

    b. Children:

19. Identify the illustrations on the following page as decerebrate posturing or decorticate posturing.

    a.

    b.

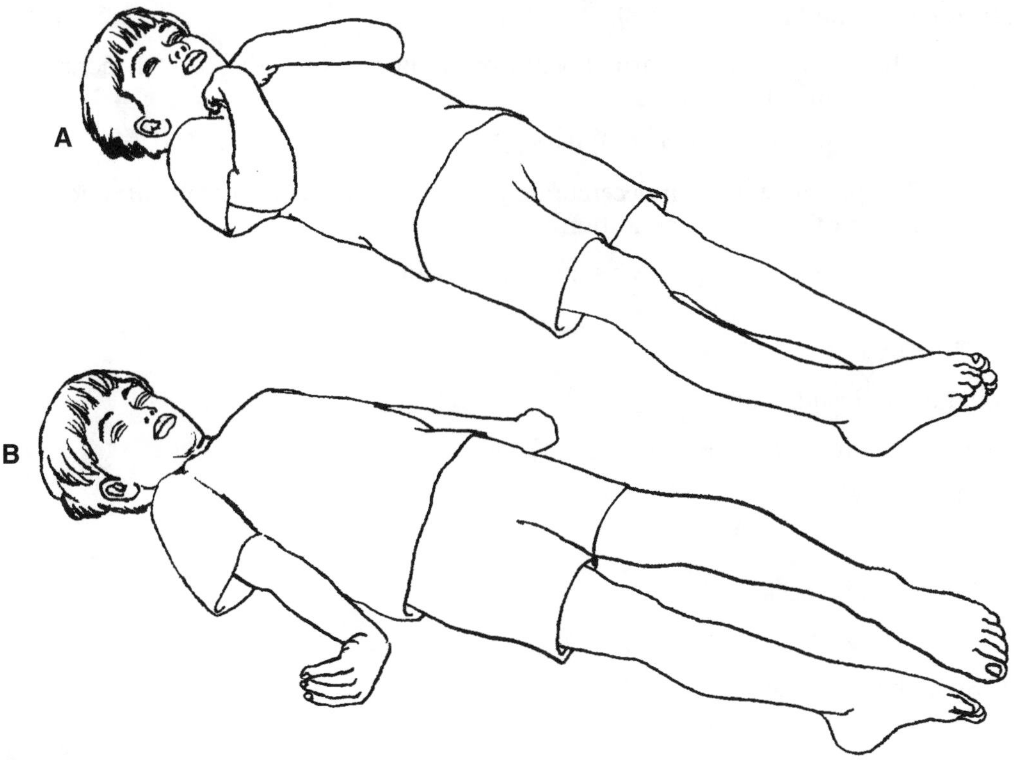

20. What three assessments are included in the Glasgow Coma Scale?

    a.

    b.

    c.

Match each level of consciousness with its description.

21. ______ Confused
22. ______ Disoriented
23. ______ Lethargic
24. ______ Obtunded
25. ______ Stupor
26. ______ Coma

a. Person requires considerable stimulation to arouse.
b. Ability to think clearly and rapidly is lost.
c. Person awakens easily but exhibits limited responsiveness.
d. Person is unable to recognize place or person.
e. Vigorous stimulation produces no motor or verbal response.
f. Person sleeps unless aroused.

Answer as either true (T) or false (F).

27. ______ Changes in a child's normal behavior are important indicators of increased intracranial pressure.
28. ______ The pupils constrict as ICP increases.
29. ______ The progression from decerebrate to decorticate posturing indicates deterioration of the child's condition.
30. ______ The appearance of the Cushing reflex is an early sign of increased ICP.

SPINA BIFIDA

31. Spina bifida results from ______________________.
32. Define the following terms.
    a. Meningocele:

    b. Myelomeningocele:

    c. Spina bifida occulta:

Answer as either true (T) or false (F).

33. ______ Degree of impairment is related to the level of the defect on the spinal cord.
34. ______ Folic acid deficiency in the mother has been linked to neural tube defects in the child.
35. ______ A child with a myelomeningocele below S3 will have serious motor impairment.
36. ______ The primary rationale for surgically closing the defect is to preserve sensory and motor function.
37. ______ Before surgery the neonate with a myelomeningocele is at risk for infection.
38. ______ Children with spina bifida are at high risk for developing a latex allergy.

HYDROCEPHALUS

39. The treatment for hydrocephalus is ______________________________.
40. How should the infant or child with hydrocephalus be positioned postoperatively?

    ____

41. What are the signs of a shunt infection?

    ____

Match each clinical manifestation with the corresponding age group. (Answers may be used more than once.)

42. ______ Full, bulging anterior fontanel
43. ______ Nausea and vomiting that may be projectile
44. ______ "Setting sun" eyes
45. ______ Shrill, high-pitched cry
46. ______ Widely separated cranial sutures
47. ______ Frontal headache in the morning relieved by vomiting or sitting upright
48. ______ Seizures

a. Infant early sign
b. Infant late sign
c. Child early sign
d. Child late sign

CEREBRAL PALSY

Answer as either true (T) or false (F).

49. ______ Almost all children with cerebral palsy will have some degree of mental retardation and other handicaps.
50. ______ In cerebral palsy, the damage to the motor system can occur in the prenatal, perinatal, or postnatal periods.
51. ______ A delay in motor development is an indicator of cerebral palsy.

HEAD INJURY

52. What is included in the initial assessment of a child with a head injury?

____

53. What guidelines should parents follow in determining when to notify the physician of a child's head injury?

____

Match each type of head injury with its description.

54. ______ Contusion
55. ______ Concussion
56. ______ Closed head injury
57. ______ Epidural hemorrhage
58. ______ Subdural hemorrhage

a. Transient and reversible neuronal dysfunction with instantaneous loss of responsiveness
b. Accumulation of blood between the dura and skull
c. Petechial hemorrhages along the superficial aspects of the brain
d. Accumulation of blood between the dura and the cerebrum
e. Nonpenetrating injury to the head

59. Describe postconcussion syndrome.

____

SPINAL CORD INJURY

Answer as either true (T) or false (F).

60. ______ Spinal shock is accompanied by flaccid paralysis.
61. ______ In a spinal cord injury, all neurons carrying sensations from parts of the body above the lesion are affected and unable to pass impulses to the brain.
62. ______ Most spinal cord injuries in children occur in the cervical spine.
63. ______ Before any attempt is made to move a child with a neck or spinal cord injury, the spine must be immobilized.

SEIZURE DISORDERS

Match each classification of seizure with its description.

64. ______ Tonic-clonic
65. ______ Atonic
66. ______ Myoclonic
67. ______ Absence
68. ______ Simple partial
69. ______ Complex partial

a. Sustained, generalized contraction of muscles followed by alternating contraction and relaxation of major muscle groups
b. Characterized by impaired consciousness, transient staring, and behaviors such as lip smacking and teeth grinding
c. Brief, random contractions of a muscle group
d. May include motor, autonomic, or sensory symptoms
e. Brief episodes of altered consciousness characterized by a blank facial expression
f. Abrupt loss of postural tone, impaired consciousness, and confusion

70. Differentiate between a seizure and epilepsy.

____

____

71. Precipitating factors in febrile seizures are the __________ and __________ of temperature elevation.

72. What information should be elicited from a parent or caregiver when a child has a seizure?

____

____

____

73. List three nursing interventions to maintain a child's safety during a generalized tonic-clonic seizure.

a.

b.

c.

74. What would the nurse teach parents about use of the antiepileptic medication phenytoin (Dilantin)?

____

____

75. Define *status epilepticus.*

____

MENINGITIS

76. What diagnostic test confirms that a child has meningitis?

77. Describe a positive Kernig's sign.

____

78. Describe a positive Brudzinski's sign.

____

79. How is acute bacterial meningitis treated?

____

Answer as either true (T) or false (F).

80. ______ Signs of meningitis in young children may be vague and nonspecific.

81. ______ The child with bacterial meningitis should be kept in isolation for 7 days.

82. ______ The treatment of viral meningitis is symptomatic and supportive.

GUILLAIN-BARRÉ SYNDROME

83. Guillain-Barré syndrome is often preceded by a(n) ______________________.

84. Most deaths from Guillain-Barré syndrome are attributed to ______________________.

HEADACHES

85. The three primary sources of recurrent headaches are:

a. ____

b. ____

c. ____

SUGGESTED LEARNING ACTIVITY

1. Assess the neurologic status of several children using the Glasgow Coma Scale.

STUDENT LEARNING APPLICATION

Enhance your learning by discussing your answers with other students.

A father brings his 4-year-old daughter Lisa to the emergency department because she has had a seizure. He explains that she became unconscious, her body became rigid, and her back began arching and relaxing. Lisa has also had a headache, stiff neck, and fever for the past day.

1. What information in this situation is suggestive of meningitis?

2. What diagnostic study would confirm this diagnosis? What would you expect an analysis to reveal?

3. What other diagnostic study might be ordered for Lisa, given her history?

4. What additional information about Lisa's seizure should you gather from her father?

5. Lisa's father then asks, "What caused the seizure?" How would you respond?

6. What is the treatment for bacterial meningitis?

7. Lisa is admitted to the hospital. As her nurse, what assessments would you make?

8. Lisa's urine output has decreased, and her urine specific gravity is 1.023. Her serum sodium level is 125 mEq/L. What do these data suggest?

9. What interventions might be initiated based on these data?

REVIEW QUESTIONS

Choose the best answer.

1. Which of the following is used to monitor brain growth?
   a. CSF analysis
   b. Head circumference measurement
   c. Electroencephalogram (EEG)
   d. CT scan

2. A clinical manifestation of increased ICP in an infant is:
   a. slurred speech.
   b. headache.
   c. double vision.
   d. bulging fontanel.

3. Raccoon eyes and clear fluid draining from the ears is suggestive of which type of head injury?
   a. Basilar skull fracture
   b. Concussion
   c. Subdural hemorrhage
   d. Contusion

4. If a child awakens easily but exhibits limited responsiveness, his level of consciousness is described as:
   a. confused.
   b. disoriented.
   c. lethargic.
   d. stuporous.

5. Which of the following is not included in the Glasgow Coma Scale?
   a. Eye opening
   b. Motor response
   c. Verbal response
   d. Neurovascular status

6. Which change in vital signs is not associated with the Cushing reflex?
   a. Increased systolic pressure
   b. Decreased heart rate
   c. Increased temperature
   d. Irregular respiratory pattern

7. A newborn has a sac in the lumbosacral area containing CSF, meninges, nerve roots, and the spinal cord. This condition is referred to as:
   a. myelomeningocele.
   b. meningocele.
   c. Arnold Chiari malformation.
   d. spina bifida occulta.

8. Before surgery, the priority for care of a newborn with a myelomeningocele is:
   a. preventing infection.
   b. preserving urinary function.
   c. promoting nutrition.
   d. maximizing motor function.

9. An early sign of hydrocephalus in an infant is:
   a. "setting sun" eyes.
   b. frontal bone enlargement.
   c. shrill, high-pitched cry.
   d. widely separated cranial sutures.

10. Which type of cerebral palsy is characterized by increased deep tendon reflexes, hypertonia, and flexion of extremities?
    a. Spastic
    b. Ataxic
    c. Athetoid
    d. Rigid

11. An expected finding in an analysis of CSF in the child with bacterial meningitis is:
    a. low protein.
    b. cloudy appearance.
    c. high glucose.
    d. increased red blood cells.

12. An appropriate nursing action during a tonic-clonic seizure is:
    a. restraining flailing extremities.
    b. placing padding between the teeth.
    c. observing the type of movements and duration of the seizure.

d. placing the child in a supine or prone position.

13. A parent describes his child as having a blank stare with eyelid twitching. This child is most likely experiencing which type of seizure?

    a. Complex partial
    b. Atonic
    c. Myoclonic
    d. Absence

14. What is the first priority when a child has sustained a spinal cord injury?

    a. Assess motor function.
    b. Assess sensory function.
    c. Immobilize the spine.
    d. Measure vital signs.

15. Which of the following statements about febrile seizures is true?

    a. The majority of children who experience febrile seizures develop epilepsy.
    b. Febrile seizures most commonly occur after 5 years of age.
    c. Seizure activity occurs during the temperature rise.
    d. A prolonged temperature elevation usually precedes the febrile seizure.

53

The Child With a Psychosocial Disorder

HELPFUL HINT

Review a psychiatric nursing textbook for additional information about psychosocial disorders and psychotropic medications.

DEFINITIONS

Complete the following crossword puzzle.

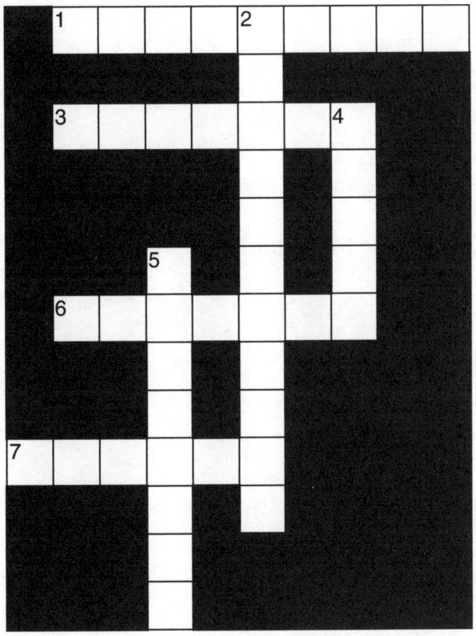

Across

1. Physical or psychological dependence on a substance even when it is known to impair cognitive or social functioning.
3. Characterized by recurrent episodes of binge eating.
6. Voluntary and intentional cessation of one's life.
7. Statement or behavior that usually occurs prior to overt suicidal activity.

Down

2. Presence of two different but interactive conditions existing simultaneously in a single individual.
4. Nonaccidental physical injury.
5. Exertion of extreme force or destructive action resulting in injury.

OVERVIEW OF CHILDHOOD PSYCHOPATHOLOGY

Answer as either true (T) or false (F).

8. ______ Cognitive development proceeds from abstract to concrete thinking.
9. ______ Significant factor affecting the impact of brain damage on the child is the maturational stage of the brain at the time the damage occurs.
10. ______ Most psychosocial disorders have a familial or biologic predisposition that may be triggered if the environment is demanding or unsupportive.

ANXIETY AND DEPRESSION

Match each disorder with its description.

11. ______ Dysthymic disorder
12. ______ Bipolar mood disorder
13. ______ Major depressive disorder
14. ______ Separation anxiety
15. ______ Posttraumatic stress disorder

a. Episode of irritable or depressed mood with disturbances in sleep, appetite, energy, and self-esteem lasting at least 2 weeks
b. Chronic mood disturbances fluctuating between depressive lows and highs for at least 1 year
c. Irritable or depressed mood for at least 1 year
d. Panic disorder following a terrifying event
e. Disabling fear about being away from parents or away from home

Answer as either true (T) or false (F).

16. ______ The most common mood disturbance in childhood is depression.
17. ______ Affective disorders have been shown to have a genetic basis.
18. ______ A child or an adolescent may have both anxiety and depression.
19. Which classification of medications is frequently prescribed for the treatment of anxiety and depression?

SUICIDE

20. Identify five manifestations that indicate a child is at risk for suicide.
    a.
    b.
    c.
    d.
    e.
21. List three questions a nurse could ask an adolescent when he says that his life is not worth living anymore.
    a.
    b.
    c.

22. Describe the best approach for the nurse to take when an adolescent has expressed thoughts of suicide.

____

____

Answer as either true (T) or false (F).

23. ______ Poor self-concept is a significant factor in suicide.
24. ______ Screening children for depression in the school system is a poor suicide prevention strategy.
25. ______ Most suicide statements by adolescents can be ignored.
26. ______ Gay and lesbian adolescents are more likely to attempt suicide than are their heterosexual peers.

EATING DISORDERS: ANOREXIA NERVOSA AND BULIMIA NERVOSA

27. Identify three distinguishing characteristics of anorexia nervosa.

    a.

    b.

    c.

28. Identify three distinguishing characteristics of bulimia nervosa.

    a.

    b.

    c.

Answer as either true (T) or false (F).

29. ______ Adolescents with eating disorders usually have a family history of affective disorders.
30. ______ Individuals with anorexia often exhibit ritualistic tendencies about food preparation and food consumption.
31. ______ Amenorrhea is commonly seen in females with bulimia.
32. ______ When assessing an adolescent with an eating disorder, it is best to use an unstructured format to elicit information.

ATTENTION-DEFICIT/HYPERACTIVITY DISORDER (ADHD)

33. Children with ADHD have problems in what three areas?

    a. ______________________________

    b. ______________________________

    c. ______________________________

34. How is a diagnosis of AHDH established?

35. The primary nursing intervention for the child with ADHD is to

    ______________________________.

Answer as either true (T) or false (F).

36. ______ Increased levels of dopamine in the brain have been associated with ADHD.

37. ______ ADHD affects boys more often than girls.

38. ______ Children with ADHD tend to have fewer behavioral problems in chaotic environments.

SUBSTANCE ABUSE

39. Describe the four phases of substance abuse.

    Phase 1:

    Phase 2:

    Phase 3:

    Phase 4:

40. List four behaviors that would alert the school nurse to a child's substance abuse.

    a.

    b.

    c.

    d.

Answer as either true (T) or false (F).

41. ______ The treatment of substance abuse includes individual, group, and family therapy.

42. ______ If the nurse is the first person to identify a substance abuse problem, the nurse should notify the adolescent's family.

43. ______ In a substance abuse treatment facility, the nurse's primary responsibility is to stabilize the child or adolescent's psychological status.

44. ______ It is important for the child or adolescent and family to identify and develop social support systems.

INFANTS OF ADDICTED MOTHERS AND INFANTS WITH FETAL ALCOHOL SYNDROME (FAS)

45. Fill in the manifestations of withdrawal for an infant born addicted to narcotics.

W: ____________________

I: ____________________

T: ____________________

H: ____________________

D: ____________________

R: ____________________

A: ____________________

W: ____________________

A: ____________________

L: ____________________

46. Identify three nursing interventions that are appropriate to decrease environmental stimuli for a newborn experiencing withdrawal.

a.

b.

c.

47. What facial characteristics are associated with FAS?

____

____

CHILDHOOD PHYSICAL AND EMOTIONAL ABUSE AND NEGLECT

48. Identify three common characteristics of the abusive family.

a. ____________________

b. ____________________

c. ____________________

49. Define *shaken baby syndrome.*

____

50. Define *Munchausen syndrome by proxy.*

____

51. How can the nurse establish trust with the child and family in suspected child abuse cases?

____

____

Answer as either true (T) or false (F).

52. ______ Family dysfunction underlies most forms of child abuse.

53. ______ In most cases a child is abused by someone who is not a family member.

54. ______ Children who are sexually abused are usually younger than 5 years at the onset of the abuse.

55. ______ When child abuse is suspected, the nurse should write down verbatim any comments made by the child.

FAILURE TO THRIVE (FTT)

56. What is the most commonly observed risk factor for nonorganic FTT?

____

57. Identify the physical indicators of FTT.

____

58. Identify the behavioral indicators of FTT.

____

Answer as either true (T) or false (F).

59. ______ Increasing caloric intake is a key feature of a treatment plan for a child with FTT.

60. ______ Brain growth and development can be affected by undernutrition in the first 2 years of life.

SUGGESTED LEARNING ACTIVITIES

1. Perform a mental status examination on a school-age child or an adolescent. Document your findings. Use the box, "Mental Status Examination of Children," on page 1534 in Chapter 53 as a guideline.

2. Complete the following table on the clinical manifestations of various forms of child abuse.

Type of Abuse	Physical Indicators	Behavioral Indicators
Physical abuse		
Physical neglect		
Emotional abuse		
Sexual abuse		

3. Complete the following tables to review the types and clinical manifestations of failure to thrive.

Type of FTT	Description	Causative Factors
Organic		
Nonorganic		
Mixed		

	Clinical Manifestations of FTT
Physical indicators	
Behavioral indicators	

STUDENT LEARNING APPLICATION

Enhance your learning by discussing your answers with other students.

Alex is a fifth-grader with ADHD who began taking Ritalin 3 times a day at the beginning of the school year. Alex is supposed to go to the school nurse's office at lunchtime for his second dose of the day. Alex's cooperation with coming for his medication has been inconsistent. He told the school nurse that he just forgets to come.

1. Could there be other reasons why Alex is not coming for his midday dose of Ritalin?

2. If you were the school nurse, what strategies might you use to help Alex remember to come for his medication every day?

3. How would you evaluate the effectiveness of Ritalin for a child with ADHD?

Alex's teacher remarks that he is a different child now that he is taking Ritalin.

4. Why would this medication make such a difference in a child's behavior?

5. Why should Alex take Ritalin after eating lunch instead of before lunch?

REVIEW QUESTIONS

Choose the best answer.

1. A parent describes her child as irritable for the past month. The child has much less energy than usual and her grades have declined. This child meets the criteria for:
   a. dysthymic disorder.
   b. cyclothymic disorder.
   c. school phobia.
   d. major depressive disorder.

2. One of the most significant risk factors for teen suicide is:
   a. poor self-concept.
   b. anxiety.
   c. heterosexual orientation.
   d. introverted personality.

3. An adolescent tells the school nurse that he has thought about killing himself. An appropriate response to the adolescent would be:
   a. "I am going to call your parents about this ASAP."
   b. "I have the number of a suicide hotline."
   c. "How are you feeling right now?"
   d. "Why would you even think about killing yourself?"

4. Which of the following is not a manifestation of anorexia nervosa?
   a. Recurring episodes of binge eating
   b. Secondary amenorrhea
   c. Extreme fear of obesity
   d. Thin extremities with muscle wasting

5. The nurse might expect a child with ADHD to be:

   a. a gifted student who is bored with school subjects.
   b. easily distracted by internal and external stimuli.
   c. able to complete one activity before moving to the next project.
   d. ritualistic about activities of daily living.

6. Which of the following family characteristics would put an adolescent at the most risk for substance abuse?

   a. Family practices an authoritarian parenting style.
   b. Family participates in school and community projects.
   c. Open communication among family members is encouraged.
   d. One parent has chronic physical and mental health problems.

7. An adolescent who uses drugs regularly and exhibits a physical dependence on the drug is considered to be in the phase of:

   a. experimentation.
   b. early drug use.
   c. true drug addiction.
   d. severe drug addiction.

8. A child has been coming to school early and staying late and is seen stealing food from the cafeteria. These behaviors are suggestive of:

   a. physical abuse.
   b. physical neglect.
   c. emotional abuse.
   d. emotional neglect.
   e. sexual abuse.

9. A 9-month-old infant hospitalized with a diagnosis of nonorganic FTT most likely:

   a. has an intense stranger anxiety.
   b. cries constantly unless held by mother.
   c. is extremely watchful of everyone in the room.
   d. is receptive to being held by the nurse.

10. Which of the following guidelines is appropriate for feeding a toddler who has not been gaining weight?

    a. Feed the child first; then allow him to attempt to feed himself.
    b. Serve different foods every day for variety.
    c. Give the child tasty "junk" food to increase calorie consumption.
    d. Try to keep meal and snack times the same each day.

54

The Child With a Cognitive Impairment

HELPFUL HINT

Review normal growth and development in Chapters 4 through 8 of your textbook.

MATCHING KEY TERMS

Match the term with the correct definition.

1. ______ intelligence
2. ______ pervasive developmental disorders
3. ______ functional age
4. ______ co-morbidity

a. Occurrence of two or more disorders in an individual
b. Disorders involving impairment in several areas of development
c. Capacity of a child to learn, think, and problem solve
d. Age equivalent at which a child is able to perform specific self-care or relational tasks

5. Children with cognitive impairments have limitations in ___________ and _______ abilities.
6. What criteria must be present for a diagnosis of mental retardation?

____

____

7. Identify four components of a developmental disability.

    a.

    b.

    c.

    d.

8. How did the Education for All Handicapped Children Act (PL 94-142) affect children with cognitive impairments?

____

9. What is an individualized education plan (IEP)?

____

COGNITIVE IMPAIRMENT

10. Why are children with developmental disabilities at risk for child abuse?

    ____

11. What is the cardinal sign of cognitive impairment?

12. Name the two most common genetic disorders in which cognitive impairment is a central feature.

    a. ____________________

    b. ____________________

Answer as either true (T) or false (F).

13. _____ Hereditary disorders are the most frequent cause of cognitive impairment in children.
14. _____ Safety is a concern for cognitively impaired children.
15. _____ Disruptive behavior disorders or other psychiatric disorders often coexist with cognitive impairment.
16. _____ The diagnosis of mental retardation is most often made during the neonatal period.
17. _____ Therapeutic management for children with cognitive impairments largely depends on community and educational resources.

DOWN SYNDROME

18. Down syndrome is also known as ________________________.
19. The most common type of living experience for a child with Down syndrome is for the child to be reared ____.
20. Down syndrome is generally diagnosed at birth as a result of the infant's ________.
21. List four areas to assess when caring for the child with Down syndrome.

    a.

    b.

    c.

    d.

Answer as either true (T) or false (F).

22. ______ Down syndrome accounts for one third of all cases of moderate to severe mental retardation.
23. ______ Most children with Down syndrome are born to women over 35 years old.
24. ______ In almost all instances, Down syndrome is the result of translocation of chromosome 21 to chromosome 14 or 22.
25. ______ When caring for a child with Down syndrome in the hospital, it is important to keep the environment and schedule as close to the child's usual environment and routines as possible.

FRAGILE X SYNDROME

Answer as either true (T) or false (F).

26. ______ Fragile X syndrome is the most common inherited cause of mental retardation.
27. ______ Children with fragile X syndrome have no distinctive physical features.
28. ______ Fragile X syndrome is 3 times more common in girls than in boys.

AUTISM

29. Autism is classified as a ________________________.
30. The ability to successfully predict short-term outcomes for children with autism is related to ____________ function rather than to ____________ behavior.
31. List four developmental areas in which qualitative impairment is seen in children with autism.

    a.

    b.

    c.

    d.

32. What is the primary characteristic of autism?

Answer as either true (T) or false (F).

33. ______ Family childrearing practices and parental personalities are the basis of the development of autism.
34. ______ The incidence of autism is equal in males and females.
35. ______ DNA testing is the definitive method of diagnosing autism.
36. ______ Autism usually becomes apparent after the age of 3 years.

Match each disorder with its characteristic clinical manifestations. (Answers may be used more than once.)

37. ______ Alzheimer's-type dementia in adulthood
38. ______ Marked distress over minor changes in environment
39. ______ Flat occiput
40. ______ Marked lack of awareness of feelings of others
41. ______ Flat feet, lax ankles, and hyperextensible fingers
42. ______ Possible presence of other medical conditions
43. ______ Prominent ears and long, narrow face
44. ______ Biting of the hands

a. Autism
b. Down syndrome
c. Fragile X syndrome

SUGGESTED LEARNING ACTIVITIES

1. Talk with parents of a child with a cognitive deficit. Discover what parental support systems they are using, within both the family and the community.

2. Arrange an interview with an occupational therapist or other member of the multidisciplinary team. Discuss early intervention programs for the child with a cognitive deficit.

STUDENT LEARNING APPLICATION

Enhance your learning by discussing your answers with other students.

Jacqui, a 4-year-old preschooler, is an outpatient at the pediatric clinic. Routine pediatric follow-up data indicate that she has consistently achieved developmental milestones, but she reaches them much later than children of the same chronologic age. Her physical appearance is normal. Jacqui's weight and height are within the normal range for a child her age. She has been healthy throughout childhood, with only minor illnesses.

1. What further assessment data would you need for Jacqui?

2. What types of assessment would you do with her family?

3. Identify potential community resources that you could use for Jacqui and her family at this stage of evaluation.

4. What would be your preliminary nursing diagnoses and interventions for Jacqui?

REVIEW OUESTIONS

Choose the best answer.

1. Which of the following is a clinical manifestation of Down syndrome?
   a. Extremely soft and smooth skin
   b. Hypertonicity of large muscles
   c. Long, narrow face with large ears
   d. Single transverse palmar crease

2. The best method of detecting mental retardation at an early age is:
   a. neuropsychologic testing.
   b. using an IQ test for cognitive abilities.
   c. developmental assessment at well-child care.
   d. radiographic evaluation of the brain.

3. The child with fragile X syndrome will likely exhibit:
   a. frustration with a change in routine.
   b. impairment in the rate of physical, social, and language skills.
   c. abnormal ways of relating to people.
   d. gaze avoidance, hand flapping, and abnormal speech patterns.

4. Which of the following questions, during a hospital admission assessment, best indicates that the nurse understands the needs of a child with Down syndrome?
   a. "Can you go over her daily routine with me?"
   b. "Does she require a special diet?"
   c. "Does she sleep through the night?"
   d. "Is she toilet trained?"

5. Injuries are less common among children with cognitive deficits during:
   a. infancy.
   b. toddlerhood.
   c. preschool age.
   d. adolescence.

6. A child with autism will display:
   a. hyperkinetic behavior, poor coordination, and cognitive deficits.
   b. absent or delayed speech and abnormal ways of relating to people.
   c. periods of remission and relapse.
   d. pubescent or adolescent onset of disorder.

7. The goal for a child with a cognitive deficit is to:
   a. find an appropriate facility to meet the long-term needs of the child.
   b. maximize the child's skill potential and provide safe, nurturing care in a supportive family.
   c. use community resources to support the family through stressful periods.
   d. assist the child to live within the child's limitations.

55

The Child With a Sensory Alteration

HELPFUL HINT

Review vision, hearing, and language development in Chapters 5 through 8 in your textbook. Also, refer to Chapter 33 Physical Assessment of Children for an overview of screening techniques.

DEFINITIONS

Complete the following crossword puzzle.

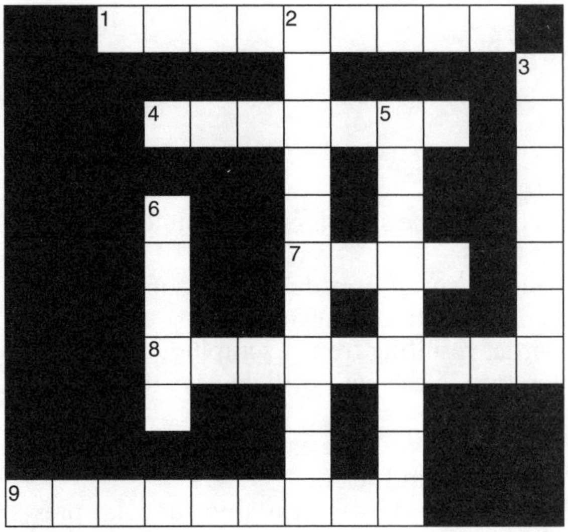

Across

1. Involuntary eye movements that make eyes appear to be darting back and forth.
4. Hearing loss resulting from damage to the conduction system between the brain stem and cerebral cortex.
7. Hearing loss characterized by the failure to hear 26 to 40 dB.
8. Eyes turn away from the midline.
9. ___________ neonatorum.

Down

2. Abnormal curvature of the cornea or the lens.
3. Hemorrhage or sanguinous exudate in the anterior chamber of the eye.
5. Reduced visual acuity not correctable by refractive means.
6. Combination of conductive and sensorineural hearing loss.

REVIEW OF THE EYE AND THE EAR

Match each part of the eye or ear with its description.

10. ______ Eustachian tube
11. ______ Malleus, incus, and stapes
12. ______ Cochlea
13. ______ Tympanic membrane
14. ______ Retina
15. ______ Iris
16. ______ Cornea
17. ______ Macula
18. ______ Sclera

a. Small snail-shaped chamber in the inner ear
b. Clear area located in the front of the eye
c. Structure that separates the outer ear from the middle ear
d. Inner area of the eye containing rods and cones
e. Structure that contains the greatest concentration of nerve endings in the eye
f. Structure that connects the middle ear with the nasopharynx
g. Bones of the middle ear
h. Colored muscular ring located behind the cornea
i. White outer covering of the eye

19. The critical period of eye development is ____________________.
20. The critical period for ear development is ____________________.
21. Binocularity is established by ______________.
22. A child usually develops 20/20 visual acuity by ______________.

DISORDERS OF THE EYE

Match each disorder with its description.

23. ______ Refractive error
24. ______ Strabismus
25. ______ Color blindness
26. ______ Glaucoma
27. ______ Cataract
28. ______ Conjunctivitis
29. ______ Orbital cellulitis
30. ______ Corneal abrasion
31. ______ Hyphema

a. Infection of the soft tissues surrounding the orbit
b. Misalignment of eyes due to lack of coordination of the extraocular muscles
c. Disorder resulting from a scraping of the lens
d. Alteration in the path of light rays through the eye
e. Inflammation of the clear membranous lining of the eyelid and sclera
f. Disorder caused by increased intraocular pressure
g. Hemorrhage resulting from a blow to the eye
h. Inability to distinguish between colors within certain groups
i. Opacity of the lens

32. Identify three behaviors indicating that a child may have a refractive error.

a.

b.

c.

33. Define legal blindness.

____

34. What complication can develop if strabismus is not treated early?

____

35. Why is eye patching used to treat strabismus?

____

36. What are the clinical signs of glaucoma?

____

37. The preferred treatment for glaucoma in children is _______________.

38. For what signs of increased intraocular pressure must a child be monitored postoperatively?

39. How should the nurse position the infant after cataract surgery?

____

40. Identify four signs and symptoms of conjunctivitis.

   a.

   b.

   c.

   d.

41. What causes conjunctivitis in the first 24 hours of life?

____

42. What infection control measures should be used when a child has conjunctivitis?

____

43. How can a parent recognize a blocked lacrimal duct in an infant?

____

44. What is the rationale for bedrest and eye patching in the treatment of hyphema?

____

____

45. A safety measure to prevent corneal abrasions and other eye injuries is _________________.

46. What assessments should the nurse making when caring for a child with a hyphema?

____

47. How should a chemical splash to the eye be irrigated?

____

Answer as either true (T) or false (F).

48. ______ A blocked lacrimal duct is usually opened surgically before 1 year of age.
49. ______ Strabismus is a normal finding up to 3 months of age.
50. ______ The child should be able to decide how long to wear the eye patch each day.
51. ______ If detected early, color blindness can be corrected.
52. ______ Intervention for the infant born with cataracts should be delayed until the infant is at least 6 months old.
53. ______ Chlamydia causes the majority of eye infections in infants.
54. ______ Untreated orbital cellulitis can result in meningitis.
55. ______ A chemical burn of the eyes should be irrigated immediately with water or saline.
56. ______ Of all sports activities, baseball and basketball are associated with the highest percentage of eye injuries.

HEARING LOSS IN CHILDREN

Match each type of hearing loss with its description.

57. ______ Central
58. ______ Conductive
59. ______ Mixed
60. ______ Sensorineural

a. Combination of conductive and sensorineural loss
b. Result of damage to the conduction system between the auditory nervous system and cerebral cortex
c. Result of damage or malformation of structures of the inner ear and/or auditory nerve
d. Sound prevented from progressing across the middle ear

61. Identify three possible causes of conductive hearing loss.

 a.

 b.

 c.

62. Name three possible causes of sensorineural hearing loss.

 a.

 b.

 c.

63. The two hearing screening tests used to identify infants with hearing deficits are ______________________ and ______________________.
64. Hearing testing in a preschool or school-age child is done by __________________.
65. List four guidelines for working with a hearing-impaired child.

    a.

    b.

    c.

    d.

Answer as either true (T) or false (F).

66. ______ The treatment for hearing loss depends on the type of loss.
67. ______ Sensorineural hearing loss is usually reversible.
68. ______ The recommended treatment for sensorineural hearing loss is a hearing aid.
69. ______ Deaf infants babble later than hearing infants.
70. ______ A child with recurrent otitis media with effusion lasting longer than 3 months should be evaluated for conductive hearing loss.

LANGUAGE DISORDERS

Match each language milestone with the age at which it normally occurs.

71. ______ Speaks first words
72. ______ Speaks first sentences
73. ______ Has a vocabulary of at least 50 words

a. 12 months
b. 18 months
c. 2 years

74. Expressive language disorders affect which three areas of speech?

    a.

    b.

    c.

75. Identify three guidelines for parents on being effective role models in the area of speech.

    a.

    b.

    c.

Answer as either true (T) or false (F).

76. ______ Girls have more rapid language development than boys until 3 years of age.
77. ______ There is strong evidence linking early talking with greater intelligence.
78. ______ Children with a receptive language disorder are unable to understand the spoken word.
79. ______ Parents should begin reading to their child during infancy.

SUGGESTED LEARNING ACTIVITIES

1. Arrange an observational experience with a pediatric ophthalmologist, audiologist, or speech therapist. What techniques do these professionals use to assess infants and children for sensory disorders? What are the most common disorders that they encounter in their practice?

STUDENT LEARNING APPLICATION

Enhance your learning by discussing your answers with other students.

Twelve-year-old Jamie is developmentally delayed and blind. He was admitted to the hospital during the night for vomiting and abdominal pain. At the moment, he is moaning in pain. His IV line is infiltrated, and he needs to have another IV line placed. Jamie's parents are not present.

1. What do you think Jamie's fears might be at this time? How would you address each of these fears?

2. Write an explanation to Jamie for the experience of placing an IV line. What factors are you considering as you do this? What makes writing this explanation for Jamie difficult?

3. You learn that Jamie is going to the operating room for an appendectomy. How might preparing him for surgery differ from preparing a sighted child?

REVIEW QUESTIONS

Choose the best answer.

1. At what age does a child normally develop 20/20 vision?
   a. 4 years
   b. 5 years
   c. 7 years
   d. 8 years

2. Which of the following is a normal finding when assessing a 5-year-old's vision?
   a. Hyperopia
   b. Myopia
   c. Astigmatism
   d. Strabismus

3. Which of the following is not a clinical sign of glaucoma?
   a. Blepharospasm
   b. Increased tearing
   c. Headache
   d. Light sensitivity

4. When several children in the same class have conjunctivitis, which type of eye drops should be used to treat it?
   a. Steroid
   b. Antibiotic
   c. Mydriatic
   d. Myopic

5. The correct technique for lacrimal massage is to:
   a. massage from the inner eye down to the nasal bone.
   b. press gently in a circular motion.
   c. massage from the lacrimal duct upward.
   d. press inward on the lacrimal duct.

6. The immediate intervention for a chemical burn to the eyes is to:
   a. flush with water and saline.
   b. apply antibiotic ointment.
   c. patch the affected eye.
   d. instill mydriatic drops to constrict the pupil.

7. During a hearing assessment, a child failed to hear higher than 65 decibels. This hearing loss is considered to be:
   a. mild.
   b. moderate.
   c. severe.
   d. profound.

8. A cause of conductive hearing loss is:
   a. ototoxic medications.
   b. exposure to loud noises.
   c. otitis media.
   d. brain tumors.

9. Which of the following is an appropriate intervention to use when working with a child who has a hearing impairment?
   a. Maintain a soft background noise.
   b. Talk extremely slowly.
   c. Speak louder than usual.
   d. Use visual aids to assist your communication.

10. A delay in language development is suggested by:
    a. babbling at 6 months.
    b. saying 3 words at 18 months.
    c. having a vocabulary of 50 words at 2½ years.
    d. beginning to use 2-word sentences at 3 years.

11. Which of the following is not an expressive language disorder?
    a. Difficulty with fluency
    b. Difficulty with articulation
    c. Problem with pitch and articulation
    d. Problem with comprehending the spoken word

Answer Key

CHAPTER 1: FOUNDATIONS OF MATERNITY AND PEDIATRIC NURSING

MATCHING KEY TERMS

1. b
2. e
3. c
4. a
5. d
6. g
7. f
8. h

HISTORICAL PERSPECTIVES

Maternity Nursing

1. Childbirth is usually a normal, healthy event in the life of a family; childbirth affects the entire family, and family restructuring is required; families are capable of making decisions about care, provided they are given adequate information and professional support.
2. a. Traditional hospital setting—labor, birth, recover, and postpartum care occur in separate rooms; delay of parent-infant contact.
   b. LDR rooms—labor, birth, and immediate recovery occur in a single room, with transfer to a postpartum room for continuing care; emphasis on keeping parents and infant together; liberal visiting.
   c. LDRP rooms—same as LDR rooms except that mother and infant remain in the same room where birth occurred.
   d. Birth centers—free-standing centers that provide antepartum, intrapartum, postpartum, and newborn care to low-risk mothers and babies; typically staffed by certified nurse-midwives.
   e. Home births—birth occurs in a familiar setting with support people the mother wants; fewer nurse-midwives now attend these births because of malpractice insurance problems.

Pediatric Nursing

1. F
2. T
3. T
4. T

CURRENT TRENDS IN MATERNITY AND PEDIATRIC CARE

1. For maternity care, prospective payment plans have resulted in shortened length of stay after delivery. This created problems for some women and infants who required readmission following early discharge. Legislation now mandates length of stay following vaginal birth as 48 hours; following cesarean birth, length of stay is 4 days. Concerns about managed care in pediatrics include delay in treatment authorization and pediatric referrals and limited coordination with community health, education, and social services.
2. F
3. T
4. F
5. T
6. T
7. F

ETHICAL PERSPECTIVES ON MATERNAL AND CHILD NURSING

1. beneficence; nonmaleficence; autonomy; justice

LEGAL ISSUES

1. duty; breach of duty; damage; proximate cause
2. client's competence to consent; full disclosure of information; client's understanding of information; client's voluntary consent

REVIEW QUESTIONS

1. b
2. c
3. a
4. c

CHAPTER 2: THE NURSE'S ROLE IN MATERNITY AND PEDIATRIC NURSING

THE ROLE OF THE PROFESSIONAL NURSE

1. T
2. T
3. F
4. care provider; teacher; collaborator; researcher; advocate; manager
5. developmental level, language, culture, previous experiences, physical environment, organization and skill of the teacher
6. a. Certified nurse-midwives—registered nurses complete a course of study and clinical experience and are certified by the American College of Nurse-Midwives; they are qualified to provide complete care during pregnancy, childbirth, and the postpartum period in uncomplicated pregnancies.
   b. Nurse practitioners—advance practice nurses who provide care to specific groups of clients in a variety of settings. They may work collaboratively with a physician or work independently, depending on the individual state's board of nursing mandates.
   c. Clinical nurse specialists—registered nurses with graduate education to be experts in the care of childbearing families or pediatric clients. Their functions may include clinical leader, role model, client advocate, and change agent.

IMPLICATIONS OF CHANGING ROLES FOR NURSES

1. Therapeutic communication is purposeful, goal directed, and focused. It requires conscious effort and practice.
2. what is being said; nonverbal clues
3. a. Block—failure to acknowledge child's feelings and providing false reassurance
   Possible response—"You will feel a prick when I give you the needle. You can cry or yell if you want. I do need you to keep your leg still. I will put a Band-Aid on it when I am done."
   b. Block—failure to acknowledge comments or feelings
   Possible response—"This pregnancy has not gone as you expected. Tell me how being on bedrest has been difficult for you."
4. To help nurses make the best clinical judgments by identifying and overcoming habits that interfere with decision-making
5. Recognize assumptions; examine personal biases; analyze the need for closure; manage data; evaluate other factors (emotions, environment) that can impede critical thinking
6. F
7. F
8. T

THE NURSING PROCESS IN MATERNITY AND PEDIATRIC CARE

1. Database assessment involves gathering data about all aspects of a client's health to identify strengths and problems. Focus assessment involves gathering additional information relevant to an actual problem or one that the client/family is at risk for acquiring.
2. Each outcome criterion is an example of how a nurse might word it; your answer may be different and still be accurate.
   a. Mrs. Lynch will ambulate in her room by 24 hours after surgery. She will ambulate the length of the hallway and back by 48 hours after surgery.
   b. By her next prenatal visit, Jane Starr will bring a diet journal for 1 day that demonstrates the correct number of servings from every food group.
   c. Andrew Franklin will be free of signs of infection, as evidenced by an afebrile state, no redness of integument, and negative cultures until his next examination in 2 weeks.

REVIEW QUESTIONS

1. b
2. c
3. b
4. a

CHAPTER 3: THE CHILD-BEARING AND CHILD-REARING FAMILY

MATCHING KEY TERMS

1. c
2. g
3. a
4. f
5. b
6. e
7. d

THE FAMILY AND NURSING CARE

1. a. stress, child care
   b. poverty, overwhelming child-rearing responsibilities
   c. differences in parenting styles, values, discipline
   d. little time to prepare for birth, little support afterward
   e. generational conflicts
   f. conflicts with community values
   g. poverty, inability to seek higher education, high infant mortality rate
   h. child neglect, risk-taking behaviors, possible criminal activity
   i. financial hardship, marital stress, sibling resentment
2. a. I
   b. I
   c. E
   d. I
   e. I
   f. E
   g. I
   h. E

CULTURAL INFLUENCES ON MATERNITY AND PEDIATRIC NURSING

1. Southeast Asians
   a. soft voice
   b. no prolonged eye contact
2. Hispanics—polite with preliminary small talk
3. African-Americans—may use idioms, colloquialisms, or speech patterns that are unfamiliar to health professionals
4. Middle-Easterners
   a. Interpreters should be from an acceptable region; information is typically only shared with friends and family.
   b. A male's opinion or permission is often required.

PARENTING

1. F
2. T
3. T
4. T
5. Distract the child with another object
6. Explains why a behavior is not permitted
7. Placing child in nonstimulating environment for about 1 minute per year of age
8. Helps children see the direct result of their misbehavior
9. A technique that rewards positive behavior and ignores negative behavior
10. A controversial form of discipline usually involving spanking

REVIEW QUESTIONS

1. b
2. b
3. a
4. d
5. c
6. a
7. a
8. c

CHAPTER 4: HEALTH PROMOTION FOR THE DEVELOPING CHILD

MATCHING KEY TERMS

1. d
2. g
3. b
4. h
5. c
6. f
7. i
8. a
9. j
10. e

TYPES OF PLAY

11. c
12. b
13. a

OVERVIEW OF GROWTH AND DEVELOPMENT

14. developmentally appropriate to meet the child's needs
15. growth
16. maturation
17. development
18. learning
19. delays
20. a. school-age; b. toddlerhood; c. adolescence; d. infancy; e. preschool age; f. newborn
21. a. weight; b. height; c. head circumference
22. 6 months; 1 year
23. head circumference
24. 20; 32

PRINCIPLES OF GROWTH AND DEVELOPMENT

25. d
26. a
27. c
28. b
29. sick or stressed
30. a block of time during which children are able to master developmental tasks
31. T
32. F
33. T
34. F
35. F

THEORIES OF GROWTH AND DEVELOPMENT

36. c
37. b
38. a
39. d
40. oral
41. phallic
42. genital
43. anal
44. latency
45. mistrust
46. autonomy
47. initiative
48. inferiority
49. identity
50. b
51. a
52. c

THEORIES OF LANGUAGE DEVELOPMENT

53. cognitive
54. understand the spoken word
55. produce meaningful vocalizations

ASSESSMENT OF GROWTH

56. Growth is an excellent assessment of physical well-being.
57. nutritional status

ASSESSMENT OF DEVELOPMENT

58. a. observation; b. interview; c. physical examination; d. standardized assessment tools
59. a. Parents' Evaluation of Developmental Status (PEDS); b. Ages and Stages Questionnaire
60. a. personal-social; b. fine motor; c. language; d. gross motor
61. T
62. F
63. T
64. F
65. F

THE NURSE'S ROLE IN PROMOTING OPTIMAL GROWTH AND DEVELOPMENT

66. basic information for parents regarding normal growth and development as the child approaches different age levels
67. predictable times when health care professionals can offer supportive help to families to diminish or prevent problems

THE DEVELOPMENTAL ASSESSMENT

68. F
69. T
70. T
71. the work of children
72. functional or sensorimotor play
73. represent an issue or a concern to be addressed
74. rules
75. e
76. c
77. b
78. d
79. a

HEALTH PROMOTION

80. T
81. F
82. F
83. T
84. T
85. T
86. F
87. gluteal
88. MMR, varicella
89. epinephrine 1:1000
90. c
91. e
92. a
93. b
94. d
95. These children require sufficient calories to support rapid growth.
96. 30
97. to avoid osteoporosis later in life
98. They do not need the added stress of unfamiliar foods.
99. a. 24-hour recall; b. Food Frequency Questionnaire; c. food diary
100. unintentional injuries

REVIEW QUESTIONS

1. a
2. c
3. d
4. d
5. c
6. b
7. b
8. d
9. d
10. c
11. a
12. d

CHAPTER 5: HEALTH PROMOTION FOR THE INFANT

MATCHING KEY TERMS

1. e
2. i
3. a
4. b
5. h
6. f
7. k
8. d
9. j
10. g
11. c

GROWTH AND DEVELOPMENT OF THE INFANT

12. 8–9 months
13. 4–5 months
14. 4–5 months
15. 3 months
16. 6–7 months
17. 10–12 months
18. 6–7 months
19. 6–7 months
20. 1–2 months
21. 4–5 months
22. 8–9 months
23. 10–12 months
24. 1–2 months
25. 6–7 months
26. tiny, collapsible air passages; immature immune systems
27. decreases; increases
28. breast milk
29. 6–9 months
30. fluid and electrolyte imbalances
31. d
32. c
33. a
34. b
35. F
36. F
37. T
38. T
39. T
40. F
41. T
42. When infants' needs are ignored or not met adequately and consistently, they perceive the environment as unsafe and develop a sense of mistrust.
43. By many mutually satisfying interactions between parent and infant. Parents adapt to their child through nurturing and by meeting the infant's needs.
44. By this age, infants have formed strong emotional attachments to their caregivers and are cognitively able to distinguish them from strangers.

HEALTH PROMOTION FOR THE INFANT AND FAMILY

45. 3
46. immunologic; digestibility
47. illegal and certain prescription and over-the-counter drugs; tuberculosis; HIV infection
48. drinking from a cup
49. vitamin C
50. F
51. F
52. F
53. T
54. T
55. holding them, speaking or humming softly to them, stroking, massaging, centering or swaddling them
56. taking them on car rides, placing them in swings, walking with them, leaving them alone to "settle down" for no longer than 15 minutes
57. rear
58. 120 degrees
59. crawl
60. hot dogs, hard candy, grapes, peanuts, raisins, chewing gum
61. back

REVIEW QUESTIONS

1. c
2. b
3. b
4. c
5. d
6. c
7. a
8. a
9. b
10. a

CHAPTER 6: HEALTH PROMOTION DURING EARLY CHILDHOOD

MATCHING KEY TERMS

1. i
2. d
3. f
4. n
5. k
6. b
7. m
8. e
9. h
10. a
11. j
12. l
13. g
14. c

GROWTH AND DEVELOPMENT DURING EARLY CHILDHOOD

15. 5
16. 2–3
17. 3
18. T
19. P
20. P
21. T
22. T
23. T
24. P
25. P
26. P
27. P
28. T
29. P
30. T
31. a
32. d
33. e
34. b
35. c

HEALTH PROMOTION FOR THE TODDLER OR PRESCHOOLER AND FAMILY

36. F
37. T
38. F
39. F
40. F
41. between about 12 and 30 months
42. They provide a sense of security and decrease the anxiety associated with increasing independence.
43. Nightmares awaken the child; night terrors do not wake the child and cannot be recalled.
44. discipline; limit setting
45. time out; time in; diversion; restricted choice
46. Never leave a child unattended in the tub; never leave buckets of water unattended; keep toilet lids closed.
47. They raise children to a level that accommodates the car's seat belt system
48. Stop. Cover face with hands. Drop to the ground. Roll until the flames are out.
49. Keep guns unloaded with trigger guards in place and locked in metal vaults that are inaccessible to all children.
50. Teach children what is appropriate touch; teach them to tell another adult, even if they are threatened; teach them to keep telling adults until the behavior stops.
51. They will be less negative and more eager to please parents.
52. Limit stress, anticipate fatigue, prevent hunger, offer choices, be consistent, avoid overprotection and excessive strictness.
53. Prior to delivery, enroll the older child in sibling preparation classes. After delivery, encourage visitors and family to pay attention to the older sibling; plan uninterrupted private time with the older child daily. Set firm limits if the older child tries to harm the baby. Praise the child for cooperative, affectionate behavior.
54. Focus on the ideas the child is expressing; do not complete words or sentences; avoid drawing attention to, criticizing, and correcting the child's speech.

REVIEW QUESTIONS

1. a
2. c
3. b
4. d
5. a
6. d
7. b
8. c
9. c
10. c
11. a
12. b

CHAPTER 7: HEALTH PROMOTION FOR THE SCHOOL-AGE CHILD

MATCHING KEY TERMS

1. e
2. b
3. a
4. d
5. c

GROWTH AND DEVELOPMENT FOR THE SCHOOL-AGE CHILD

6. F
7. T
8. F
9. F
10. F
11. Active play increases coordination, refines motor skills, serves as a foundation for physical fitness as an adult, improves cardiovascular fitness, increases strength and flexibility, and aids in the prevention of obesity.
12. Children have higher metabolic rates and limited ability to sweat.
13. actions
14. weight; volume
15. Cognitively, they are able to arrange things in logical order and are able to recall similarities and differences.
16. Children learn that friendship is more than just being together. They begin to share problems and give each other emotional support. They develop a sense of loyalty.
17. Their eustachian tubes have grown.
18. by learning to do new things and by learning to do them well
19. As children learn to do things well, they become more confident and feel good about themselves.
20. Rules provide predictability and security. By conforming to external rules, children learn self-discipline and internalize values.
21. a. Child obeys to avoid punishment; b. Child obeys to avoid disapproval or to please others; c. Child obeys out of respect for authority.
22. a. expectations; b. rewards, punishments

HEALTH PROMOTION FOR THE SCHOOL-AGE CHILD AND FAMILY

23. a. 6–11, b. 3–5, c. 2–4, d. 2–3, e. 2–3
24. 12; 9–10
25. by making children accountable for their actions and by allowing them to experience the consequences of their actions
26. Positively reinforce for effort, encourage self-discipline and good study habits, ensure adequate sleep, communicate with and support teachers; provide a quiet well-lighted study area.
27. by knowing laws related to self-care children, by teaching specific strategies for staying safe at home alone, and by working to develop expanded after-school programs in their communities.
28. They can set consistent times for meals and snacks; only offer nutritious food options; role model good nutrition and exercise habits; plan physical activities for their child; limit TV and computer game time; avoid fast food restaurants; not use food as a reward.

REVIEW QUESTIONS

1. b
2. d
3. a
4. d
5. b
6. b
7. b
8. c
9. d
10. c

CHAPTER 8: HEALTH PROMOTION FOR THE ADOLESCENT

MATCHING KEY TERMS

1. e
2. d
3. i
4. b
5. f
6. j
7. c
8. a
9. h
10. k
11. g

ADOLESCENT GROWTH AND DEVELOPMENT

12. menstruation
13. peak height velocity (PHV)
14. breast buds (thelarche)
15. gynecomastia

16. Tanner staging or SMR
17. testicular enlargement
18. estrogen; testosterone
19. assure confidentiality, be patient, be flexible, remain nonjudgmental, assume nothing, use open-ended questions, encourage problem solving and analysis, be an advocate, do not side against parents
20. period granted to teens as they are experimenting with roles and not yet ready to make permanent commitments
21. It provides safety and validation as teens emotionally move away from the family and experiment with new roles.
22. early
23. early
24. late
25. middle
26. middle
27. late
28. early, middle
29. middle
30. T
31. F
32. T
33. F
34. T
35. T
36. T
37. 46%
38. poor impulse control, poor school performance, poor mental health, family disorganization, conduct disorders, substance abuse, homosexuality, stress
39. sexual abstinence
40. T
41. F
42. T
43. T
44. F
45. T

REVIEW QUESTIONS

1. d
2. d
3. c
4. c
5. b
6. d
7. c
8. b

CHAPTER 9: HEREDITARY AND ENVIRONMENTAL INFLUENCES ON CHILDBEARING

MATCHING KEY TERMS

1. c
2. e
3. i
4. d
5. a
6. b
7. h
8. j
9. g
10. f

HEREDITARY INFLUENCES

1. DNA is the basic building block of genes. Specific segments of DNA form a gene and many genes form a chromosome.
2. an international effort to map all genes contained in the 46 human chromosomes
3. a. Genetic information about an individual has implications for other family members. Should this information be shared with family, health insurance providers, employers?
   b. A person with a genetic problem may feel inferior or guilty about passing it on to children.
   c. A person with a genetic abnormality who is currently asymptomatic may experience long-term anxiety waiting for the disease to occur.
   d. A person with a genetic abnormality may be denied insurance coverage or be forced to pay exorbitant premiums.
4. a. Child must receive a copy of autosomal recessive gene from both parents; no sex difference.
   b. Child may receive a copy of autosomal dominant gene from either parent; no sex difference.
   c. Because females are carriers, child receives abnormal gene from mother. Males are affected because they do not have a compensating normal X chromosome. Affected fathers will pass on abnormal genes to their daughters who become carriers but not to their sons.
5. T
6. F
7. F
8. T
9. F

MULTIFACTORIAL DISORDERS

1. They are present and detectable at birth. They tend to be single, isolated defects.
2. number of affected close relatives, severity of disorder in other family members, sex of affected person, geographical location, season of year

ENVIRONMENTAL INFLUENCES

1. at least 3 months before a pregnancy
2. the woman's need for the therapeutic effects of the drug and how the drug will affect the fetus

3. protected by a lead apron
4. Maternal hyperthermia is a teratogen.

GENETIC COUNSELING

1. family
2. nondirective

NURSING CARE OF FAMILIES CONCERNED ABOUT BIRTH DEFECTS

1. a. Identify women who may benefit from genetic counseling.
   b. Identify women who may benefit from genetic counseling; provide support if they receive abnormal results; support their decisions; teach.
   c. Evaluate family's perception of the problem; explain diagnostic tests and results; make referrals.
   d. Support family; make referrals.

REVIEW QUESTIONS

1. b
2. d
3. b
4. c
5. b

CHAPTER 10: MANAGEMENT OF FERTILITY AND INFERTILITY

MATCHING KEY TERMS

1. d
2. c
3. f
4. e
5. g
6. a
7. b

KEY CONCEPTS

1. The typical failure rate reflects the way real people use a contraceptive and includes mistakes or inconsistencies of use. It is most meaningful when counseling clients.
2. Be sensitive to their feelings; accept them; maintain confidentiality.
3. Pregnancy is rare after age 50 or if menstruation has ceased for at least 2 years.
4. Sperm may be in the ductal system, distal to the ligation of the vas deferens, and able to impregnate a woman.
5. Menstrual irregularities, weight gain, headaches, depression, hair loss and decreased bone density.
6. They prevent secretion of follicle-stimulating and luteinizing hormones, thus preventing ovulation; they also make the cervical mucus too thick for sperm to penetrate and the endometrium less hospitable for implantation.
7. They thicken cervical mucus to inhibit sperm penetration and make the endometrium less hospitable.

8. a. Have a backup method readily available for side effects with discontinuance or missed doses.
   b. Take at the same time of day to maintain constant blood levels, maximize effectiveness, and reduce breakthrough bleeding.
   c. Stop pills and use a backup if pregnancy is suspected; get a sensitive pregnancy test.
   d. Low-estrogen oral contraceptives do not interfere with nutritional status
   e. Combination pills reduce milk production, and small amounts are transferred to milk; use after lactation is well established.
   f. Interactions may alter the effectiveness of each medication; inform health care provider of all medications.
9. Pelvic examination, Pap smear, breast examination, blood pressure check. Evaluate for side effects or adverse reactions.
10. High doses of oral contraceptive within 72 hours of unprotected intercourse, with a second dose 12 hours later; high doses of progestin-only contraceptives; insertion of the copper T 380A intrauterine device within 5 days; mefepristone
11. Pelvic infections associated with the IUD are usually due to STDs. If the woman and her partner are mutually monogamous, the risk of STDs is low, thus reducing the risk of IUD-associated infection.
12. Check for the tail weekly for 4 weeks, then monthly after the menstrual period and if you have signs of expulsion (cramping or unexpected bleeding). See your health care provider if strings are longer or shorter than before. Report signs of infection or pregnancy. Return yearly for a Pap smear and check for anemia.
13. avoidance of systemic hormones, protection from sexually transmissible diseases
14. The spermicide adds a chemical barrier to the mechanical barrier of the condom and lubricates the condom to reduce tearing.
15. Avoid douching for at least 6 hours to avoid washing the protection away.
16. Natural membrane condoms do not protect from sexually transmitted diseases, including HIV.
17. It is less effective (typical failure rate of 21%), and many women do not like its appearance.
18. She should have it checked yearly, after a weight gain or loss of more than 10 pounds, or after any pregnancy or abortion.
19. Any error in predicting ovulation or safe times for intercourse may result in pregnancy.
20. Complete this table as you read the text in this chapter.
21. abnormal hormone stimulation, acute or chronic illness, infections of the genital tract, anatomic abnormalities, exposure to toxins, therapeutic treatments for cancer or other illness, excessive alcohol intake, illicit drug ingestion, elevated scrotal temperature, antibodies produced by the man or the woman that alter function
22. disorders of the central or autonomic nervous system, spinal cord disorders, peripheral vascular disease, drugs
23. diabetes, neurologic disorders, surgery that affects sympathetic nerve function, drugs (therapeutic or illicit), some spinal cord injuries, anatomical abnormalities, excessive alcohol intake, psychological factors
24. obstruction, inflammation, or infection in the genital tract
25. cranial tumors, stress, obesity, anorexia, systemic disease, ovarian or endocrine abnormalities
26. cancer chemotherapy, excessive alcohol intake, cigarette smoking
27. infections, endometriosis or surgery that causes adhesions, congenital anomalies
28. polyps or cervical damage from surgical procedures, hormonal imbalances
29. abnormalities in the fetus or placenta; maternal factors.
30. Refer to Table 10-4 in your textbook to complete this exercise.
31. The risk for multifetal pregnancies increases because multiple ova may be released and thus fertilized. Ovarian hyperstimulation syndrome may cause exudation of fluid into the woman's peritoneal and pleural cavities.

32. low sperm count, genetic defect carried by the male, woman's desire for a biological child without having a male partner
33. A personal and family health history is taken; questions are asked about social habits and personality. Other tests include a physical examination and laboratory studies, including those for genetic defects. Donor sperm is frozen and held for 6 months before use.
34. Refer to text, "Advanced Reproductive Techniques," to complete this exercise.

REVIEW QUESTIONS

1. b
2. d
3. a
4. c
5. b
6. a
7. c
8. d
9. b
10. b
11. d
12. a
13. c
14. b

CHAPTER 11: REPRODUCTIVE ANATOMY AND PHYSIOLOGY

MATCHING KEY TERMS

1. a
2. b
3. e
4. c
5. d
6. d
7. c
8. a
9. a
10. h
11. e
12. i
13. f
14. b
15. g

KEY CONCEPTS

1. An unknown area of the brain prevents the young child's hypothalamus from responding to estrogen and testosterone secretion by the ovaries or testes. Without gonadotropin-releasing hormone from the hypothalamus, further estrogen or testosterone secretion ceases.
2. Puberty; 8–13; 9½–13½

3. breast development, growth of the testes and penis
4. 2 to 2½ years
5. Boys begin puberty slightly later than girls. Also, testosterone's effect on closing the epiphyses of the long bones is not as strong as estrogen's. Thus boys start puberty later (and taller) and continue growing in height longer than girls.
6. a. Longitudinal fibers
   importance—expel the fetus at birth
   location—fundus
   b. Interlacing fibers (Fig. 11-4)
   importance—compress blood vessels to prevent hemorrhage after birth
   location—middle layer
   c. Circular fibers
   importance—prevent reflux of menstrual blood from the uterus into the tubes, control entry of the embryo into the uterus for implantation, and retain the fetus until proper time for birth
   Location—constriction around fallopian tubes and internal cervical os
7. fallopian tubes
8. a. Female ova are produced only during prenatal life.
   b. Male spermatozoa are produced continuously after puberty.
9. a. Estrogen and progesterone fall just before menstruation, causing increasing secretion of FSH and LH by the anterior pituitary; follicles mature with increasing estrogen secretion until one follicle outgrows all others.
   b. Marked increase in LH secretion, a slight fall in follicular estrogen, and a rise in follicular progesterone secretion; final maturation and release of the most mature ovum.
   c. The corpus luteum secretes progesterone to prepare the endometrium for a fertilized ovum; corpus luteum will persist and continue to secrete progesterone if it receives a signal (human chorionic gonadotropin) from a fertilized ovum. Otherwise, progesterone secretion falls and menstruation occurs.
10. a. Cells of the basal layer of the endometrium multiply; endometrial glands form; spiral arteries and endometrial veins elongate.
    b. Endometrium continues to thicken; substances are secreted to nourish an embryo if one implants.
    c. Vasospasm occurs if the corpus luteum stops producing estrogen and progesterone, causing the endometrium to become necrotic; the necrotic layer separates from the basal layer to produce the menstrual flow.
11. Tight underwear keeps the testes near the body, possibly overheating them and preventing normal sperm formation.

REVIEW QUESTIONS

1. b
2. d
3. b
4. b
5. d
6. a
7. c
8. d
9. d
10. a
11. b
12. c

CHAPTER 12: CONCEPTION AND PRENATAL DEVELOPMENT

MATCHING KEY TERMS

1. c
2. a
3. g
4. b
5. d
6. i
7. h
8. j
9. f
10. e

KEY CONCEPTS

1.

	Mitosis	Meiosis
Type of cell involved	Somatic cell	Gamete (reproductive cell)
Number and type of chromosomes in each resulting cell	46 Chromosomes (44 autosomes and 2 sex [X and Y or 2 X] chromosomes)	23 Chromosomes (22 autosomes and an X plus either a Y [sperm] or an X [female])

2. See Table 12-1 of your textbook, to complete this exercise.
3. The zona pellucida prevents other sperm from entering, and the ovum completes its second meiotic division.
4. Good blood supply, thick uterine lining, and muscles to limit postbirth blood loss
5. See Table 12-3 of your textbook, to complete this exercise.
6. a. 4 weeks
   b. 8 weeks
   c. 10 weeks
   d. 10 weeks
   e. 26 weeks
   f. 6 weeks
   g. 12 weeks
   h. 16–24 weeks
   i. 24 weeks
7. a. creamy skin covering to lubricate and protect fetal skin from amniotic fluid
   b. fine, downy hair that helps vernix adhere to the skin
   c. heat-producing fat found in back of the neck, behind sternum, and around kidneys
   d. surface-active lipid substance that helps alveoli remain slightly open between breaths to ease the work of breathing
8. Fertilization age is calculated in weeks from the actual time of conception. Gestational age is calculated from the first day of the woman's last menstrual period. Gestational age is about 2 weeks longer than fertilization age.
9. a. High fetal hemoglobin and hematocrit give the fetus more oxygen-carrying capacity; fetal hemoglobin also can carry 20% to 50% more oxygen than adult hemoglobin.
   b. Fetal carbon dioxide quickly diffuses into the mother's blood, causing her blood to become more acidic and fetal blood to become more alkaline; this allows fetal blood to combine with oxygen more readily.

10. a. Provides the newborn with temporary passive immunity to diseases to which the mother is immune.
    b. Maternal blood-type antibodies may cross the placenta and destroy incompatible fetal erythrocytes.
11. a. Causes persistence of the corpus luteum to maintain estrogen and progesterone secretion during early pregnancy and causes fetal testes to secrete testosterone to stimulate development of normal male reproductive structures
    b. Promotes normal growth and nutrition of the fetus, stimulates maternal breast development, and makes more glucose available to fetus by reducing maternal insulin sensitivity and glucose utilization
    c. Causes uterine and breast enlargement, growth of the breasts' ductal system, and enlargement of fetal external genitalia
    d. Changes endometrium into decidua to nourish conceptus before placenta is established, reduces uterine contractions, and stimulates breast growth and development of the breast alveoli and ductal system
12. Cushions fetus from impacts; provides stable temperature; promotes normal fetal growth and development (promotes symmetrical development, preventing membrane adherence, and allows fetal movement)
13. a. Carries oxygenated blood and nutrients from the placenta to the fetus.
    b. Carries deoxygenated blood and waste products from the fetus to the placenta
    c. Protects the cord vessels from stretching or pressure that would interrupt flow
14. a. As infant breathes, resistance to blood flow to lungs falls and the foramen ovale closes; tissue proliferation causes it to fill in the septum between the right and left atria.
    b. Rising arterial oxygen levels cause constriction; becomes a ligament.
    c. Cessation of umbilical cord blood flow with birth causes it to become nonfunctional; becomes a ligament.
15.

	Monozygotic	**Dizygotic**
Number of ova and sperm involved	1 Ovum and 1 sperm	2 Ova and 2 sperm
Genetic component	Identical genes	Like any other siblings
Sex	Same sex	May be same or different sex
Hereditary tendency	No hereditary influence known	Hereditary (and ethnic) tendency often found
Number of amnion(s) and chorion(s)	Varies according to time when inner cell mass divides in two, but most often 2 amnions and 1 chorion	Always has 1 amnion and 2 chorions

REVIEW QUESTIONS

1. c
2. a
3. c
4. b
5. d

CHAPTER 13: PHYSIOLOGIC ADAPTATION TO PREGNANCY

MATCHING KEY TERMS

1. f
2. b
3. c
4. a
5. e
6. d

KEY CONCEPTS

1. a. 12 weeks
   b. 16 weeks
   c. 20 weeks
   d. 36 weeks
2. a. bluish color that often extends to the vagina and labia; cause is hyperemia
   b. cervical, uterine, and vaginal softening with increased vascularity and softening of the connective tissue
   c. plug caused by increased secretion of mucus from cervical glands that blocks ascent of bacteria from the vagina
   d. mixture of cervical mucus and a small amount of blood; disruption of mucous plug and small capillaries of cervix
3. a. bluish color (as in Chadwick's sign), thickening of vaginal mucosa, prominence of rugae, heightened sexual interest
   b. greater pliability and distensibility of vagina
   c. increased acidic vaginal discharge that retards growth of bacteria, but favors growth of *Candida albicans* (yeast)
4. Pregnancy cannot be maintained without progesterone.
5. corpus luteum; placenta
6. The high levels of estrogen and progesterone inhibit FSH and LH.
7. darkening of the areolae, increased nipple and areolae size, areolae become more erect, Montgomery's tubercles become prominent
8. Changes in heart sounds begin between 12 and 20 weeks and end 2 to 4 weeks after birth. They may include splitting of the first heart sound and a systolic murmur.
9. See "Cardiovascular System" in your text to complete this chart. See also Appendix A.
10. Lying in the supine position places the heavy uterus over the aorta and inferior vena cava, which temporarily occludes these vessels. Signs and symptoms include faintness, lightheadedness, dizziness, agitation, and sometimes brief unconsciousness. This position can reduce placental blood flow. Prevention/treatment is to position woman on her side or with a pillow under one hip.
11. Increased fibrinogen levels offer protection from excess blood loss but also predispose the woman to thrombus formation.
12. Vasocongestion from estrogen's effects causes increased vascularity and edema, leading to nasal stuffiness, nosebleeds, and voice changes. It may also result in ear fullness or earaches.
13. The growing uterus eventually lifts the diaphragm and reduces lung expansion. Because the respiratory center becomes more sensitive to carbon dioxide, the minute volume increases and the partial pressure of carbon dioxide falls.
14. Hypotonia prolongs emptying time and allows bile to become thicker.
15. Although parathyroid hormone usually acts to increase absorption of calcium from the intestine, reduce renal losses, and mobilize bone, estrogen and calcitonin interfere with its effects on bone mobilization during pregnancy.

16. The fetus draws on maternal glucose and amino acids, which reduces the mother's glucose levels and her ability to synthesize glucose. During the first trimester, the lower maternal blood glucose causes the pancreas to secrete less insulin. During the second trimester, hormones (human placental lactogen, prolactin, progesterone, and cortisol) reduce the maternal tissue sensitivity to insulin. Thus the mother's blood glucose levels rise to make more available for the fetus. The woman normally responds by increasing insulin production.
17. Edema of the legs and feet is not uncommon. Edema above the waist (face and fingers) may be an indication of pregnancy-induced hypertension and should be reported.
18. Presumptive: some signs are amenorrhea, nausea, vomiting, fatigue, frequency, breast and skin changes. Probable: some signs are abdominal enlargement, cervical softening, ballottement, Braxton-Hicks, pregnancy test. Positive: Fetal heart sounds, fetal movements felt by examiner, visualization of fetus. The difference among the indications is that presumptive indicators are the least reliable because they are often caused by other conditions; probable indicators are stronger evidence but still may have other causes; positive indicators are those caused only by pregnancy.
19. Instructions not followed, too early, urine too dilute, ectopic pregnancy
20. a. 10 weeks, b. 18–20 weeks
21. a. November 11, b. May 9
22. Later in the pregnancy risk factors may appear that were not apparent at previous assessments.
23. Protein, glucose, ketones
24. a. Uterine size is larger than expected for the length of gestation.
    b. Fetal movements are more numerous, which the woman who has had a previous pregnancy is more likely to notice.
    c. Greater weight gain occurs because of greater uterine growth, increased blood volume and amniotic fluid, and presence of two or more fetuses.
25. a. There is a 500-ml increase in blood volume over the singleton pregnancy.
    b. Cardiac workload is higher due to increased blood volume.
    c. Greater diaphragm elevation increases dyspnea.
    d. Greater compression of aorta and inferior vena cava causes earlier and more pronounced supine hypotension.
    e. Greater ureter compression increases edema and proteinuria.
    f. Pressure on bowels increases constipation.
26. See "Women Want to Know," pp. 275–276 in your textbook, to complete this exercise.
27. See pp. 278–279 in your text to complete this exercise. Practice how you would really say this teaching in real life.

CRITICAL THINKING EXERCISES

1. Spasm of the endometrial spiral arteries, which supply the placenta, narrows them and reduces the blood volume that would otherwise be contained within the placenta. This increases the volume in the rest of the mother's circulation.

CASE STUDY

1. Gravida 5, para 3, abortions. T=2; P=1; A=1; L=4
2. January 12
3. 19 weeks
4. Katherine's fundal height at the umbilicus is expected at 20 weeks and her gestation is 19 weeks by dates. It is possible that her pregnancy is more advanced than dates would indicate, she may have hydramnios, or she could be carrying twins again.

5. The demands of her children are a probable cause for the delay in seeking prenatal care. Also, she may feel that she knows from experience and does not feel the need for earlier prenatal care. She may feel that, since pregnancy is not an illness, it does not demand special care.
6. Hemoglobin and hematocrit (H&H) or complete blood count; blood typing and Rh factor with antibody screen; rubella titer; urinalysis (or just a screen ["Dipstick"] for protein, glucose, and ketones). Other tests may be done, based on Katherine's ethnicity (such as for sickle cell trait), risk factors, and medical and obstetric history.

REVIEW QUESTIONS

1. b
2. b
3. d
4. b
5. d
6. a

CHAPTER 14: PSYCHOSOCIAL ADAPTATIONS TO PREGNANCY

MATCHING KEY TERMS

1. a
2. f
3. c
4. e
5. d
6. b

KEY CONCEPTS

1. a. Anxious to find confirmation of pregnancy, ambivalence, focus on self
   b. Physical evidence of pregnancy, focus on fetus, narcissism, introversion, body image, sexual interest
   c. Feelings of vulnerability replaced by coming to terms with the situation, fantasies or nightmares, increased dependence, desire to see the baby, dread about labor or being anxious for the pregnancy to end
2. Increase in uterine size, weight gain, breast changes, fetal movements (quickening)
3. Sexual interest and activity may be heightened or reduced. The woman may be more responsive because pelvic vasocongestion heightens sensitivity and lubricates the vaginal area. Fear of miscarriage, harming the fetus, or causing discomfort may suppress sexual desire in either partner. The woman may feel less attractive, or her partner may find her less attractive at this time.
4. a. Fetus seems vague and unreal, rather than seeming like a baby to her
   b. Perceives fetus as real and needing her protection, growing sense of fetus as a separate person
   c. Wants to see her baby on the outside and as a separate being
5. It makes the fetus seem much more like a separate being rather than a part of the woman's body.
6. Grief may be caused by feelings of giving up life as a carefree woman and loss of spontaneity to go places and do things.

7. Seeking safe passage for herself and baby; securing acceptance of herself and baby; learning to give of herself; developing attachment to the unknown child
8. Grappling with reality of pregnancy and a new child; struggling for recognition as a parent; desire to be seen as relevant to the childbearing process
9. Age—including whether they are still working and whether they believe they are "old enough" to be grandparents; other grandchildren—excitement about the first, but less enthusiasm for subsequent grandchildren; perception of their role as grandparents—a source of information and support, or are professionals the experts?
10. a. Make any changes in sleeping areas before the infant arrives; may feel displaced; prepare others for feelings of resentment and jealousy
    b. May look forward to a brother or sister and how the baby is born and grows but have little perception of how small and helpless the infant will be; need assurance of parents' love
    c. Enjoy preparing for the baby, want information about growth and changes in the fetus; enjoy time alone with parents
    d. May be embarrassed by their parents' obvious sexuality, preoccupied with their own issues, and/or look forward to the infant; involve them to the extent they are comfortable
11. a. Have difficulty putting aside her own desires for the well-being of an infant; must give of herself before developmentally prepared to do so
    b. May be poor and have late prenatal care; must enlist others to provide support that a partner would provide
    c. May grieve for the exclusive relationship with first child; concern about having enough time and energy to spread around; concern about acceptance of new infant by other child or children
12. a. Wearing proper clothing to ensure safe birth; extreme modesty, do not want male health care providers; may consult curanderas
    b. Avoid tying knots to prevent complications with umbilical cord; will not eat berries because believe it will cause birth marks
    c. Strong belief in fate so may not seek prenatal care
    d. Modesty dictates female care providers; need permission from husband for any treatment
13. a. Low-income women may not be able to pay for classes. They may enter prenatal care late, or have none, and miss opportunities even for free classes.
    b. Some want education so they can participate fully in all decisions related to childbearing.
    c. Some want to obtain skills to help them cope with the pain and demands of birth.
14. a. Dealing with discomforts common in early pregnancy, what to expect, value of prenatal care, avoiding hazards
    b. Body mechanics, working during pregnancy, childbirth choices, postbirth needs of mother and infant
15. Warm-up exercise; low-impact activities; avoid excessive heart rate elevation
16. a. Indications, options, surgical procedure, postoperative course
    b. When VBAC is possible, extra precautions, what to expect during labor, coping techniques, possibility of a repeat cesarean birth

CASE STUDY

1. Inadequate financial resources may have been the chief reason Sara delayed prenatal care, because she has limited income of her own and may be unable to depend on her parents for money. Also, she has no partner support and apparently feels isolated. Embarrassment and fear of her family's response, especially since she has five siblings, may also play a part. Since she did not know what to do, she may have simply done nothing.

2. Altered health maintenance and body image disturbance are the priority nursing diagnoses this situation suggests. Other nursing diagnoses might include altered family processes and knowledge deficit because they contribute to the priority nursing diagnoses.
3. Potential conflicts include Sara's probable late entry into prenatal care, erratic clinic visits, and noncompliance with professionals' recommendations.
4. Financial assistance, nutritional consultation and assistance, transportation, and other social services
5. Sara is more likely to be poor because she ended her education early. She is likely to have more children in her lifetime, and her children also have a greater likelihood of ending their education early and being poor. Although Sara has a higher risk for these problems, they do not have to occur.

REVIEW QUESTIONS

1. b
2. c
3. a
4. d
5. d
6. a
7. c

CHAPTER 15: NUTRITION FOR CHILDBEARING

MATCHING KEY TERMS

1. d
2. e
3. b
4. i
5. k
6. j
7. a
8. f
9. c
10. h
11. g

KEY CONCEPTS

1. Low birth weight, preterm birth, increased risk of fetal and newborn morbidity and mortality
2. Macrosomia, labor abnormalities (often resulting in cesarean birth), and meconium staining of the amniotic fluid
3. a. Gain 25 to 35 pounds.
   b. 28-40 lb
   c. 15-25 lb
   d. Gain at least 15 pounds.
4. 3.5 pounds; 1.6 kg; just under 1 pound; 0.44 kg
5. a. 4
   b. 4
   c. 9

6. 300
7. 46; 71
8. A, D, E, and K
9. legumes, nuts, dried fruits, dark green leafy vegetables, broccoli
10. Excessive amounts of one vitamin or mineral may reduce absorption of others; high doses of some (such as vitamin A) are toxic; a false sense of security may develop that causes the woman to eat a less healthy diet.
11. 8 to 10; 8 ounces each. Limit fluids low in nutrients such as carbonated drinks, coffee, tea, and high-sugar "juice" drinks.
12. a. 7
    b. 3-5 vegetables, 2-4 fruits
    c. 3
    d. 7+ ounces
    e. 3 teaspoons unsaturated fat; rest sparingly
13. Yin (cold) and yang (hot) applies to foods and conditions in many cultures, influencing what the woman eats during her pregnancy. She will balance a "hot" condition such as pregnancy by eating "cold" foods, and vice versa.
14. a. Sour foods, fruits, noodles, sweets
    b. Fish, excessively salty or spicy foods, alcohol, rice, and unfamiliar foods
    c. "Hot" foods, such as rice with fish sauce, broth, salty meats, fish, eggs, and hot drinks
    d. May be deficient in calories, calcium, iron, zinc, magnesium, vitamins B_6 and D; high in sodium
    e. Increase in dark green leafy vegetables increases calcium, iron, magnesium, folic acid; tofu or broth from vinegar-soaked pork or chicken bones increases calcium and iron; increase in meat or poultry intake increases vitamin B_6 and zinc
15. a. Pregnancy is considered "hot" and postpartum period is considered "cold," so diet is adjusted to balance.
    b. Foods include dried beans, rice, beef, pork, chicken, corn, chili peppers, tomatoes and tortillas.
    c. Diet is high in fiber and complex carbohydrates but also high in fat and calories (overweight is a problem); low in vitamins A and D, iron, and calcium.
16. Income lower than 185% of the federal poverty level; eligible throughout pregnancy and for 6 months postpartum if formula feeding or 1 year if breast feeding
17. Vitamins C and A, folic acid, calcium, iron, zinc
18. Focus only on necessary changes; ask for the teenager's input; help her make changes that still keep her diet similar to that of her peers.
19. a. Combine vegetable foods that have complementary amino acids or eat small amounts of complete protein foods (such as cheese) with vegetables
    b. Calcium-fortified soy products or supplement
    c. B_{12}-fortified foods or supplement
20. Have frequent small meals; reduce fatty foods; drink liquids between meals; eat protein snack at bedtime; eat carbohydrate food before getting out of bed in the morning
21. May begin pregnancy with a nutritional deficit if she has had several pregnancies (usually more than five), especially if they are closely spaced. Meeting nutritional and other needs of her family may take priority over her own needs.
22. She needs to eat enough to supply all the fetuses as well as meet her own needs. Supplementation with calcium, iron, and folic acid may be needed.
23. a. Obtaining substance is more important than eating well
    b. Metabolic rate increases and appetite decreases. Decreases availability of some vitamins and minerals
    c. Deficient use of protein, thiamine, folic acid, zinc; impaired metabolism; alcohol may replace food in the diet

24. a. Increases appetite, but women may not take in foods of good quality
    b. Interferes with insulin response to glucose and metabolism
    c. Appetite suppressant; tendency to drink more alcohol or caffeine-containing beverages
    d. Depresses appetite
25. a. Pregnancy could deplete her own stores; could interfere with the recovery process and establishing a milk supply; she should not take appetite suppressants.
    b. Adolescents may be deficient in many nutrients; they may lack iron and vitamin A.
    c. The woman may have inadequate B_{12}, D, or calcium.
    d. Prolonged lactation may result in removal of calcium from bones; must have adequate intake and/or supplementation.
26. a. Occasional single glass of alcoholic beverage may not be harmful; larger amounts may reduce milk-ejection reflex and be harmful to infant.
    b. Limit intake to the equivalent of two cups of coffee; excess can make the infant irritable and reduce the iron content of milk.
    c. Drink 8 to 10 glasses or more according to thirst (excluding caffeinated beverages).

CASE STUDY

1. Low hemoglobin (10.5 g/dL)
2. Anemia (hemoglobin of 10 g/dL or less) is a possibility because of Carmen's low hemoglobin at her initial visit and the close spacing of her children. Inadequate calcium intake is another because she may be lactose intolerant. Excess weight gain may occur because her current weight gain is about 8.5 pounds more than would be expected at this point in her pregnancy. Refer to the text for food sources of iron and nondairy calcium.
3. In addition to discussing her likes and dislikes, the nurse should consider common low-cost foods. The nurse should also consider whether Carmen adheres to "hot" and "cold" foods during childbearing. If Carmen does not speak and read English, a fluent Spanish-speaking professional is ideal to help her understand her nutritional needs.

REVIEW QUESTIONS

1. c
2. b
3. a
4. d
5. c
6. b
7. a
8. c
9. d

CHAPTER 16: PRENATAL DIAGNOSTIC TESTS

MATCHING KEY TERMS

1. h
2. g
3. d
4. e
5. f
6. c
7. b
8. a

KEY CONCEPTS

1. a. Confirm pregnancy, its location, gestational age, and determine whether it is multifetal; confirm fetal viability; adjunct to chorionic villus sampling
   b. Fetal viability, evaluate fetal anatomy, estimate gestational age, locate placenta, determine fetal presentation, evaluate amniotic fluid volume and fetal movement, adjunct to amniocentesis.
2. Transabdominal; it elevates the uterus and displaces the gas-filled intestines
3. An accurate gestational age is needed for accurate maternal serum alpha-fetoprotein evaluation, to identify intrauterine growth restriction, or if there is a question about the expected date of delivery. It is most accurately assessed by measuring the crown-to-rump length at 6 weeks' gestation. During the last half of pregnancy, it is assessed by several measurements, including the biparietal diameter, femur length, and abdominal circumference. From 12 to 20 weeks, the biparietal diameter is most accurate (±7 days).
4. a. Chromosomal abnormalities
   b. Open defects such as open neural tube defect
5. Triple-marker screening includes maternal serum alpha-fetoprotein, human chorionic gonadotropin, and unconjugated estriol; it increases detection of trisomies 18 and 21. Follow-up may include amniocentesis with karyotyping.
6. 10
7. Pregnancy loss, infection, limb reduction defects, Rh sensitization
8. a. To detect fetal genetic abnormalities; detect AFP levels, evaluate fetal condition with Rh incompatibility
   b. Evaluate fetal lung maturity, identify fetal hemolytic disease
9. Ratio of 2:1; diabetes mellitus
10. Presence of these substances in the amniotic fluid confirms fetal lung maturity.
11. 2 or more weeks
12. VST identifies whether fetal heart rate accelerations occur in response to sound stimulation; it shortens non-stress test (NST) or confirms a nonreactive NST.
13. Fetal heart rate; uterine contractions
14. Nipple stimulation, oxytocin infusion
15. Negative—normal (no late decelerations); positive—abnormal (late decelerations following 50% or more of the contractions); suspicious or equivocal—intermittent late or variable decelerations; Equivocal-hyperstimulation—late decelerations with excessive contractions; unsatisfactory—fewer than 3 contractions within 10 minutes or a poor quality tracing
16. Nonstress test, fetal breathing movements, gross fetal movements, fetal tone, amniotic fluid volume
17. During fetal hypoxemia, blood is shunted away from the kidneys and lungs and toward the brain, resulting in a lower amniotic fluid volume.

CRITICAL THINKING EXERCISES

Figure 16-8 A:

a. 125 to 130 bpm
b. 10 minutes
c. 7 total, 4 occurring with marked fetal movement (FM)
d. None
e. 25 to 30 bpm; duration 20 to 30 seconds
f. Probably reactive: In this 10-minute period, there are at least 2 accelerations of at least 15 bpm that have a duration of at least 15 seconds.

Figure 16-8 B:

a. 140 to 145 bpm
b. 10 minutes
c. None
d. None
e. No accelerations to analyze
f. The test is incomplete because less than 20 minutes has elapsed. However, if there are still no accelerations during the next 30 minutes, the test will be nonreactive.

Note that the variability in both strips is only 5 bpm. If this low variability continues throughout the remainder of the testing period, the test illustrated in Figure 16-8 A will be equivocal. It is also possible that these strips have caught the fetus in a sleep cycle.

CASE STUDIES

1. a. Pregnancy-induced hypertension may reduce placental perfusion, and delivery of the baby is its only real cure. The amniocentesis is most likely being done to assess fetal lung maturity. If the lungs are mature, induction of labor is likely.
   b. Care before amniocentesis: displacement of uterus with a rolled towel under the right hip; assessment of maternal blood pressure and fetal heart rates; ultrasound location of fetus, placenta, and largest pockets of amniotic fluid. Care after amniocentesis: maternal rest for 30 to 60 minutes with electronic fetal monitoring; caution to avoid strenuous activity for a day or two; teach to report uterine contractions, vaginal bleeding, leaking amniotic fluid, fever.
2. a. Diabetes is a disorder involving the blood vessels, and there is a possibility that the placental function is impaired because of this maternal condition.
   b. Findings that suggest normal placental function through the non-stress test include a normal baseline FHR with long-term variability of at least 10 bpm and two or more FHR accelerations of at least 15 bpm for at least 15 seconds within a 20-minute time period.
   c. The test will probably be repeated at least weekly.

REVIEW QUESTIONS

1. b
2. d
3. a
4. c
5. b

CHAPTER 17: GIVING BIRTH

MATCHING KEY TERMS

1. h
2. f
3. j
4. b
5. c
6. k
7. e
8. I
9. g
10. d
11. a

KEY CONCEPTS

1. a. Contractions must be stronger in the upper uterus than in the lower uterus to propel the fetus toward to outside.
   b. Woman cannot consciously cause labor to start or stop. Otherwise, many infants would be born early as the woman became tired of being pregnant, or labor might be suspended when it became intense.
   c. Intervals between contractions allow resumption of blood flow to placenta to supply oxygen and remove wastes for the fetus.
2. The upper uterus contracts actively to push the fetus downward, while the lower uterus is more passive to reduce resistance to fetal passage. Any other pattern would be ineffective at pushing the fetus out.
3. A full bladder increases pain and interferes with fetal descent.
4. Any maternal condition that reduces perfusion of the placenta, such as diabetes or hypertension, or fetal anemia, which reduces oxygen-carrying capacity, can reduce tolerance even for normal labor contractions.
5. In pregnancy, production of fetal lung fluid decreases and absorption into interstitium of the lungs increases. During labor, absorption of lung fluid intensifies and compression of head and thorax causes expulsion of additional fluid. After birth, the remainder is absorbed into pulmonary and lymphatic circulations.
6. Uterine contractions—first stage; uterine contractions and maternal pushing—second stage
7. They allow molding to adapt the fetal head to the size and shape of the maternal pelvis.
8. a. Longitudinal (common) or transverse (rare)
   b. Flexion (common) or extension (uncommon)
   c. Cephalic (common), breech, or shoulder (rare, less than 0.2%)
9. Refer to Figure 17-9 to complete this exercise. Frank breech is most common.
10. a. Occiput
    b. Chin (mentum)
    c. Sacrum
11. They promote relaxation and ability to work with her body's efforts rather than working against the natural forces.
12. a. Increased fetal glucocorticoid and androgens reduce placental progesterone production (which relaxes uterus) and increase prostaglandin production (which stimulates uterus).
    b. Higher estrogen levels make the uterus more sensitive to substances that stimulate it to contract, while lower progesterone levels allow it to be stimulated more easily.

13. *Braxton Hicks contractions*—irregular, mild contractions intensify near term; more noticeable in parous women; *lightening*—descent of fetus toward pelvic inlet increases pressure on bladder but allows easier breathing; more noticeable in nulliparas; *increased vaginal secretions* with congestion of vaginal mucosa caused by fetal pressure; *bloody show*—mixture of cervical mucus and blood as the mucous plug is released; seen earlier and in greater quantity in nulliparas; *energy spurt*; *weight loss* of 1 to 3 pounds
14. Refer to Figure 17-12 to complete this exercise.
15. After the fetal head is born, the fetal shoulders are transverse (crosswise) in the pelvis and must rotate to pass under the pubic arch.
16. Latent phase—up to 3 cm dilation; active phase—4 to 7 cm; transition phase—8 to 10 cm
17. First stage: nullipara—8 to 10 hours (range 6 to 18 hours); parous woman—6 to 7 hours (range 2 to 10 hours). Second stage: nullipara – 50 minutes; parous – 20 minutes.
18. Uterus has spherical shape, uterus rises upward in abdomen, cord descends further from vagina, gush of blood
19. Firm uterine contraction compresses bleeding vessels at the placental site to prevent hemorrhage.
20. Refer to Table 17-1 in your textbook to complete this exercise.
21. Condition of the mother and fetus; establishing a therapeutic relationship
22. Vaginal examination should not be performed if the woman is bleeding actively (not bloody show) because the examination may increase bleeding.
23. Time of rupture; whether rupture was spontaneous or artificial; quantity; FHR for at least 1 minute; color (clear, possibly with bits of vernix, is normal; green indicates fetal meconium passage; yellow suggests infection); other characteristics (cloudy appearance suggests infection); odor (foul or strong odor suggests infection)
24. To prevent supine hypotension from aortocaval compression by the heavy uterus
25. a. Blood pressure higher than 140/90
    b. Temperature of 38° C (100.4° F) or higher
26. Use soft, indirect lighting. Keep the temperature comfortable with a fan or damp, cool washcloths. Have the woman wear socks for cold feet. Keep the woman reasonably clean by changing her disposable underpad as often as needed. Offer ice chips or a wet washcloth to wet her lips. Remind her to empty her bladder at least every 2 hours. Encourage her to change positions frequently, assuming the position of comfort (except the supine position). Offer a shower, whirlpool, or other water therapy.
27. Cardiopulmonary; thermoregulatory; identification bands
28. Hemorrhage; discomfort
29. Full bladder interferes with the contraction of the uterus

CRITICAL THINKING EXERCISES

2. Cervical dilation is 4 cm; effacement is 75%; presentation is cephalic; membranes are ruptured; fluid is normal. The woman is beginning the active phase of first stage labor.

CASE STUDY

1. Regular contractions that have increased in duration, intensity, and frequency suggest true labor. Irregular contractions and those that do not intensify suggest false labor. In addition, discomfort is usually felt in her back or sweeping around to her lower abdomen. Erin should be instructed to come to the birth center if she thinks her membranes may have ruptured, even if she is not having contractions.

2. Priorities are to (a) assess the fetal heart rate and the color, odor, and character of the amniotic fluid; (b) assess Erin's vital signs; and (c) determine the nearness to birth by evaluating contractions and cervical dilation.
3. Either the nitrazine paper or the fern test, or both, may be used to evaluate whether the membranes have ruptured.
4. Active phase of first stage labor
5. The FHR is normal for a term fetus, and it is reassuring that the FHR accelerates with fetal movement.
6. Except for the greenish color, the amniotic fluid is normal. The amniotic fluid is green because the fetus passed meconium before birth.
7. Cephalic; right occiput posterior (ROP)
8. Assuming any of several upright positions and leaning forward during contractions; hands and knees; firm sacral pressure
9. Erin should avoid prolonged breath-holding. She can be taught to take a deep breath and exhale it, then take another deep breath and push for 4 to 6 seconds at a time while exhaling. A final breath at the end of the contraction helps her relax.
10. The exact time to position Erin for birth will depend on how fast she has labored thus far. In general, a woman having her first baby is positioned for the birth when the fetal head crowns and remains visible between contractions.
11. The 1-minute Apgar score will be 9, with 1 point deducted for the baby's bluish hands and feet.
12. a. Suction to remove excess secretions; position on one side on a flat surface
    b. Dry the baby quickly, particularly the head; place in a prewarmed radiant warmer or in skin-to-skin contact with a parent. Use a cap on the baby's dry head to reduce heat loss from that area when not in the radiant warmer.
13. The first 1 to 4 hours after the placenta delivers is the fourth stage of labor.
14. Firmness, height, and position of the uterine fundus; vital signs; amount of lochia. Observing and intervening for a full bladder helps prevent hemorrhage due to the bladder's interference with uterine contraction.
15. Cold packs to the perineal area; analgesics; a warm blanket to limit the common post-birth chill

REVIEW QUESTIONS

1. b
2. d
3. c
4. b
5. b
6. c
7. a
8. a
9. d
10. b
11. d
12. a
13. c
14. d
15. b
16. d
17. a
18. b
19. d

CHAPTER 18: INTRAPARTUM FETAL MONITORING

MATCHING KEY TERMS

1. e
2. c
3. b
4. d
5. g
6. f
7. a

KEY CONCEPTS

1. Adequacy of maternal blood volume and flow to the placenta, normal maternal blood oxygen saturation, adequate exchange of oxygen and carbon dioxide in the placenta, open circulatory path between the placenta and fetus through umbilical cord vessels, normal fetal circulatory and oxygen-carrying functions
2. a. Sympathetic stimulation increases the heart rate and strengthens the heart contractions to increase cardiac output by releasing epinephrine and norepinephrine.
   b. Baroreceptors sense blood pressure changes in the carotid arch and major arteries to slow the heart and reduce the blood pressure, thus reducing cardiac output.
   c. Chemoreceptors in the medulla oblongata, aortic arch, and carotid bodies sense changes in oxygen, carbon dioxide, and pH to increase the heart rate.
   d. Adrenal glands secrete epinephrine and norepinephrine in response to stress and release aldosterone to cause retention of sodium and water, thus increasing the blood volume.
   e. The fetal cerebral cortex causes the fetal heart rate to increase during fetal movement and decrease during fetal sleep. The hypothalamus coordinates the branches of the autonomic nervous system. The medulla oblongata maintains balance between forces that speed and slow the fetal heart rate.
3. Refer to text, "Pathologic Influences on Fetal Oxygenation," to complete this exercise.
4. Refer to text, "Auscultation and Palpation" and "Electronic Fetal Monitoring," to complete this exercise.
5. The solid intrauterine pressure catheter must be zeroed at the beginning of monitoring and cannot be rezeroed later. Its pressures are also slightly higher than those of the fluid-filled catheter. The fluid-filled catheter is sensitive to height of the catheter tip in relation to the transducer.
6. a. 110 to 160 bpm
   b. rate less than 110 bpm that persists for at least 10 minutes
   c. rate greater than 160 bpm that persists for at least 10 minutes
   d. changes of the FHR from one beat to the next
   e. broader fluctuations in the FHR over 1-minute intervals
7. narcotics or sedatives; fetal sleep; tachycardia; prematurity; decreased central nervous system oxygenation; abnormalities of the central nervous system, heart, or both.
8. Variability reflects normal function of the autonomic nervous system, which helps the fetus adapt to the stress of labor.
9. Refer to text, "Periodic Patterns in the Fetal Heart Rate" and Table 18-1, to complete this exercise.
10. fetal scalp stimulation, vibroacoustic stimulation, fetal scalp blood sampling, fetal oxygen saturation monitoring
11. 7.25; 7.35

12. a. Check blood pressure to identify hypotension or hypertension, contractions to identify uterine hyperactivity, and recent maternal medications to identify sedative effects; perform vaginal examination to identify prolapsed cord; initiate internal monitoring to provide more accuracy
    b. Change position to displace uterus, decreasing aortocaval compression; discontinue oxytocin and/or administer tocolytics to reduce uterine activity
    c. Administer oxygen at 8 to10 L/min through a snug face mask
    d. Reposition or perform amnioinfusion to reduce umbilical cord compression
13. Add fluid to create a cushion around the umbilical cord; dilute thick meconium to reduce the effects of possible aspiration at birth

REVIEW QUESTIONS

1. c
2. b
3. a
4. d
5. b
6. a
7. d

CHAPTER 19: PAIN MANAGEMENT FOR CHILDBIRTH

MATCHING KEY TERMS

1. e
2. d
3. b
4. a
5. f
6. c

KEY CONCEPTS

1. Childbirth pain is a normal process; the woman has several months to prepare; labor pain has a foreseeable end; labor pain is not constant, labor pain ends with the birth.
2. Excess pain can result in fear and anxiety, which stimulate the sympathetic nervous system to release substances that simultaneously cause vasoconstriction and pooling of maternal blood in her vascular system, plus a higher uterine muscle tone with reduction of effective contractions. The net effect is that blood flow to and from the placenta falls and labor contractions are less effective, thus prolonging labor.
3. The fetal occiput is pushed against the woman's sacral promontory with each contraction, causing intense back pain. In addition, the fetus must usually rotate into the occiput anterior position to be born, so labor is often longer.
4. relaxation, cutaneous stimulation, mental stimulation, breathing
5. Direct—FHR has a decrease variability; Indirect—maternal hypotension will decrease fetal blood flow
6. The test dose is done to identify inadvertent subarachnoid or intravascular injection of the drug. Evidence of these problems includes rapid and intense motor and sensory block (subarachnoid injection) or numbness of the tongue and lips, lightheadedness, dizziness, and tinnitus (intravascular injection).

7. a. Inadvertent dural puncture may allow spinal fluid to leak, causing intense headache that is worse when sitting or standing. A blood patch may give prompt relief. Lying flat and adding hydration helps rebuild the spinal fluid.
   b. Prehydration with warmed intravenous solution (500 to 1000 ml or more) and avoiding aortocaval compression reduce hypotensive effects.
   c. Regularly assess the bladder and have the woman void at least every 2 hours.
   d. Coach the woman to push with contractions if she cannot feel them. Forceps or vacuum extraction may be necessary.
8. The subarachnoid block punctures the dura and arachnoid membranes, entering the space that contains cerebrospinal fluid, which confirms the correct location for injection of the anesthetic drug for this block.
9. Consult your text, "Pharmacologic Pain Management," to complete this exercise.
10. Bedrest with oral or intravenous hydration; blood patch
11. These drugs have combined opioid agonist-antagonist effects and should not be given to a woman who has had a recent dose of a pure opioid agonist (may reverse effectiveness of first drug) or to a woman who is addicted to opiates such as heroin (may precipitate acute withdrawal).

CASE STUDY

1. The nurse must be careful to avoid assumptions such as that the pregnancy was unplanned, that Alice did not have prenatal care, and that she and her husband cannot learn nonpharmacologic pain management methods. You can probably think of other assumptions that nurses should avoid.
2. Initial interventions are to tell Alice and her husband kindly that her labor pattern is normal right now and show them data that indicate that mother and fetus are doing well. The nurse should speak calmly and in a soothing voice, conveying to Alice and her husband that they can have confidence in their caregivers and that Alice is capable of giving birth.
3. The nurse should teach Alice simple breathing and relaxation techniques between contractions. Say something like, "I'm going to teach you how to breathe so that you can cope with labor better" in a positive manner that conveys the expectation that the techniques *will work*, rather than doing the teaching in a tentative manner. Give liberal positive feedback when Alice uses the techniques taught and give her husband positive feedback for his coaching.
4. It would be better for Alice to delay taking medication until labor is in the active phase. Administration of analgesics too early can slow labor progress. However, this fact must be balanced against the adverse effects of excessive pain and anxiety.
5. At this point, Alice could probably receive either an opioid analgesic or an epidural block.
6. The nurse must prehydrate Alice with 500 to 1000 ml of warmed IV solution, check her blood pressure frequently to detect hypotension, and observe the FHR for signs of reduced placental perfusion that can occur with maternal hypotension. The nurse must also observe for bladder distention related to loss of sensation and high volumes of intravenous fluids. Alice may need coaching to push during the second stage if she cannot feel the urge. Additionally, the nurse must be alert for signs of catheter migration.
7. The nurse must continue to observe for bladder distention, which can result in poor uterine contraction and postpartum hemorrhage. Return of sensation must be documented. The nurse must assist Alice to the bathroom at first in case she still has reduced sensation or hypotension that could result in a fall.

REVIEW QUESTIONS

1. b
2. d
3. c
4. a
5. b
6. d
7. c

CHAPTER 20: NURSING CARE DURING OBSTETRICAL PROCEDURES

MATCHING KEY TERMS

1. a
2. c
3. d
4. b

KEY CONCEPTS

1. prolapse of the umbilical cord, infection, and placental abruption
2. Obtain baseline FHR prior and compare FHR after procedure; assess temperature every 2 hours; keep woman clean and dry.
3. Have the woman lie flat for 15 to 20 minutes to reduce gel leakage. Observe the FHR for changes that may occur with uterine contractions. Assess for excessive contractions that can reduce fetal oxygen supply (see Chapters 17 and 18).
4. Assess the FHR every 15 minutes during first-stage labor and every 5 minutes during second-stage labor. Problems include tachycardia (>150 to 160 bpm), bradycardia (<110 to 120 bpm), late decelerations, and reduced FHR variability. Assess uterine activity for contractions that are too frequent or too long or a uterus that does not relax for at least 60 seconds between contractions. Blood pressure and pulse identify changes from the baseline; temperature assessment identifies infection that may occur with ruptured membranes. Intake and output, assessment for headache, blurred vision, behavioral changes, increased blood pressure and respirations, decreased pulse, rales, wheezing, and coughing identify possible water intoxication. Postpartum hemorrhage may occur if an overstimulated uterus cannot contract effectively.
5. In addition to identifying the true cause of the nonreassuring assessments, interventions may include stopping the oxytocin infusion, increasing the rate of the nonadditive infusion, positioning to avoid aortocaval compression, and giving oxygen by face mask. Internal monitoring may be initiated if not already in place. The physician may also order a tocolytic drug if uterine hyperactivity is the problem.
6. a. A nonstress test evaluates placental function and apparent fetal health to avoid stressing a fetus that may already be compromised.
   b. Ultrasound guides the version and helps monitor the fetal heart rate. Also will confirm fetal age and presentation and adequacy of amniotic fluid.
   c. A tocolytic drug relaxes the uterus to make the version easier to perform.
   d. Administering Rh immune globulin destroys fetal Rh-positive RBCs that might stimulate anti-Rh antibodies in the Rh-negative woman. These may enter the mother's bloodstream because of tiny placental disruptions during the version.
   e. FHR monitoring evaluates how the fetus is tolerating the version and when the fetal condition returns to baseline afterward.
   f. Uterine activity monitoring identifies persistent contractions that may herald the onset of labor.

7. Add a catheter to the delivery table to empty the mother's bladder, making more room for the instrument-assisted birth. Postpartum, observe for trauma, usually lacerations (bright red bleeding with a firm fundus) or hematoma (pain, edema, discoloration). Cold packs to the perineal area limit bruising and edema. Observe for reddening, mild bruising, or small lacerations where forceps were applied. A chignon is typical if a vacuum extractor is used. Explain that these minor problems usually resolve quickly. Facial asymmetry, usually seen when crying, suggests nerve damage that resolves more slowly.
8. Infection, pain, increase blood loss, decrease sexual satisfaction.
9. Upright position with pushing, delay pushing until the urge is felt, use of open-glottis technique with pushing; daily perineal massage during the last 3 weeks of pregnancy.
10. The infant may be born preterm if a cesarean birth is scheduled. Absorption of lung fluid may be delayed, resulting in transient tachypnea. Injury can occur, such as laceration or bruising.
11. a. to reduce gastric secretions
    b. Wedge under hip avoids aortocaval compression by the heavy uterus.
    c. These tests identify reserve to tolerate blood loss, risk for poor blood clotting to control hemorrhage, blood type for possible transfusion, and prepare blood to be immediately ready if the need for transfusion arises.
    d. reduces risk for postpartum infection
    e. Keeps bladder out of the way of uterine incision.

CASE STUDY

1. Postterm gestation is the probable reason for induction.
2. Tests for fetal lung maturity, such as the lecithin/sphingomyelin (L/S) ratio, and for presence of phosphatidylglycerol (PG) and phosphatidylinositol (PI) may be done. Even though Linda is 42 weeks, incorrect dates could mean that her fetus is actually younger.
3. Set up as a secondary infusion, regulated by a pump, start and increase the rate slowly, and add to the primary infusion line at the lowest possible port. This technique ensures that the oxytocin can be quickly stopped if the need arises. The pump controls the infusion precisely. See also Drug Guide 16-1. Observe the FHR and uterine activity for nonreassuring signs or uterine hyperstimulation.
4. Before the amniotomy, obtain baseline information about the fetal heart rate. Place absorbent underpads under Linda's hips. After the amniotomy, assess the fetal heart rate for at least 1 minute and report nonreassuring signs or significant changes from baseline; observe and chart the quantity, color, clarity, and odor of the amniotic fluid.
5. No change in the oxytocin is needed at this time, although amniotomy may increase contractions enough to allow a dosage reduction.
6. The oxytocin infusion should be stopped because some contractions have only a 30-second resting interval. This could exhaust the fetal oxygen reserve and lead to distress. Additionally, labor is now well established and dilation is progressing, so stimulation does not appear to be warranted.
7. Actual care depends on how quickly the surgery must take place. Provide emotional support to reduce anxiety. Keep the partners together as much as possible. Provide preoperative teaching, abbreviated as necessary for the actual situation. Perform preoperative procedures such as indwelling catheter and abdominal shave. Explain who will be present at birth and their responsibilities. Explain recovery room care. Pad bony prominences. Secure legs with a safety strap. Tilt the table or place a wedge under one hip to avoid aortocaval compression. Apply the grounding pad and other monitors. Clean the incision line and apply a sterile dressing.

8. Take vital signs every 15 minutes for 1 to 2 hours. Observe uterus for firmness and position, lochia, urine output, intravenous infusion, abdominal dressing, and pain relief needs. Observe for return of motion and sensation (for regional block anesthesia) or level of consciousness (for general anesthesia or if sedative drugs were given).

REVIEW QUESTIONS

1. b
2. d
3. a
4. c
5. d
6. a
7. c
8. b
9. c
10. d

CHAPTER 21: POSTPARTUM ADAPTATIONS

MATCHING KEY TERMS

1. h
2. k
3. c
4. j
5. m
6. i
7. l
8. b
9. f
10. a
11. e
12. d
13. g

KEY CONCEPTS

1. a. Stretched uterine muscle fibers contract and gradually regain their former size and contour.
   b. Number of uterine muscle cells remains the same, but each cell decreases in size through catabolism.
   c. Outer area of endometrium (decidua) is expelled with the placenta. Remaining decidua separates into two layers: the superficial layer is shed in lochia and the basal layer regenerates new endothelium.
2. Lochia rubra contains blood, mucus, and bits of decidua; is red in color; and has a duration of about 3 days. Lochia serosa contains serous exudate, erythrocytes, leukocytes, and cervical mucus; it is a pinkish color; and its duration is from the 4th to the 10th day. Lochia alba contains leukocytes, decidual cells, epithelial cells, fat, cervical mucus, and bacteria; it is white or colorless; its duration varies from 11th day until the 3rd to 6th week.

3. a. Breast feeding stimulates release of oxytocin from the pituitary gland, which tends to intensify afterpains but also maintains better uterine contraction. This facilitates involution.
   b. Lactation suppresses ovulation and estrogen secretion, causing more vaginal dryness than nonlactating mothers have. This may cause painful sexual intercourse unless lubrication is added.
4. Blood volume and cardiac output increase as blood from the uteroplacental unit returns to the central circulation and as excess extracellular fluid enters the vascular compartment for excretion. Because stroke volume increases, pulse decreases.
5. Pregnant and postpartum women have higher fibrinogen levels, which increase the ability to form clots. Factors that lyse clots are decreased, however. Some women have another risk in addition to this baseline risk: those who have varicose veins, a history of thrombophlebitis, or a cesarean birth.
6. Leukocytes can increase up to $30{,}000/mm^3$. Refer to Appendix D to answer the second question.
7. A full bladder interferes with the ability of the uterus to contract firmly and occlude open vessels at the placental site. This allows them to bleed freely.
8. Estrogen and progesterone prepare the breasts for lactation. Prolactin initiates milk production in the alveoli. Oxytocin causes milk ejection from the alveoli into the lactiferous ducts.
9. Rho(D)—mother is Rh–, newborn is Rh+; Rubella vaccine—if her prenatal rubella antibody screening showed non-immune
10. Refer to Procedure 21-1 to complete this exercise.
11. Refer to text, "Focused Assessments After Vaginal Birth," to complete this exercise.
12. The answer to this exercise should be in your own words and should fit the women you care for in your clinical setting.
13. a. Observe respiratory rate and depth (every 30 minutes to 1 hour if epidural narcotics were used); monitor apnea for epidural narcotic administration; auscultate breath sounds for retained secretions; assist the mother to turn, cough, and deep-breathe; use incentive spirometer.
    b. Assess for return of peristalsis by auscultating bowel sounds; observe for abdominal distention; observe surgical dressing for intactness and drainage; observe incision line after dressing removal for signs of infection (REEDA); palpate fundus gently.
    c. Monitor IV for rate of flow and site condition; observe urine for amount, color, and clarity.
14. Increase activity progressively, drink adequate fluids (at least 8 glasses of water), and add dietary fiber (found in fruits and vegetables, whole grain cereals, bread, and pasta) to prevent constipation. Prunes are a natural laxative.
15. Fever; localized area of redness, swelling, or pain in the breasts that is unrelieved by support or analgesics; persistent abdominal tenderness or feelings of pelvic fullness or pelvic pressure; persistent perineal pain; frequency, urgency, or burning when urinating; change in lochia character (increased amount, return to red color, passage of clots, or foul odor); localized tenderness, redness, or warmth of the legs.
16. Bonding describes the initial, rapid attraction felt by parents toward their newborn infant. It is a one-way process, from parent to infant. Attachment describes a longer-term, two-way process that binds parent and infant. Attachment is facilitated by positive feedback from the infant and by mutually satisfying experiences.
17. Maternal touch progression is from fingertipping to palm touch to enfolding the infant and bringing him or her close to the body.
18. The mother progresses from calling the infant "it" to referring to the infant as "he" or "she" to using the infant's given name.
19. Refer to the text, "The Process of Maternal Role Adaptation," to complete this exercise.

20. "Postpartum blues" describes a mild, transient depression that affects more than 70% of American women. It has an onset within the first week after birth and is characterized by fatigue, weeping, mood instability, and anxiety. The mother may not be able to define why she is upset. The primary nursing care is to give the woman empathy and support and let her know that the condition is usually self-limiting.
21. The nurse should involve the father in infant care teaching and decisions. Fathers may not know what to expect from newborns and benefit from information about growth and development. A review of any prenatal teaching is helpful as well.
22. The nurse should help the parent or parents acknowledge their feelings and deal with them to facilitate their attachment with the child.
23. The nurse should help parents interact with each twin individually rather than interacting with them as a "package." It is essential to point out essential qualities and characteristics of each infant individually.
24. Avoidance cues include looking away, splaying the fingers, arching the back, and fussiness. These are clues that the infant needs some quiet time.

CASE STUDY

1. Nita's fundus is not well contracted, probably due to a full bladder since it is positioned to the right of the umbilicus. Her multifetal birth and multiparity increase the risk for postpartum hemorrhage.
2. Massage the uterus to cause it to contract firmly and control bleeding. The next intervention should be to assist Nita to empty her bladder or catheterize her if she is unable to void. Otherwise, the uterus will relax again.
3. You should immediately teach Nita how to assess her uterus for firmness and the relationship between a full bladder, her multiparity, and her multifetal birth to uterine contraction.
4. No interventions are needed. Bradycardia and a slight elevation in temperature are common at this time.
5. The best nursing response is to reassure Nita that the afterpains are typically short-term and that analgesics can ease them. Also teach her that a full bladder will worsen afterpains.
6. Two factors increase afterpains in Nita's case: multiparity and uterine overdistention with two fetuses.
7. Analgesics taken at least 30 minutes before the expected time of breast feeding can decrease afterpains. Lying in a prone position with a small pillow or folded blanket under the abdomen often helps.
8. Teach Nita to gradually increase her ambulation, drink additional fluids (at least 8 glasses of water daily), and increase dietary fiber. Prunes are a natural laxative, and she can consult her birth attendant for recommended laxatives if natural remedies do not work.
9. RhoGAM is given to the Rh-negative mother if her infant is Rh positive and if she has not previously built up anti-Rh antibodies. Rubella vaccine is given to the nonimmune postpartum woman because it is highly unlikely that she will get pregnant soon.
10. Nita should be cautioned to avoid another pregnancy for at least 3 months.
11. Nita's fundus is slightly higher than usual, but this is explained by her multiparity and delivery of twins.
12. Lochia flow should be rubra (possibly changing to serosa), scant, and free of foul odor or clots.
13. Slight reddening is typical of normal healing at this early stage. Close approximation of the edges and lack of drainage confirm that healing seems to be taking place normally. Proper perineal cleansing and pad application should be reinforced. The nurse should also review signs and symptoms of infection to report.

REVIEW QUESTIONS

1. a
2. b
3. c
4. d
5. a
6. b
7. d
8. a
9. c
10. d
11. a
12. d
13. a
14. c

CHAPTER 22: THE NORMAL NEWBORN: ADAPTATION AND ASSESSMENT

MATCHING KEY TERMS

1. f
2. h
3. b
4. e
5. d
6. c
7. g
8. a
9. *b
10. d (females)
11. c (*abnormal if present before than 24 hours)
12. i
13. *h
14. a
15. *j
16. *f
17. *d (males)
18. g
19. a
20. c (*suggests infant is preterm if excessive)
21. b
22. d (females)
23. *j
24. *k
25. *e
26. *g
27. *d (males)
28. c (*suggests infant is preterm if excessive)

KEY CONCEPTS

1. a. Decreased blood oxygen level and blood pH and an increased blood carbon dioxide level stimulate the respiratory center in the medulla. Occlusion of the umbilical cord vessels may end the flow of a placental substance that inhibits respirations.
   b. The sudden change in environmental temperature at birth stimulate skin sensors, which then stimulate the brain's respiratory center.
   c. Fetal chest compression during vaginal birth forces additional lung fluid from the chest. Added stimuli to breathe include suctioning, drying, holding, sounds, and light.
2. Residual air in the lungs allows the alveoli to remain partly expanded after exhalation. This reduces the work necessary to expand the alveoli with subsequent breaths.
3. a. 4
   b. 2
   c. 8
   d. 6
   e. 1
   f. 3
   g. 7
   h. 5
4. Thin skin; blood vessels near the surface; little insulating subcutaneous fat; heat readily transferred from internal organs to skin; greater ratio of surface area to body mass
5. Evaporation occurs when wet surfaces are exposed to air and dry conditions. Conduction occurs when the infant is exposed to direct contact with a cool surface. Convection refers to heat loss by air currents near the infant. Radiation refers to heat loss when the infant is near a cold surface. All methods except evaporation can also be a source of heat gain, such as contact with warm blankets, warmed air currents near infant, or warm incubator walls.
6. Brown fat is metabolized to generate heat, which is transferred to the blood vessels running through it and then circulated to the rest of the body. Infants that may have inadequate brown fat include preterm infants, those with intrauterine growth restriction, and those exposed to prolonged cold stress.
7. Heat production requires oxygen for metabolism, which can exceed the infant's capacity to supply the oxygen. Glucose use is accelerated when the metabolic rate rises to produce heat, possibly depleting these stores and resulting in hypoglycemia. Metabolism of glucose and brown fat without adequate oxygen causes increased production of acids. These acids interfere with transport of bilirubin to the liver, where it can be conjugated and excreted, thus causing jaundice.
8. Values for all three are higher in the newborn than in the older infant or adult. The fetus needs these higher levels to supply adequate oxygen to the tissues. Fetal hemoglobin (hemoglobin F) carries more oxygen than adult hemoglobin.
9. Vitamin K is produced in the intestines by the normal intestinal flora. Newborns cannot produce this flora until a few days after starting to eat. Vitamin K is necessary to activate the clotting factors.
10. Refer to the text, "Stools," to complete this exercise.
11. Glucose lower than 40 mg/dl
12. Preterm or small-for-gestational-age infants are at risk because adequate glycogen and possibly fat may not have accumulated. Postterm infants may have used up their stores of glycogen before birth as a result of deteriorating placenta function. Large-for-gestational-age infants may produce excessive insulin that quickly consumes their glucose; this is particularly true if the mother is diabetic. In addition, stress or hypothermia may consume all available glucose.

13. a. Newborns have more erythrocytes for their size and these break down faster than adult erythrocytes, producing a greater quantity of bilirubin to be excreted.
    b. The liver is immature and does not immediately produce enough glucuronyl transferase to conjugate bilirubin as quickly as it is produced.
    c. Lack of normal intestinal flora prevents reduction of conjugated bilirubin to urobilinogen for excretion. Large amounts of beta-glucuronidase in the intestines convert conjugated bilirubin back into the unconjugated form.
    d. Feeding helps establish normal intestinal flora.
    e. Birth trauma may cause added hemolysis of erythrocytes, adding to the bilirubin load.
    f. Metabolism of brown fat for heat production and asphyxia, which results in anaerobic metabolism, both produce fatty acids. The fatty acids bind more readily to albumin than bilirubin, resulting in more unconjugated and unbound bilirubin in the circulation. Prevention of cold stress and asphyxia and the time of first feeding may be altered by nursing interventions.
14. Pathologic jaundice has any of these characteristics: appears before 24 hours of age; direct bilirubin level above 2 mg/dl; rate of bilirubin increase greater than 5 mg/dl/day; bilirubin level higher than 12 mg/dl in a term infant or 10 to 14 mg/dl in a preterm infant; jaundice that persists after the second week of life
15. a. Inadequate intake of colostrum causes retention of meconium, which is high in bilirubin. High levels of beta-glucuronidase in the intestine deconjugate bilirubin in the meconium, adding to the load on the liver. Poor intake reduces the milk supply, worsening the problem. Nursing measures and teaching to stimulate the infant to nurse better and thus increase milk production are appropriate treatment.
    b. True breast milk jaundice is characterized by rising bilirubin levels after the first 3 to 5 days of life; levels peak at 5 to 10 mg/dl 2 weeks after birth and takes several months to reach normal levels. Treatment may include phototherapy, temporarily discontinuing breast feeding for 24 to 48 hours, or both.
16. The proportion of extracellular water in newborns is double that of adults.
17. a. A newborn's kidneys are not well equipped to handle a large load of fluid, possibly resulting in fluid overload.
    b. Newborns have half the adult's ability to concentrate urine, and thus cannot conserve fluid efficiently.
18. Leukocytes respond slowly to the site of infection and are inefficient in destroying invading organisms. The usual inflammatory response and fever are often not present because of the immature hypothalamus.
19. a. IgG is received from the mother to provide passive antibodies to viruses and bacteria to which the mother has immunity. It also protects against bacterial toxins. The infant increases production of his or her own IgG beginning at 3 to 4 weeks of age.
    b. IgM is produced by the infant to protect against gram-negative bacteria.
    c. IgA is produced by the infant and is received in colostrum and breast milk to protect against infections of the respiratory and gastrointestinal systems.
20. Newborns during the first period of reactivity are wide awake and active. Respirations may be as high as 80 bpm, and the heart rate may be as high as 180 bpm. Respiratory assessments show nasal flaring, crackles, retractions, and increased mucous secretions. This is an ideal time to facilitate parent-infant acquaintance because both are highly interested in each other. After the first sleep period following the first period of reactivity, infants are alert, interested in feeding, and often pass meconium. The pulse and respiratory rates may increase, and some infants may have cyanosis or periods of apnea. Mucous secretions increase. The nurse must be alert for respiratory complications during this stage.
21. Refer to text, "Behavioral States," to complete this exercise.

22. Respiratory problems; obvious anomalies
23. Caput: cause – pressure; features – crosses suture line; teaching – disappears within 12 hours to several days. Cephalhematoma: cause – pressure; features – does not cross suture line; teaching – may take weeks to months to resolve, may be higher risk for jaundice
24. a. Associated with other anomalies; assess infant carefully
    b. Single palmar crease that often occurs in infants that have chromosomal abnormalities such as Down syndrome
    c. May indicate spina bifida occulta or failure of the vertebra to close fully
    d. Associated with chromosomal disorders
    e. Indicates facial nerve injury with paralysis during birth
25. Refer to Table 22-1 to complete this exercise.
26. Refer to Procedure 22-2 and Table 22-1 to complete this exercise.
27. Tachypnea (sustained), retractions that continue after the first hour, nasal flaring after the first hour, cyanosis involving the lips, tongue, and trunk (central cyanosis), grunting, seesaw respirations, asymmetry of chest expansion
28. Jitteriness, poor muscle tone, sweating, respiratory signs (dyspnea, apnea, cyanosis), hypothermia, high-pitched cry, lethargy, seizures, eventually coma; some show no signs of hypoglycemia
29. Female: labia majora darker than surrounding skin and completely cover the clitoris and labia minora; white mucous discharge or pseudomenstruation; hymenal or vaginal tags; patent urinary meatus and vagina. Male: pendulous scrotum that is darker than surrounding skin and covered with rugae; testes palpable in the scrotal sac; meatus centered at the tip of the glans penis; prepuce covering the glans and adherent to it
30. a. Suggests polycythemia; may contribute to higher bilirubin levels as the excessive erythrocytes break down, so observe for more severe jaundice and emphasize to parents
    b. Indicates meconium passage in utero; observe infant for associated respiratory difficulties
    c. Erythema toxicum; differentiate from infection; teach parents that rash is self-limiting
    d. Mongolian spots; more common in dark-skinned infants; most disappear during early childhood; teach parents who are unfamiliar with these
    e. Nevus flammeus (port-wine stain); large or obvious ones can later be removed by laser surgery
    f. Cafe-au-lait spots; more than 6 spots or spots larger than 1.5 cm are associated with neurofibromatosis and should be reported to the physician
31. Bruises on the face or upper body are often present when the infant had a nuchal cord at birth.

CASE STUDIES

1. Total maturity score is 43.
2. The infant's maturity rating is between 40 and 42 weeks (approximately 41 weeks).
3. Weight is 3005 g; length is 48 cm; head circumference is 33 cm. The infant is appropriate for gestational age (AGA) in all measurements.
4. All measurements fall near the 25th percentile, which means that 75% of infants of this gestational age are larger, and 24% are smaller. The nurse would not anticipate the need for additional care or expanded assessments or care on the basis of the gestational age assessment alone.

REVIEW QUESTIONS

1. b
2. d
3. a
4. b
5. d
6. a
7. c
8. d
9. b
10. d
11. c
12. c
13. d
14. a
15. d
16. a
17. d
18. b
19. b
20. a
21. d

CHAPTER 23: THE NORMAL NEWBORN: NURSING CARE

KEY CONCEPTS

1. Suction the mouth first and then the nose (if needed). The infant might gasp when the nose is suctioned, drawing any secretions that are in the mouth into the airway.
2. The head is about one fourth of the newborn's total body surface area and is thus a large surface for heat loss. Damp hair presents a continuing source for evaporative heat loss.
3. If the infant's temperature has dropped significantly, the nurse may wish to confirm it with a rectal temperature. Look for and correct sources of heat loss, such as wet clothing or exposed skin. Wrap the flexed infant snugly in warm blankets. A radiant warmer, regulated by a skin probe, may be needed for very low temperatures. Teach parents about maintaining the infant's temperature, particularly if their actions have contributed to the low temperature.
4. a. Conduction
   b. Conduction
   c. Radiation
   d. Evaporation
   e. Convection
5. Base your answer on the following: when blood glucose levels decrease permanent brain damage may occur. Feeding the infant will help maintain appropriate glucose levels. Repeating the glucose level screenings will confirm that appropriate blood levels are being maintained in order to prevent brain damage.
6. When the temperature is stable.
7. For bleeding and urination
8. Notify physician if there is no urinary output within 6 to 8 hours, bleeding more than a few drops with first diaper changes, or displacement of the Plastibell. Apply

pressure if any bleeding occurs. Report signs of infection, such as redness, edema, tenderness, and discharge (a yellow exudate that dries is normal). Apply petrolatum gauze to the site of a Gomco circumcision.

9. Signs of infection include redness at the cord base, exudate or failure to dry, and odor. To prevent infection, apply alcohol to the cord and its base about three times per day. Keep the cord area dry by keeping the diaper low. Delay tub bathing until the cord has detached and the area is fully healed.
10. Identification is accomplished by matching the imprinted numbers on the adult's wrist band with the infant's identification band. The numbers should be matched *every* time the infant is reunited with the parent. The nurse should visually match the numbers or have the parent read the imprinted numbers from his or her band.
11. Low or elevated temperature; signs of localized infection, such as redness, edema, discharge, foul-odored drainage; lethargy; poor feeding; periods of apnea without obvious cause; any unexplained change in behavior
12. a. Vitamin K, which is necessary for normal blood coagulation, is given because the infant's gastrointestinal tract is sterile at birth and temporarily lacks the microorganisms that will make it.
    b. Erythromycin ointment is used to prevent eye infections acquired in the mother's birth canal, such as gonorrhea.
    c. Hepatitis B immunization is given to promote the infant's manufacture of antibodies against this viral infection of the liver.
13. Mothers who are positive for hepatitis B (carriers) may transmit the organism to their infant at birth. A dose of hepatitis B immune globulin within 12 hours of birth, in addition to the vaccine, provides passive antibody protection until the infant manufactures his or her own active antibodies to the virus.
14. Refer to text, "Follow-up Care," to complete this exercise.

REVIEW QUESTIONS

1. c
2. b
3. a
4. d
5. b
6. a
7. d
8. a

CHAPTER 24: NEWBORN FEEDING

MATCHING KEY TERMS

1. c
2. d
3. b
4. a

KEY CONCEPTS

1. 400 to 440 calories per day; 20 to 22 ounces of breast milk or formula daily; 360 to 544 ml of fluid per day

2. Colostrum, which is produced during the first week, is a thick, yellow substance rich in immunoglobulins, especially IgA. It has laxative effects and is high in protein, fat-soluble vitamins, and minerals. It is lower in calories, fat, and lactose. Transitional milk begins 7 to 10 days after lactation begins; immunoglobulins and proteins decrease; lactose, fat, and calories increase. Mature milk begins 2 weeks after onset of lactation; it has a bluish color and provides 20 calories per ounce.
3. Refer to text, "Breast Milk and Formula Composition," to complete this exercise.
4. Prolactin stimulates the breasts to produce milk. It is enhanced by suckling and removal of milk from the breasts, and it is inhibited by estrogen, progesterone, and placental lactogen during pregnancy and by inadequate removal of milk after nursing begins. Oxytocin stimulates the milk-ejection reflex. It is enhanced by comfort, thinking about the infant, and the stimulation of suckling. It is inhibited by discomfort or inadequate suckling.
5. Breast shells used in late pregnancy can draw nipples out.
6. a. Feel like a cheek
   b. Slightly firmer than a cheek
   c. Hard, shiny, taut tissue
7. a. The mother cups the breast in a "C" position, with her thumb on top and the fingers underneath. This is preferred because her fingers are less likely to slip toward the nipple than with the scissors position.
   b. In the scissors position, the mother guides her nipple by securing it between her index and middle finger.
8. Nutritive suckling is evidenced by smooth, continuous movements with only occasional pauses to rest. Swallowing may follow each suck or after two or three sucks. Nonnutritive suckling produces fluttery or choppy motions without the sound of swallowing. Infant swallowing has a soft "ka" or "ah" sound.
9. Break suction before removing the infant from the breast by inserting a finger between the infant's gums or indenting the breast tissue near the infant's mouth.
10. 2; 3; 8
11. Frequent nursing stimulates peristalsis, which increases the rate of excretion of bilirubin in stools.
12. After a feeding or at night
13. Serious infections such as tuberculosis, HIV infection, maternal cancer, maternal substance abuse
14. a. Use rigid polypropylene plastic containers.
    b. Milk may be stored in the refrigerator for 48 hours (preferred) or in the refrigerator's freezer for 1 month; it can be kept at a deep freeze at 0°F for 6 months.
    c. Do not microwave. Thaw in the refrigerator or by holding under running water.
15. a. Wash the top of the can and the can opener just before opening and pouring into washed bottles and capping. Refrigerate an open can and discard any remaining milk after 48 hours.
    b. Dilute the concentrated liquid with an equal part of water. Do not over- or underdilute. Fill clean bottles with diluted formula as in ready-to-feed.
    c. Dilute formula in a clean bottle exactly as directed, usually one scoop for each 2 ounces of water. As in concentrated liquid formula, do not over- or underdilute.
16. a. Feed the infant every 3 to 4 hours, but do not adhere to a rigid schedule.
    b. Do not prop the bottle. To do so may cause aspiration of formula. Bottle propping is associated with dental caries when the primary teeth erupt and with ear infections.
    c. Do not microwave formula because it may have "hot spots" that would burn the infant.
    d. Discard all remaining formula after 1 hour of use.

CASE STUDY

1. A good initial action would be to help Margaret calm her fussy baby so that the infant will be more likely to nurse. This action accomplishes two goals: (1) it helps Margaret learn the skill of comforting her infant and (2) it increases the likelihood that the infant will nurse well when positioned well at the breast.
2. After the infant is calmer, suggest positions that Margaret might use to begin nursing. Support her arm in the chosen position with pillows or blankets. Explain the basics of helping her infant latch on to the breast: stimulating the infant's mouth until it opens wide, then drawing the infant close; inserting the nipple and areola well back into the mouth; checking to see that the lips are flared on the breast tissue. Describe and have Margaret observe for typical patterns that indicate nutritive suckling: smooth rhythmic suckling, interrupted by swallowing with a soft "ka" or "ah" sound.
3. Teach Margaret that the milk-ejection reflex may take as long as 5 minutes to occur and that nursing periods that are too short will only provide the foremilk, which has a lower fat content, is less satisfying, and does not promote the infant's growth. If the infant receives only the foremilk regularly, she will want to nurse often and will be less satisfied. Engorgement is also more likely. Teach her to break the suction before removing the infant from the breast. Positioning the infant to avoid pulling on the nipple and making sure that the areola is well into the infant's mouth will help reduce nipple soreness, although it will not totally prevent it.
4. Infants usually feed every 2 to 3 hours and should not sleep longer than 5 hours without nursing. Teach the mother to plan on nursing 8 to 12 times in each 24-hour period. Duration is generally about 10 to 15 minutes on each breast. The infant should nurse on the first breast until nonnutritive suckling begins; then the mother should change to the other breast. Switching back and forth between breasts several times during feedings reduces the amount of hindmilk secreted.
5. Wear a well-fitting bra day and night. Avoid creams, ointments, or soaps on the breasts. Clean with plain water. Express colostrum and rub it into the breasts. Wear absorbent pads in the bra if breasts are leaking, but do not allow the wet pad to have prolonged contact with the breast. Leave bra flaps down after nursing. See also Nursing Care Plan 22-3 and Mothers Want to Know: Solutions to Common Breast Feeding Problems in your textbook.
6. Refer to Mothers Want to Know: Is My Baby Getting Enough Milk? in your textbook.

REVIEW QUESTIONS

1. b
2. a
3. d
4. a
5. c
6. b

CHAPTER 25: THE CHILDBEARING FAMILY WITH SPECIAL NEEDS

MATCHING KEY TERMS

1. e
2. a
3. c
4. f
5. d
6. b

KEY CONCEPTS

1. a. Development of independence from parents is interrupted. The teenage girl usually becomes more dependent on them, rather than becoming more independent of her family home.
   b. Education is often interrupted and may never be completed. Overall educational level is lower.
   c. Reliance on welfare system is more likely because of incomplete education and limited job skills.
2. Pregnancy-induced hypertension, anemia and nutritional deficiencies, UTIs, depression, and high incidence of sexually transmissible diseases
3. a. There is a higher incidence of chromosome abnormalities such as Down syndrome.
   b. Older women are more likely to have underlying chronic medical conditions that complicate pregnancy, such as diabetes or hypertension.
   c. There is a higher incidence of multifetal gestation, preterm labor, dysfunctional labor, vaginal bleeding, preeclampsia, gestational diabetes and cesarean birth. Infants are more likely to be small for gestational age.
4. a. She may have less energy to cope with the demands of an infant plus the day-to-day activities of living.
   b. She may have less peer support because most other women her age have teenagers or young adults.
5. Most substances ingested by the mother cross the placenta and enter the fetal circulation. The fetus cannot metabolize the substance as quickly, so the substance lingers for a prolonged time in the fetal body.
6. Refer to textbook, Table 25-1, to complete this exercise.
7. Cocaine directly stimulates uterine contractions. Preterm labor contractions are rarely abrupt and intense at their onset. The fetus or neonate may have problems related to the maternal cocaine, such as abruptio placentae, premature rupture of the membranes, precipitous birth, stillbirth, tachycardia, irritability, muscular rigidity, hypertension, and an exaggerated startle reflex.
8. Withdrawal of heroin can be fetal for the fetus. The mother can be put on Methodone during the pregnancy, but the neonate will need to withdraw from that medication after birth.
9. a. Late prenatal care, failing to keep appointments, and not following recommendations
   b. Poor grooming, inadequate weight gain, weight gain pattern that does not conform to that expected for the gestational age
   c. Spontaneous abortions, premature births, abruptio placentae, stillbirths
   d. Anger or apathy toward pregnancy, particularly if these are evident at a time when the normal ambivalence of early pregnancy should be resolved
10. a. Profuse sweating, hypertension, irregular respirations, lethargic response to labor, lack of interest in interventions, dilated pupils, increased body temperature, sudden onset of severely painful contractions, emotional lability and paranoia, fetal tachycardia, and fetal hyperactivity

b. Withdrawal symptoms such as yawning, diaphoresis, rhinorrhea, restlessness, and excessive tearing

11. Facial abnormalities cause parental concerns about how others will accept their child because the defect is obvious. Genital defects cause ambiguity and anxiety about the child's identity—is the baby a boy or a girl? How should the baby be dressed?
12. Parents must grieve for the expected normal child before they can detach from this fantasy and move on to accepting the child they have.
13. The father as well as the mother must be assisted to deal with the shock and sadness, rather than all attention being focused on the mother's grief. Only when the father deals with his emotions can he support his partner and explain the loss to the couple's family and friends.
14. Woman: multiple injury sites; late entry into prenatal care; increased risk for low maternal weight gain and anemia; more substance abuse. Fetus: prematurity, low birth weight, and neonatal death
15. Tension-building: when threats and angry behaviors escalate; increased use of alcohol and drugs; the woman tries to avoid or placate her abuser.
    Battering: with hitting, burning, beating, or raping the woman. The woman often simply endures the abuse.
    Honeymoon phase: when the abuser is overly solicitous and tries to make up with his partner. He often insists on having intercourse to prove that she forgives him. The woman wants to believe that he will never abuse her again.

REVIEW QUESTIONS

1. c
2. d
3. b
4. c
5. a

CHAPTER 26: THE PREGNANT WOMAN WITH COMPLICATIONS

MATCHING KEY TERMS

1. e
2. d
3. c
4. f
5. b
6. g
7. a

KEY CONCEPTS

1. Termination of a pregnancy without action taken by the woman or any other person
2. Refer to text, "Spontaneous Abortion," to complete this exercise.
3. Fibrinogen and platelets—decreased; prothrombin, partial thromboplastin time—prolonged; fibrin degradation products—increased
4. The nurse can explain that most spontaneous abortions occur because of factors or abnormalities that could not be avoided. Also, allow the client the opportunity to express her feelings.

5. Abrupt onset of shoulder pain may occur with a ruptured ectopic pregnancy because blood accumulated in the abdomen irritates the diaphragm.
6. Explain the side effects, such as nausea and vomiting. Teach the woman to refrain from drinking alcohol, ingesting vitamins containing folic acid, or having sexual intercourse until hCG is not detectable in the serum (usually 2 to 4 weeks).
7. Elevated hCG; vaginal bleeding that varies in amount and color; uterine enlargement greater than expected for the gestation; nondetectable fetal heart activity; excessive nausea and vomiting; early onset of pregnancy-induced hypertension
8. Most molar tissue is benign, but choriocarcinoma is a possibility. Serum hCG will be evaluated every 1 to 2 weeks. Pregnancy must be avoided until normal prepregnancy levels of hCG are attained.
9. Foods high in iron should be emphasized to aid in restoring hemoglobin levels. These include liver, red meat, spinach, egg yolks, carrots, and raisins. She should also include vitamin C foods which increase the utilization of iron. Use the information in the text to formulate your explanation.
10. Refer to the text, "Hemorrhagic Conditions of Late Pregnancy," to complete this chart.
11. The woman and her family should be taught to assess the vaginal discharge, fetal movement counts, and uterine activity. She should be given guidelines for what to report. Curtailment of sexual intercourse should be discussed.
12. Cocaine is a vasoconstrictor, including constriction of the uterine endometrial arteries, which leads to premature placental separation.
13. Much or all of the blood may be trapped by the placenta, which may remain attached at the edges.
14. Early signs: tachycardia, diminished peripheral pulses, normal or slightly decreased blood pressure, tachypnea, pallor and coolness of the skin and mucous membranes. Late signs: falling blood pressure, pallor, skin that is cold and clammy, urine output less than 30 ml/hr, restlessness, agitation, decreased mentation.
15. Lateral positioning with the head flat to increase cardiac return and enhance circulation to the placenta and vital organs; restricted maternal movement to reduce demand for oxygen; provide explanations, reassurance, and emotional support to reduce anxiety that would increase demand for oxygen
16. a. Reduced blood flow causes a reduced glomerular filtration rate, which causes a rise in blood urea nitrogen (BUN), creatinine, and uric acid. Glomerular damage due to reduced perfusion allows protein to leak across the glomerular membrane, resulting in interstitial fluid accumulation, hypovolemia, and increased blood viscosity and hematocrit (hemoconcentration). Angiotensin II and aldosterone are secreted in response to hypovolemia, further increasing the blood pressure.
    b. Reduced perfusion decreases liver function. Hepatic edema and subcapsular hemorrhage may occur. Serum may have elevated liver enzymes.
    c. Vasoconstriction leads to pressure-induced rupture of small capillaries, resulting in small cerebral hemorrhages. Symptoms such as headache and visual disturbances may result.
    d. Reduced osmotic pressure may result in pulmonary edema.
    e. Reduced perfusion may cause infarctions or abruptio placentae. The risk of DIC is also higher. The fetus may have growth restriction and persistent hypoxemia.
17. Edema of preeclampsia typically occurs above the waist: face and fingers. A sudden weight gain often precedes visible edema.
18. Epigastric pain occurs with liver capsule distention, which often heralds an imminent convulsion.
19. Central nervous system depression results in diminished deep tendon reflexes and respiratory depression. Reduced urinary output can cause magnesium to accumulate to unsafe levels.
20. calcium gluconate

21. Chronic hypertension is present before 20 weeks of gestation.
22. a. The woman must have Rh-negative blood because she will not make anti-Rh antibodies if she is also Rh positive.
    b. The newborn must have Rh-positive blood because Rh-negative blood cannot induce development of anti-Rh antibodies in the woman.
    c. Indirect Coombs' test should be negative, indicating that the woman has not made anti-Rh antibodies (become sensitized) to Rh-positive blood during the pregnancy.
    d. The direct Coombs' test identifies maternal antibodies in the newborn's blood and should be negative.
23. ABO incompatibility may occur if a type O mother has a fetus that is type A, B, or AB because these blood types contain an antigen that is not present on type O erythrocytes. Many type O people have developed high levels of antibodies to blood types A, B, or AB, and the antibodies can cross the placenta and damage fetal erythrocytes that are one of these types. The effects are usually less severe than Rh incompatibility.
24. Polydipsia (excess thirst), polyuria (excess urine output), polyphagia (excess appetite), weight loss
25. Hypoglycemia and hyperglycemia are associated with more spontaneous abortions and congenital malformations.
26. With no vascular impairment, hyperglycemia can lead to macrosomia. Vascular impairment limits glucose and oxygen transport to the fetus and may result in intrauterine growth restriction.
27. a. They decrease in the first trimester because of reduced maternal food intake and uptake of glucose by embryo/fetus.
    b. They increase in the second and third trimesters because of maternal insulin resistance and greater food intake.
    c. They usually decrease during labor because of exertion and lack of food intake. Euglycemia is maintained with IV infusion of insulin and glucose.
    d. They decrease in the postpartum period because of loss of hormones from placenta that caused insulin resistance.
28. If her glucose challenge test (a screening test) is 140 mg/dl or higher, she needs the diagnostic 3-hour oral glucose tolerance test.
29. To increase her sense of control and the likelihood that she will adhere to the therapeutic recommendations
30. Releasing tissue after needle insertion; injection over 2 to 4 seconds; quick needle withdrawal
31. These sugars raise blood glucose levels quickly to high levels and alter glucose control for many hours.
32. rales, dyspnea on exertion, cough, hemoptysis, progressive edema and tachycardia.
33. class III
34. Heparin is the anticoagulant of choice because it does not cross the placenta.
35. Each labor contraction causes up to 500 ml of blood to be shifted from the uterus and placenta to the central circulation. About 500 ml of blood returns to the central circulation when the placenta delivers. The added blood volume increases the diseased heart's workload and can result in congestive heart failure.
36. Her excess weight gain may be caused by excess food, fluid retention from cardiac decompensation or excess salt intake, or preeclampsia (see Chapter 25). Thus you must assess her diet and assess for other signs and symptoms of cardiac decompensation and preeclampsia.
37. Folic acid is needed for cell duplication and the growth of the fetus and placenta. Folic acid deficiency is associated with a higher incidence of neural tube defects. It is difficult to get the required pregnancy amount by diet alone, and folic acid is often destroyed by cooking.

38. Placental infarctions occur that decreases the exchange surface of the placenta
39. pain (abdomen, chest, vertebrae, joints, extremities); pallor; signs of cardiac failure
40. fetal loss, prematurity, preeclampsia, renal complications
41. Many anticonvulsants are associated with significant fetal abnormalities. Yet, without the drugs, grand mal seizures are more likely to occur, which can cause fetal hypoxia, acidosis, and death.
42. Early, acute stage—flu-like symptoms for a few weeks, followed by seroconversion a few weeks or months later
    Middle, asymptomatic period—low-level viral replication and loss of CD4 cells
    Transitional period—symptomatic disease
    Late, crisis period—symptomatic disease
43. Use the information in the text, pp. 661–665, to complete this table.
44. AIDS is said to occur when the immune system does not protect the person and opportunistic infections occur.
45. Zidovudine (recommended for pregnant women); protease inhibitors such as saquinavir (Invirase)
46. Support grieving and retention of client control; promote wellness (nutrition, rest, activity, avoidance of crowds and poor sanitary conditions, skin care); teach that breast feeding is contraindicated; reinforce medication information
47. Use the information in the text, pp. 666-667, to complete this table.

CASE STUDIES

1. The main objective of the nurse's assessment is to identify why Patricia had a sudden excessive weight gain. Pregnancy-induced hypertension is a likely suspect, but the nurse must assess for other possible causes, such as a substantially increased food intake.
2. The staff must determine if Patricia's weight gain is the result of pregnancy-induced hypertension (PIH) and take steps to treat it.
3. The nurse should assess for other signs and symptoms of PIH: hypertension; urine protein; edema, particularly of the face and fingers; epigastric pain; visual disturbances such as spots or blurring; severe and unrelenting headache; dyspnea.
4. A dipstick test to identify proteinuria would be done to identify excessive levels in the urine. Reduced kidney perfusion causes glomerular damage, causing the protein to be lost.
5. The nurse needs Patricia's past pattern of weight gain and her previous vital signs to evaluate today's information more accurately.
6. The nurse should ask Patricia if her rings are tight (finger edema), if she sees spots in front of her eyes or has blurring of vision, or if she has had severe headaches (cerebral edema), if she has upper abdominal pain or nausea (distended liver capsule), and if she has difficulty breathing (pulmonary edema).
7. Refer to Table 25-4 to complete this exercise.
8. Patricia's PIH is mild and the fetal signs are favorable. Because the fetus is 34 weeks, delay of birth would be good unless the PIH worsens. In that case, poor placental perfusion is likely to cause the fetus more problems, including possible fetal demise, than preterm delivery.
9. Teaching involves activity restrictions, including how to achieve them, assessment of fetal activity, maternal blood pressure, weight, and urine protein. The woman and family must be taught what signs and symptoms to report and when to return for fetal surveillance studies and regular prenatal visits.
10. During early pregnancy, fetal demand for glucose tends to cause maternal hypoglycemia. Debra is near the beginning of the second trimester, so increasing resistance to insulin in her cells and more rapid breakdown of insulin occur to make more glucose available to her fetus.

11. Debra will probably need increasing amounts of insulin as her pregnancy progresses. Also, the goal is to keep her blood glucose level as near to normal as possible, so she will need to test her blood glucose as many as five to seven times each day and may take more frequent insulin doses (regular and intermediate-acting). Her diet should have about 2200 to 2400 calories per day distributed among three meals and two to four snacks.
12. Routine prenatal visit testing includes vital signs and fetal heart rate, assessment of her blood glucose levels (including her daily logs), and urinalysis for protein, glucose, and ketones. Glycosylated hemoglobin testing is done as needed.
13. Tests needed as pregnancy progresses are designed to evaluate placental function and fetal health and maturity. These include maternal serum alpha-fetoprotein, ultrasound, fetal echocardiography, "kick counts," nonstress or contraction stress test, biophysical profile, amniotic fluid index, or amniocentesis to evaluate fetal lung maturity. Doppler velocimetry may be performed.
14. Possible fetal effects include congenital defects, large or small fetal size, and persistent fetal hypoxia.
15. Labor may be induced or cesarean delivery performed if the fetus shows signs of decreased placental perfusion with hypoxia. While in labor, Debra will have hourly blood glucose evaluations to determine her need for insulin. Tight glucose control during labor minimizes newborn hypoglycemia.
16. The neonatal nurse should anticipate possible newborn hypoglycemia if the newborn was exposed to high maternal blood glucose in utero, with high fetal insulin secretion to metabolize the glucose. After birth, the glucose supply is cut off while the pancreas continues to secrete large quantities of insulin temporarily
17. The newborn will need frequent blood glucose monitoring for the first few hours after birth. See Chapter 30 for more information about caring for the infant of a diabetic mother.

REVIEW QUESTIONS

1. b
2. d
3. a
4. d
5. c
6. b
7. d
8. b
9. a
10. d
11. c
12. b
13. b
14. a
15. d
16. a
17. c
18. d
19. a
20. b
21. d
22. c
23. b

CHAPTER 27: THE WOMAN WITH AN INTRAPARTUM COMPLICATION

MATCHING KEY TERMS

1. b
2. c
3. d
4. a
5. e

KEY CONCEPTS

1. Uterine contractions must be coordinated, strong enough, and numerous enough to propel the fetus through the woman's pelvis.
2. Use Table 27-1 in the text to complete this exercise.
3. Amniotomy and oxytocin augmentation.
4. All nursing actions center on helping the woman make each push most effective.
5. They add the force of gravity to maternal pushes.
6. a. Help the woman understand that her tissues can distend to accommodate the fetus; apply warm compresses to the perineum.
   b. Teach the woman to push only when she feels the urge or with every other contraction; administer fluids as ordered; offer reassurance.
7. Upright positions favor fetal descent (gravity), and with that descent, fetal head rotation.
8. Uterine overdistention with hypotonic dysfunction, abnormal fetal presentation(s), fetal hypoxia, postpartum hemorrhage due to uterine overdistention
9. a. dilation at least 1.2 cm/hr; descent at least 1.0 cm/hr
   b. dilation at least 1.5 cm/hr; descent at least 2.0 cm/hr
10. For mother: promotion of comfort, conservation of energy, emotional support, position changes that favor normal progress, and assessments for infection; for fetus: observation for signs of intrauterine infection and for compromised fetal oxygenation
11. a. Place her in a side-lying position, administer oxygen, maintain blood volume with nonoxytocin IV fluids, stop oxytocin if in use, administer terbutaline or other tocolytic drug that may be ordered.
    b. Help woman focus on nonpharmacologic pain control methods if analgesia is not possible; remain with the woman.
12. Urinary incontinence, increased vaginal discharge, loss of the mucous plug
13. Points to include are: avoid sexual activity, take temperature 4 times a day and report if >100° F (37.8° C), report contractions.
14. Side effects of beta-adrenergic drugs include maternal and fetal tachycardia, decreased blood pressure, wide pulse pressure, dysrhythmias, myocardial ischemia, chest pain, pulmonary edema, hyperglycemia and hypokalemia, tremors, and restlessness. Propranolol (Inderal), a beta-blocking drug, should be available to reverse the effects.
15. a. Prostaglandin synthesis inhibitors block the action of prostaglandins, which stimulate uterine contractions; an example is indomethacin.
    b. Calcium antagonists block the action of calcium, which is necessary for muscle contraction; an example is nifedipine.
16. In addition to text, refer also to a drug reference manual.
    a. Observe maternal blood pressure, pulse, and respirations and fetal heart rate to identify tachycardia or hypotension; assess lung sounds; assess for presence of dyspnea or chest pain to identify pulmonary edema or myocardial ischemia; obtain ordered glucose and potassium levels; have propranolol available.

b. Observe for urine output of at least 30 ml/hour, presence of deep tendon reflexes, and respirations of at least 12/min; assess heart and lung sounds; observe bowel sounds and assess for constipation; have calcium gluconate available.
c. Observe for nausea, vomiting, and abnormal bleeding; check fundal height; have woman do kick counts to identify fetal movements.
d. Teach about flushing of the skin and headache; observe maternal pulse(report if >110/minute) and fetal heart rates and maternal blood pressure; warn of postural hypotension, and teach to assume a sitting or standing position gradually after lying down.
e. Assess lung sounds; teach woman to report chest pain or heaviness or any difficulty breathing.

17. Complete: cord visible at vaginal opening. Occult prolapsed cord cannot be seen or felt on vaginal examination but is suspected based on fetal heart rate. The cord may slip into the vagina, where it can be felt as a pulsating mass. It may slip outside the vagina, where it is visible.
18. Relieve pressure on the cord with position changes; increase oxygen delivery to the placenta.
19. Complete rupture—open communication between the uterine and peritoneal cavities; incomplete rupture—rupture into the peritoneum or broad ligament but not into the peritoneal cavity; dehiscence—partial separation of a previous uterine scar
20. Pushing on an uncontracted uterus to expel clots after birth may result in uterine inversion. Massage the uterus until it is firm before expelling clots with fundal pressure.
21. Amniotic fluid is rich in thromboplastin, initiating uncontrolled clotting that consumes normal clotting factors.
22. If the mother's condition deteriorates, the fetal condition will inevitably deteriorate also because the fetus is totally dependent on the woman for oxygen, nutrients, and waste removal.
23. Despite stable maternal and fetal vital signs, an enlarging uterus following trauma suggests possible abruptio placentae. Notify the physician promptly.

CASE STUDIES

1. The nurse must (a) attempt to verify whether Ann's membranes have ruptured, but without performing a vaginal examination; (b) determine when they ruptured; (c) assess maternal vital signs and fetal heart rate, looking specifically for signs of infection; (d) assess for contractions that may indicate preterm labor as well as preterm PROM.
2. Fluid draining from the vagina; positive Nitrazine and fern test; cloudy fluid; fetal tachycardia; occasional contraction
3. The vaginal fluid drainage and the positive Nitrazine and fern tests suggest that Ann's membranes have ruptured. Infection is suggested by the cloudy fluid and fetal tachycardia. Contractions suggest possible preterm labor.
4. A vaginal examination is not advised because the vaginal discharge is typical of amniotic fluid (meaning that membranes are truly ruptured), there already appears to be an infection, Ann's gestation is preterm, and she is already having contractions. Little information is likely to be gained from the examination, and it might introduce more microorganisms into the uterus.
5. Starting intravenous fluids should be the top priority because (a) hydration with fluids may stop preterm labor contractions and (b) venous access may be needed quickly for emergency procedures.
6. A side-lying position with the head of the bed low increases placental blood flow and reduces pressure of the fetal presenting part on the cervix. Bedrest may reduce uterine activity.

7. Urine output of at least 30 ml/hour, presence of deep tendon reflexes, and respiratory rate of at least 12/minute suggest that the magnesium is within safe limits. Serum drug levels will also be ordered (see Chapter 26 for additional information).
8. Teach her the importance of maintaining even spacing of the drug; set her alarm clock to take terbutaline during the night; expect side effects such as palpitations, tremors, restlessness, weakness, or headache. Report heart rate over 110/minute, chest pain, or dyspnea.
9. Explain the activity restrictions her doctor recommends, and explore with her how she can maintain them. Teach signs and symptoms of recurrent preterm labor, and tell her to return to the hospital if they occur. Teach her the relationship of hydration and uterine irritability, and tell her to drink at least 8 full glasses of water each day. Teach her signs of urinary tract infection to report—urgency, increased frequency, and pain.

REVIEW QUESTIONS

1. c
2. b
3. d
4. a
5. c
6. a
7. d
8. b
9. d
10. b
11. c
12. d
13. a

CHAPTER 28: THE WOMAN WITH A POSTPARTUM COMPLICATION

MATCHING KEY TERMS

1. c
2. b
3. e
4. d
5. f
6. a

KEY CONCEPTS

1. Early postpartum hemorrhage occurs within 24 hours of birth; late hemorrhage occurs after this time. More than 500 ml of blood after vaginal birth or more than 1000 ml of blood after cesarean birth constitutes postpartum hemorrhage.
2. Uterine atony occurs when the figure-8 muscle fibers of the uterus do not contract firmly to compress bleeding endometrial vessels at the placental site.
3. The uterus is difficult to locate, and when found it is soft rather than firm and higher than the expected level near the umbilicus. It may become firm with massage but fails to remain firm. Lochia is excessive, more than one *saturated* pad per hour.

4. Support the lower uterus with one hand while gently but firmly massaging the fundus until it contracts. Push on the fundus *after the uterus is firm* to express clots that have accumulated in the uterine cavity and could interfere with continued uterine contraction. Check for a distended bladder, often indicated when the uterus is displaced to one side (usually the right). Have her urinate or catheterize her if necessary. Drugs such as oxytocin or methylergonovine may be needed to maintain uterine contraction. Maintain intravenous access.
5. Excess, usually brighter red, bleeding in the presence of a firmly contracted uterus that is in the expected location suggests a laceration.
6. Pain is the greatest distinction because confined bleeding exerts pressure on sensory nerves. The uterus is firm, excluding uterine atony as the cause. Lochia is normal because the bleeding is concealed, excluding a bleeding laceration. A rising pulse and respiratory rate and falling blood pressure are signs of hypovolemia that may occur with any type of hemorrhage.
7. a. Stimulation of baroreceptors and release of catecholamines result in vasoconstriction of peripheral blood vessels and rising heart rate and blood pressure. Gradual tachycardia is typically the earliest sign of hypovolemia. Respirations increase as the woman attempts to increase her intake of oxygen. The skin is pale and cool, and capillary refill is prolonged.
   b. Inadequate perfusion results in buildup of lactic acid and metabolic acidosis, resulting in vasodilation, which accelerates blood loss. The skin becomes cold and clammy. Urine output falls or even stops as circulation to the kidneys is reduced. When blood volume is inadequate to perfuse the brain and heart, death results.
8. Women should be told the normal sequence, amount, and duration of lochia. They should be taught assessment and expected descent of the fundus. Guidelines should be provided for reporting deviations from normal.
9. They have higher levels of clotting factors (fibrinogen, factors III, VIII, and X) and suppression of factors that prevent clot formation (plasminogen activator and antithrombin III). Also, venous stasis occurs and possible blood vessel injuries.
10. Refer to "Thromboembolic Disorders" in the text to complete this chart.
11. Heparin: activated partial thromboplastin time (aPTT). Warfarin: prothrombin time and International Normalized Ratio (INR).
12. Teach heparin injection technique to client and a family member, as appropriate. Teach client to report unusual bruising or petechiae, nosebleeds, bloody urine, bleeding gums, or increased vaginal bleeding; use a soft toothbrush; and do not go barefoot. Teach side effects of the specific anticoagulant. Caution about drugs or alcohol, which should not be taken with the specific anticoagulant. Teach when to return for laboratory studies.
13. Signs and symptoms vary according to the degree of pulmonary blood flow obstruction but include sudden sharp chest pain, tachycardia, dyspnea, tachypnea, pulmonary rales, cough, hemoptysis, decreased partial pressure of oxygen (arterial blood gases), and atelectasis and pleural effusion seen on x-ray.
14. A temperature of 38° C (100.4° F) or higher after the first 24 hours, occurring on at least 2 days during the first 10 days following birth
15. All the parts of the female reproductive tract are connected to each other and to the peritoneal cavity. The area is richly supplied with blood vessels and lymphatics, providing a well-nourished, dark, warm environment that favors bacterial growth.
16. Amniotic fluid, blood, and lochia make the normally acidic vagina more alkaline, fostering growth of organisms. The necrotic endometrial lining with lochia promotes growth of anaerobic organisms. Small areas of trauma allow microorganisms to enter the tissues. However, granulocytes in the endometrium and lochia help prevent infection. Aseptic technique and careful handwashing avoid transfer of organisms to the mother.
17. These signs suggest a paralytic ileus caused by spread of the infection into the peritoneal cavity. The nurse should assess bowel sounds and report all findings to the physician.

18. edema, warmth, redness, pain, separation of edges, seropurulent drainage
19. Apricot, plum, prune, and cranberry juices help acidify urine, which makes the urine less friendly to microorganisms.
20. Stasis of milk promotes growth of infecting microorganisms, possibly leading to abscess.
21. Septic thrombophlebitis also involves infection and usually affects the ovarian, uterine, or hypogastric veins. It requires antibiotic and anticoagulant treatment.
22. Postpartum depression symptoms include *persistent* loss of interest in surroundings and loss of loving or pleasurable feelings; *persistent* fatigue, complaints of ill health, and difficulty concentrating; *persistent* loss of interest in food; and *persistent* sleep disturbances. It is the persistence of these behaviors and feelings that marks the difference.
23. Bipolar disorder is characterized by both manic episodes (with irritability, hyperactivity, euphoria, grandiosity, little sleep, and poor judgment) and depressive episodes (characterized by tearfulness, preoccupations of guilt, feelings of worthlessness, sleep and appetite disturbances, and inordinate concern with the baby's health or delusions about the baby's being dead or defective). Major depression has only the depression features, not the manic features.

CASE STUDY

1. The medication could be taking longer than usual to exert its analgesic properties, it could be outdated, Jana's pain tolerance at this time could be very low, or other birth trauma may have occurred. In addition, although Jana's fundal height is appropriate, she may need to urinate since it has been 1½ hours since birth and her bladder may be fuller than it seems.
2. The nurse needs more information about the pain: location, intensity on a 1 to 10 scale (comparing its present level with the level before she took the analgesic), character, and if anything worsens or improves it. In addition, the nurse must look at Jana's perineal area for evidence of a hematoma.
3. If Jana still has not voided, the nurse should carefully assess her bladder and place her on the bedpan to void. However, Jana's symptoms suggest a concealed hemorrhage with early hypovolemia: unrelieved pain and a rising pulse in the presence of a firm fundus and normal lochia. Unrelieved pain is not typical of a full bladder, although it may worsen the pain of a hematoma. Therefore, Jana should not ambulate to the bathroom because of the higher risk of fainting. If she does not void promptly, it would be appropriate to catheterize her (assuming there is an order), both to see if emptying her bladder relieves the pain and to determine her urine output, which is a significant indicator of fluid volume status. The physician or nurse-midwife should be promptly notified of all assessments and interventions.

REVIEW QUESTIONS

1. c
2. a
3. b
4. d
5. b
6. a
7. c
8. d
9. a
10. c

CHAPTER 29: THE HIGH-RISK NEWBORN: PROBLEMS RELATED TO GESTATIONAL AGE AND DEVELOPMENT

MATCHING KEY TERMS

1. d
2. e
3. c
4. b
5. a
6. a
7. b or c
8. c
9. b or c
10. a
11. c
12. a
13. c
14. b or c
15. c
16. a or c
17. b or c
18. a
19. c
20. a
21. b
22. b or c
23. a
24. b or c

KEY CONCEPTS

1. a. born before the 38th week of gestation begins
   b. birth weight 2500 g (5 pounds, 8 ounces) or less
   c. birth weight 1500 g (3 pounds, 5 ounces) or less
   d. birth weight 1000 g (2 pounds, 3 ounces) or less
   e. birth weight less than expected for duration of gestation
2. Periodic breathing is cessation of breathing for 5 to 10 seconds without other changes; apneic spells last over 15 seconds and/or are accompanied by cyanosis and bradycardia.
3. The prone position is associated with an increased incidence of sudden infant death syndrome (SIDS). However, the prone position allows the immature preterm infant to use respiratory muscles more efficiently, reduces respiratory effort, and increases oxygenation and lung compliance.
4. Hydration keeps secretions thin so they are more easily removed.
5. Thin skin with little insulating fat, less heat-producing brown fat accumulation, poor flexion to reduce exposed body surfaces, immature temperature control center in the brain
6. Radiant warmers, incubators, warmed oxygen, measures to reduce air currents, transparent plastic blanket over the radiant warmer bed, keeping portholes of incubators closed as much as possible, heated blankets and hats when out of the incubator or radiant warmer, padding surfaces with warmed blankets when procedures are done
7. Greater water loss through the thin, permeable skin, nonflexed positioning that increases insensible losses, drying effects of outside heat sources, rapid respiratory

rate and use of oxygen, poor ability of kidneys to concentrate or dilute urine before 35 weeks of gestation, and poor ability of kidneys to regulate electrolytes
8. Weighing diapers to determine the difference between the dry weight and the wet weight; collecting urine with cotton balls at the perineum to check specific gravity; weighing the unclothed infant daily or twice daily on the same scale at the same time of day
9. Dehydration: decreased urine output, increased weight loss, increased urine specific gravity, dry skin or mucous membranes, sunken fontanel, poor tissue turgor, increased blood sodium, protein, and hematocrit; overhydration: increased urine output with below-normal specific gravity, edema, too-rapid weight gain, bulging fontanel, decreased blood sodium, protein, and hematocrit
10. Maternal infection, incomplete passive antibody transfer from the mother during the third trimester, immature immune response, therapeutic procedures that are often invasive and damage their delicate skin
11. Poor suck, swallow, and breathing coordination; immature gag reflex; high expenditure of energy for sucking related to the nutrients ingested
12. Aspirate for residual from previous feeding, measure abdominal circumference to identify distention, test stool for reducing substance with Clinitest tablet, and test for occult blood in stool.
13. Association of the comfort of fullness with sucking; preparation for nipple feeding.
14. Breast milk has immunologic benefits; it is more easily digested; it provides enzymes, hormones, and growth factors; it causes less stress because the baby can better regulate respirations and suckling; the mother's body keeps the baby warm.
15. Tachypnea, nasal flaring, retractions, cyanosis, grunting on expiration, decreased or wet breath sounds, acidosis with hypoxemia; chest x-ray showing "ground-glass" appearance or atelectasis
16. bronchopulmonary dysplasia and retinopathy of prematurity.
17. Placental deterioration with chronic hypoxia, weight loss, oligohydramnios, and meconium passage into the amniotic fluid; continued placental function, with continued growth that increases the risk for birth injury or cesarean birth
18. a. poor glycogen stores at birth
    b. little insulating subcutaneous fat
    c. Polycythemia secondary to intrauterine hypoxemia, with more erythrocyte breakdown after birth
19. Symmetrical: infant is smaller than normal for gestation but head, chest, length, and weight are proportionate; problem began early in pregnancy. Asymmetrical: head, chest, and length are normal but weight is decreased; problem began during second half of pregnancy. Infants that have symmetrical growth retardation are more likely to have long-term consequences.
20. Fractures of the clavicle, damage to brachial plexus or facial nerve, cephalhematoma, and bruising.

CASE STUDY

1. The most likely nursing diagnoses are ineffective infant feeding pattern related to fatigue when nursing; risk for ineffective thermoregulation related to immaturity of temperature regulation and minimal body fat; knowledge deficit (parents) related to special needs of the preterm infant
2. Point out how Kaylee has begun to gain weight. Emphasize the benefits of the mother's breast milk for a preterm infant, even if some must be given by gavage. Encourage the parents to hold and stroke Kaylee to the limits of her tolerance, and point out when she responds positively to them. Involve the parents in her care. Gradually have the parents take over more of her care while observing unobtrusively. Place her name on the incubator to personalize it. Note her individual responses to

care, such as likes and dislikes or amusing habits. Provide visual stimulation (as tolerated), as you would for other newborns. Give parents the telephone number to the nursery, and encourage them to call at any time. If available, refer them to a parental support group.

REVIEW QUESTIONS

1. b
2. c
3. a
4. d
5. b
6. a
7. c

CHAPTER 30: THE HIGH-RISK NEWBORN: ACQUIRED AND CONGENITAL CONDITIONS

MATCHING KEY TERMS

1. c
2. a
3. e
4. b
5. d

KEY CONCEPTS

1. In primary apnea, the infant may respond to stimulation when respirations cease. In secondary apnea, the infant does not respond to stimulation and loses consciousness. Secondary apnea is more ominous because stimulation is not enough to reverse it, blood oxygen levels decrease further, and the infant loses consciousness.
2. Refer to text, under each of the titles to complete this exercise.
3. Bilirubin is the waste product of excess erythrocyte breakdown after birth. Jaundice is the staining of the skin and sclerae by bilirubin. Kernicterus occurs when the bilirubin levels are high enough to stain the brain tissue. Bilirubin encephalopathy is an extension of kernicterus to include damage to brain tissue by the bilirubin staining.
4. Bilirubin encephalopathy is more likely to occur at lower bilirubin levels in the preterm infant than in the term infant.
5. Refer to text, Nursing Care Plan 30-1, and "Parents Want to Know: Home Care for the Infant Receiving Phototherapy," to formulate your explanation.
6. Exchange transfusion replaces the infant's blood that has high levels of bilirubin, low erythrocytes, and many sensitized erythrocytes with blood that has normal levels of these components. Also, the blood that replaces the infant's blood is not sensitive to the circulating antibodies from the mother that have destroyed the infant's own erythrocytes.
7. a. hepatitis B, rubella
   b. candidiasis, which may also occur in the infant with AIDS
   c. cytomegalovirus, herpes (with disseminated infection), rubella, toxoplasmosis
   d. group B streptococcal infection
   e. gonorrhea, Chlamydia
   f. human immunodeficiency virus/AIDS

8. immune system immaturity, with a slower reaction to invading organisms; poor localization of infection that allows more extensive spread of infection; less effective blood-brain barrier
9. Early-onset sepsis is related to prolonged rupture of membranes, prolonged labor, or chorioamnionitis; it begins within 24 hours of birth and progresses more rapidly. Mortality is 5% to 20%. It often involves the respiratory system or central nervous system. Late-onset sepsis develops after 1 week and is caused by exposure to organisms after birth. It usually involves the central nervous system. Mortality is 5% with frequent long-term effects.
10. Signs of infection are often subtle. They include temperature instability, respiratory problems, and changes in feeding habits or behavior. Septic shock can develop quickly.
11. Blood is analyzed at the highest (peak) and lowest (trough) levels to provide a basis for any needed changes in dosage and to prevent toxic effects on body tissues.
12. If the diabetic woman has vascular changes, placental blood flow may be reduced, interfering with fetal growth. If the diabetic woman does not have vascular changes and her glucose levels are poorly controlled, she transfers large amounts of nutrients to the fetus. The fetus secretes large amounts of insulin to metabolize these nutrients, resulting in macrosomia.
13. a. High fetal insulin levels interfere with surfactant production.
    b. Maternal glucose supply ends, but the infant temporarily continues a high level of insulin production.
    c. Parathyroid hormone production is reduced.
    d. Poor oxygenation requires that the fetus make more erythrocytes.
14. Length and head circumference are usually normal for the gestational age. The face is round and red, the body is obese, and muscle tone is poor. The infant is irritable and may have tremors when disturbed.
15. Signs include jitteriness, tremors, diaphoresis, rapid respirations, low temperature, poor muscle tone.
16. to prevent sluggish blood flow and ischemia to vital organs
17. Infants appear hungry, but suck and swallow are poorly coordinated; frequent regurgitation, vomiting, and diarrhea; signs typical of hypoglycemia but with a normal blood glucose level; restlessness; failure to gain weight. Frequent regurgitation, vomiting, diarrhea.
18. The infant has poor coordination of suck and swallow, reducing actual milk intake. At the same time, energy expenditure is high because of excess activity.
19. mental retardation

CASE STUDY

1. The positive Coombs' test done on cord blood obtained at birth indicates that antibodies from the mother have attached to the infant's red blood cells.
2. Monitoring of Steven's bilirubin level and skin color for jaundice are essential related assessments.
3. Phototherapy is the appropriate treatment at this time. The light causes bilirubin in the skin to change into a water-soluble form that can be excreted.
4. Nursing interventions related to phototherapy include the following:
    - Cover the infant's closed eyes with patches to prevent light damage. Check placement of the patches hourly. Cover the reproductive organs with a diaper or other covering.
    - Change the infant's position every 2 hours to distribute light exposure evenly over the skin surface. Check the fiberoptic blanket at the same intervals to ensure maximum exposure of the skin surface.

- Check the infant's temperature every 2 to 4 hours. Place a skin probe on the infant if in an incubator.
- Monitor intake and output. Weighing diapers is the most accurate output measurement.
- Remove the infant from the lights as little as possible, such as for feeding or other care. This will not be necessary if a phototherapy blanket is used.

5. Side effects may include frequent loose, green stools; a tanned appearance in dark-skinned infants; skin rash; or temporary lactose intolerance.
6. High bilirubin levels may cause kernicterus, with possible bilirubin encephalopathy as bilirubin deposits cause staining of the brain. Bilirubin encephalopathy has a high mortality, and survivors may suffer cerebral palsy, mental retardation, hearing loss, or other neurologic and developmental problems.
7. Steven should have an exchange transfusion to replace blood that has a high bilirubin level because of massive erythrocyte destruction with blood that is not affected by maternal antibodies in Steven's system. It is essential to prevent kernicterus and possible encephalopathy.
8. Type O Rh-negative blood that is cross-matched to be compatible with the mother's is transfused. The transfused blood is not affected by the maternal antibodies circulating in Steven's system.
9. The exchange transfusion is performed by removing 5 to 10 ml of Steven's blood and replacing it with an equal amount of donor blood. This process is continued until about twice his blood volume has been exchanged.
10. The expected results are that about 85% of Steven's erythrocytes will be replaced and the bilirubin will be reduced to about 45% of the pre-exchange level.
11. Complications of exchange transfusion may include infection, hypervolemia, hypovolemia, cardiac arrhythmias, hypocalcemia.
12. The nurse's role in the procedure is to prepare equipment and the blood, assess the infant during and after the procedure, and keep accurate records of blood withdrawn and infused. The transfusion is done under a radiant warmer with a cardiac monitor in place.

REVIEW QUESTIONS

1. b
2. d
3. a
4. d
5. b
6. b
7. d

CHAPTER 31: WOMEN'S HEALTH CARE

MATCHING KEY TERMS

1. h
2. a
3. b
4. g
5. e
6. c
7. f
8. d

KEY CONCEPTS

1. obesity, inactivity, and smoking
2. Monthly by all women older than 20 years; 1 week after the menstrual period begins or on a specific day of the month if she is not menstruating
3. Yearly starting with women at the age of 40. Earlier screenings may be recommended for women at high risk for breast cancer.
4. Monthly for women over age 18 and by those under age 18 if sexually active
5. Schedule the examination about 2 weeks after her menstrual period; do not douche or have sexual intercourse for at least 48 hours before the examination; do not use vaginal medications, sprays or deodorants.
6. a. Firm, hard, freely movable nodules that may or may not be tender and do not change during the menstrual cycle; observation with possible excision and pathologic analysis
   b. Thickening or multiple smooth, well-delineated nodules; tenderness and pain noticeable during the latter half of the menstrual cycle; fine needle aspiration with possible open biopsy if fluid is bloody; drugs not usually prescribed
   c. Firm, irregular mass with enlarged axillary nodes and nipple retraction and discharge; surgical biopsy; no treatment if ductal ectasia is confirmed
   d. Serous or serosanguineous discharge from the nipple; excision of mass and duct with analysis of discharge to rule out malignancy
7. Surgical therapy removes part or all of the breast. Adjuvant therapy may include radiation, chemotherapy, immunotherapy and hormone therapy. Breast reconstruction assists in the psychologic recovery.
8. a. Absence of menses by the normal age of menstruation if the girl has breast or pubic hair development. Causes: Turner's syndrome (single X chromosome) exposure to diethylstilbestrol, abnormal reproductive tract development, hormonal imbalances, systemic disease, hypothalamic-pituitary abnormalities, excessive exercises or eating disorders.
   b. Cessation of menses for 6 months in a woman who has established menstruation. Causes: systemic disease, hormonal imbalances, strenuous aerobic exercise, poor nutrition, oral contraceptives, and ovarian tumors; pregnancy is a normal cause.
9. Pregnancy complications, anatomic lesions (benign or malignant), drug-induced bleeding, systemic disorders, failure to ovulate
10. Urge the woman to seek medical help. Help the woman record bleeding episodes and associated symptoms. Teach about needed lifestyle changes.
11. a. Mild analgesics and reassurance about the cause of the discomfort
    b. Oral contraceptives and prostaglandin-inhibiting drugs such as NSAIDs
    c. Medications to suppress endometrial tissue proliferation. Medication to suppress ovarian hormones; hysterectomy with bilateral salpingo-oophorectomy; lysis of adhesions and laser vaporization of the lesions
12. Urge the woman to seek a thorough examination to diagnose her problem properly. Teach dietary changes, exercises, stress management, and techniques to promote sleep and rest (refer to "Women Want to Know: How to Relieve Symptoms of PMS").
13. Refer to "Medical Termination of Pregnancy" in your textbook to complete this exercise.
14. Postmenopausal bleeding suggests endometrial cancer.
15. Estrogen alone would cause endometrial hyperplasia if the woman has her uterus.
16. Breast cancer, heart disease
17. Initially, no signs occur. When they appear, they include loss of height, back pain, the "dowager's hump," disappearance of the waistline, and abdominal protrusion. Fractures of the hip, vertebrae, and wrist are the most common osteoporosis-associated breaks.
18. Periodic pelvic examinations, Pap tests, ultrasonography, and tests for tumor markers

19. Refer to your text, "Infectious Disorders of the Reproductive Tract" to complete this exercise.
20. Bacteria, often *C. trachomatis* and *N. gonorrhoeae*, ascend through the cervix into the upper reproductive tract and pelvic cavity. Here the organisms cause a chronic inflammatory response that causes scarring of the fallopian tubes and adhesions near the tubes. Infertility is a common result.

REVIEW QUESTIONS

1. c
2. d
3. a
4. c
5. b
6. a
7. d
8. d
9. c

CHAPTER 32: COMMUNICATING WITH CHILDREN AND FAMILIES

MATCHING KEY TERMS

1. c
2. f
3. e
4. d
5. a
6. b
7. g

COMPONENTS OF EFFECTIVE COMMUNICATION

8. T
9. F
10. T
11. F
12. T
13. F
14. T
15. F

FAMILY-CENTERED COMMUNICATION

16. Family-centered care emphasizes that the family is intricately involved in the care of the child. Health care professionals and families become partners in the care of the child. Family-centered care recognizes that the family has a right to participate in planning, implementing, and evaluating the child's plan of care.
17. Include all family members; encourage families to write down their questions; remain nonjudgmental; give families both verbal and nonverbal messages that convey openness and availability; respect and encourage feedback from families; avoid assumptions about core family beliefs and values; and respect family diversity.

18. Convey genuine respect and concern during the first encounter.
19. Understand the parents' perspectives; determine a common goal and stay focused on it; seek win-win solutions; listen actively; openly express your feelings; avoid blaming; and summarize the decision.
20. As demographics change, nurses face the challenge of providing culturally competent care. Culture influences a family's values and beliefs, as well as communication style, methods of decision making, and other behaviors related to health care practices.

THERAPEUTIC RELATIONSHIPS: DEVELOPING AND MAINTAINING TRUST

21. Buying gifts for certain children, giving out a home telephone number, competing with other staff for the child/family's affections, inviting child/family to social gatherings, accepting invitations to family gatherings, visiting child/family during off-duty time, revealing personal information, loaning money, and making decisions for the family about the child's care.

NURSING CARE: COMMUNICATING WITH CHILDREN AND FAMILIES

22. T
23. T
24. F
25. F
26. Something along the lines of: "I am going to take off the old bandage and put on a new one."
27. Something along the lines of: "I am going to take you to a different room now. You can stay in this room while you are at the hospital."
28. Something along the lines of: "I am going to give you medicine through a small needle."
29. Something along the lines of: "I am going to measure your temperature" or "I am going to listen to your heart beating with my stethoscope."

COMMUNICATING WITH CHILDREN WHO HAVE SPECIAL NEEDS

30. Assess the child's self-help skills, orient child to surroundings, encourage parents to stay with child, keep furniture and objects in same places, explain sounds that child may hear, identify yourself when entering room, explain all procedures, keep call light in same place, and allow child to handle equipment.
31. Assess the child's self-help skills, identify family's method of communicating and adopt it, encourage parents to stay with child, learn the child's sign language, develop a communication board, make sure hearing aids work, enter room cautiously and touch child gently before speaking, face child when speaking, do not shout or exaggerate speech, use play to communicate and demonstrate procedures, have another person stand in front of the child if a procedure requires standing behind the child.
32. Assume the child can see, hear, and comprehend something in what is said; use a friendly tone of voice; address the child when entering and leaving the room; gently touch child when saying his name; speak softly and slowly; do not talk as if the child were not there; explain all procedures as they are being done; talk to the child about activities and objects in the room; allow adequate time for child to respond to simple questions; ascertain child's ability to respond to simple questions; be attentive for signs and gestures that indicate likes or dislikes; and document techniques that work.

REVIEW QUESTIONS

1. b
2. b
3. d
4. b
5. a
6. d
7. c

CHAPTER 33: PHYSICAL ASSESSMENT OF CHILDREN

MATCHING KEY TERMS

1. g
2. d
3. i
4. l
5. j
6. a
7. m
8. e
9. h
10. k
11. c
12. f
13. b

GENERAL APPROACHES TO PHYSICAL ASSESSMENT

14. T
15. T
16. F
17. F
18. T
19. T

TECHNIQUES FOR PHYSICAL EXAMINATION

20. indirect
21. fingertips
22. back of the hand
23. dull
24. bell
25. b
26. a
27. c
28. T
29. T
30. F
31. T
32. T

33. Use a measuring board or use a tape measure with the infant lying flat.
34. It provides some indication of nutritional status and may detect tumor growth or an abnormal rate of development.
35. balanced
36. nipple line
37. muscle mass; fat
38. 22
39. a. age, gender; b. horizontal; c. vertical; d. intersect; e. percentile
40. vitiligo
41. abdomen; upper arm
42. alopecia; hirsutism
43. hair
44. 1 to 2
45. V (trigeminal); VII (facial)
46. allergies
47. notch between the nose and upper lip
48. Ask the child to stick out the tongue as though licking a lollipop and observe for any deviation of the tongue to one side.
49. X (vagus)
50. b
51. e
52. d
53. a
54. f
55. c
56. F
57. T
58. F
59. T
60. F
61. T
62. F
63. when they have reached menarche
64. so that auscultation is not affected by percussion and palpation
65. At a site away from the tenderness, place your hand perpendicular to the abdomen, press down slowly and deeply, then lift your hand quickly.
66. Explain procedures, be honest and direct, and use a matter-of-fact approach.
67. to screen for testicular cancer, which has a high incidence in young men
68. b
69. a
70. d
71. e
72. c
73. T
74. F
75. T
76. F
77. T
78. T
79. T
80. F

REVIEW QUESTIONS

1. d
2. c
3. b
4. a
5. b
6. d
7. d
8. a
9. b
10. c

CHAPTER 34: EMERGENCY CARE OF THE CHILD

MATCHING KEY TERMS

1. b
2. d
3. h
4. c
5. e
6. g
7. a
8. f

GENERAL GUIDELINES FOR EMERGENCY NURSING CARE

9. Communicate an attitude of calm confidence, establish a trusting relationship with the child and family, try to avoid separating the child and parents, designate one staff member as caretaker of the child and liaison to the parents, tell the truth, provide incentives and rewards, and assess the child's unspoken thoughts and feelings.
10. Encourage the family members to move to a quiet place; encourage them to talk about their feelings as opposed to the facts and to use reflective statements; avoid defensiveness, explanation, or justification of your own or others' behaviors; speak in simple sentences;
11. f
12. b
13. d
14. g
15. c
16. a
17. e

GROWTH AND DEVELOPMENT ISSUES IN EMERGENCY CARE

18. c
19. b
20. e
21. a
22. d

The Family of a Child in Emergency Care

23. fear; anxiety

Emergency Assessment of Infants and Children

24. The triage nurse performs the initial observation in the emergency setting and decides the level of care needed for the child.
25. respiratory rate and effort, skin color, response to the environment
26. A: airway assessment; B: breathing assessment; C: cardiovascular assessment; D: disability (neurologic assessment); E: exposure
27. T
28. T
29. F
30. T
31. F
32. measuring of vital signs; assessment for pain; history and head-to-toe assessment, and inspection
33. respiratory rate, pulse, temperature, blood pressure
34. A: allergies; M: medications taken, immunization history; P: prior illness or injuries, L: last meal, eating habits, E: events leading up to this illness or injury
35. complete blood count with differential count, serum electrolytes, glucose, and urinalysis
36. All medication dosages and fluid amounts are calculated according to the child's weight in kilograms.

Cardiopulmonary Resuscitation of the Child

37. shock and respiratory failure
38. 20 per minute; 3
39. Perform the Heimlich maneuver.
40. Perform abdominal thrusts. The lay rescuer should use CPR.
41. A blind finger sweep is not performed because of the risk of forcing the object farther down into the airway.
42. Place infant in downward-slanting position and administer five back blows, alternating with five chest thrusts.
43. brachial artery; carotid artery
44. 100 compressions per minute
45. epinephrine

THE CHILD IN SHOCK

46. H
47. C
48. D
49. D
50. C
51. C
52. H
53. F
54. F
55. F

PEDIATRIC TRAUMA

56. F
57. T
58. T
59. T
60. F
61. T
62. Assess and manage life-threatening injuries.
63. assessment and management of airway, breathing, circulation, and disability (neurologic deficits)
64. Assess for pain, inspect and document any and all signs of injury by performing a head-to-toe assessment, and obtain a history of the injury.
65. Motor vehicle: Was child wearing a seat belt or sitting in a child's car safety seat? What type of seat belt? What was the speed of the vehicle? With what did the vehicle collide? At what point on the motor vehicle was the location of impact? Where was the victim seated in the vehicle? How much damage was done to the vehicle? Fall: How far did the child fall? How did the child land? On what type of ground did the child land? Did any objects "break" the child's fall? Penetrating injury: How long and wide was the blade of the knife? How far away was the gun when it was fired? What type of gun was used? What was the caliber of the gun?
66. Indicators: history inconsistent with physical findings; activity leading to the trauma inconsistent with the child's age and condition; delay in seeking treatment for the trauma; history of other emergency visits. Physical findings: bruises and fractures in various stages of healing, injuries that are unusual for children, patterns of injury indicating a specific object caused the injury
67. continuous assessment of the child's respiratory, circulatory, and neurologic status

INGESTIONS AND POISONINGS

68. oral ingestion
69. removing the toxic substance, diluting the toxin, performing gastric lavage, administering activated charcoal, giving specific antidote for the toxic substance
70. F
71. T
72. T
73. T
74. T
75. F
76. T
77. F
78. T
79. What substance was ingested? How much was ingested? What was the approximate time of ingestion? Has the child's condition changed from the time of ingestion? What treatment was administered at home?

ANIMAL, HUMAN, AND SNAKE BITES

80. bite marks that look like fangs, burning at the site, ecchymosis and erythema, pain or numbness, and edema
81. wound irrigation and debridement; tetanus prophylaxis if not current; antibiotics if there is a high probability of infection

SUBMERSION INJURIES

82. hypoxia
83. The diving reflex is stimulated when the face is submerged in cold water. Blood is shunted away from the periphery, increasing blood flow to the brain and heart.
84. respiratory system
85. hope

HEAT-RELATED EMERGENCIES

86. Moving the child to a cool place, and starting additional cooling measures.
87. Move the child to a cool place; start additional cooling measures such as loosening/removing wet clothes, and applying cool, dry clothes. Offer oral fluids if there is no alteration in mental status or vomiting.
88. hot, dry, red skin; change in level of consciousness or coma; rapid, weak pulse; rapid, shallow breathing; elevated core body temperature (>105° F)

DENTAL EMERGENCIES

89. F
90. T

REVIEW QUESTIONS

1. c
2. c
3. d
4. a
5. b
6. c
7. d
8. d
9. a
10. a
11. c
12. a
13. c
14. c
15. a

CHAPTER 35: THE ILL CHILD IN THE HOSPITAL AND OTHER CARE SETTINGS

MATCHING KEY TERMS

1. e
2. d
3. f
4. c
5. a
6. b

SETTINGS OF CARE

7. hospital (including 24-hour observation, emergency hospitalization, outpatient/day facilities, medical-surgical unit, intensive care unit, and rehabilitative care), school-based clinics, community clinics, and home care
8. T
9. T
10. F
11. F
12. T
13. T
14. T
15. T

STRESSORS ASSOCIATED WITH ILLNESS AND HOSPITALIZATION

16. child's age, cognitive development, preparation, coping skills, culture, previous experiences with the health care system, and parents' reactions to the illness
17. infant; toddler
18. Protest: Child is agitated, resists caregivers, cries, and is inconsolable. Denial: Child is hopeless, quiet, withdrawn, and apathetic. Detachment: Child may ignore parents but is interested in environment, plays, and seems to form relationships with caregivers and other children.
19. The child does not wish to be separated from parents, and acting out is a way of expressing these feelings.
20. The nurse should ask parents about the toddler's home routines (feeding, bathing, bedtime) and try to adapt hospital routines to what the toddler is accustomed.
21. Because preschoolers lack an understanding of body integrity, they fear mutilation and are afraid of bodily harm from invasive procedures.
22. Involving the school-age child in his/her care may promote a sense of control. This may include making menu selections, keeping the room neat, playing with younger children, and assisting with treatments.
23. They do not want to draw attention to themselves. So they may eat the wrong foods or skip their medications or glucose monitoring.
24. regression in toileting or self-feeding skills; temper tantrums; clinging; crying

FACTORS AFFECTING A CHILD'S RESPONSE TO ILLNESS AND HOSPITALIZATION

25. child's age, level of cognitive development, parent's response to illness or hospitalization, preparation, and coping skills
26. Blowing bubbles or blowing on a pin wheel to promote relaxed breathing, using imagery for the older child, using distraction techniques such as singing, playing games, and reading books
27. increased self-confidence and self-esteem, mastery of self-care skills, learning new information, and an increase in coping skills.

PLAYROOMS IN HEALTH CARE SETTINGS

28. They differ in design and intent. Therapeutic play is guided by health team members to help meet the physical and psychologic needs of the child.
29. Dramatic play in which the child acts out or dramatizes real-life physical or emotional stressors.
30. The playroom should have no association with unpleasant experiences. The child should not receive any treatments (including medications) in the playroom.

31. A reward system can be used in which the child receives a reward when a goal is met. Another example is allowing the child to blow bubbles or a whistle as a fun way to do deep breathing exercises.

ADMITTING THE CHILD TO A HOSPITAL SETTING

32. Admission should not be a series of questions directed at the child and family but a time of collaboration between nurse and family. The nurse should be aware of the child's and family's needs and should structure the admission process to meet those needs.
33. nutrition, elimination, sleep, self care and emotional status

THE ILL CHILD'S FAMILY

34. Parents may experience a loss of control in the unfamiliar environment of the hospital. Parents may be confused as to what they can and cannot do for their child.
35. Siblings may experience jealousy, insecurity, resentment, confusion, and anxiety.

DEVELOPMENTAL APPROACHES TO THE HOSPITALIZED CHILD

36. c
37. f
38. d
39. d
40. e
41. b
42. a

REVIEW QUESTIONS

1. b
2. c
3. d
4. d
5. a
6. c
7. d
8. c
9. d
10. d

CHAPTER 36: THE CHILD WITH A CHRONIC CONDITION OR TERMINAL ILLNESS

MATCHING KEY TERMS

1. e
2. g
3. d
4. c
5. a
6. b
7. f

8. A chronic illness is long term. It usually does not have a complete cure and it frequently limits activities of daily living (ADL).
9. Children with chronic illness are living longer. Advances in medicine have led to children living with illnesses that were previously fatal. Both quality of life and longevity have been enhanced by improvements in diagnostic testing and treatment.
10. Children with special health care needs are those who have, or are at risk for, a chronic physical, developmental, behavioral, or emotional condition and who also require health care and related services of a type and amount beyond that required for children generally.

THE FAMILY OF THE CHILD WITH SPECIAL HEALTH CARE NEEDS

11. A situational crisis is an unexpected crisis for which the family's usual problem-solving abilities are not adequate.
12. family cohesiveness
13. balances illness with other family needs, maintains clear family boundaries, develops communication competence, attributes positive meaning to the experience, maintains family flexibility, maintains commitment to family as a unit, engages in active coping efforts, maintains social integration, and develops collaborative relationships with health care professionals
14. F
15. T

THE GRIEVING PROCESS

16. not only the child but the entire family
17. denial and isolation, anger and resentment, bargaining, sadness or depression, and acceptance
18. F
19. T

THE CHILD WITH SPECIAL HEALTH CARE NEEDS

20. age at onset of the disorder; growth and development
21. self-esteem; autonomy
22. T
23. F

THE CHILD WITH A CHRONIC ILLNESS

24. to achieve and maintain the highest level of physical, emotional, and psychosocial health and function possible.
25. remaining intact, maintaining normalization, maximizing functioning
26. child's condition
27. communication
28. obtaining information about the child's condition and future services; receiving support through reading material related to parents with similar children; more time for themselves; opportunities to meet and talk with parents of similar children; help in locating child care or respite care providers; assistance in paying for food, medical expenses, and clothing; help in discussing problems and reaching solutions
29. T
30. T
31. F

NURSING CARE: THE CHILD WITH A CHRONIC CONDITION IN THE COMMUNITY SETTING

32. Risk for delayed growth and development related to the effects of chronic illness or disability, Disturbed body image related to actual or perceived physical differences or disabilities resulting from a chronic illness, Interrupted family processes related to intermittent situational crisis of chronic illness
33. Autonomy is often lost as a result of limitations imposed by the condition or treatment. Opportunities for autonomy can facilitate a positive sense of self-esteem.
34. The child will exhibit minimal disturbance of body image and will adapt to changes in physical appearance caused by alopecia, as evidenced by stating or demonstrating acceptance of loss of hair.

THE TERMINALLY ILL OR DYING CHILD

35. c
36. a
37. b
38. d
39. T
40. F
41. T

CARING FOR THE DYING CHILD

42. meeting with spiritual counselor; participating in staff support groups; participating in patient care conferences or ethics committee meetings
43. whether or not to inform the child of the prognosis
44. T
45. T
46. T
47. F
48. F
49. F
50. F
51. T
52. T

REVIEW QUESTIONS

1. a
2. b
3. a
4. a
5. b
6. c
7. d
8. a

CHAPTER 37: PRINCIPLES AND PROCEDURES FOR NURSING CARE OF CHILDREN

MATCHING KEY TERMS

1. c
2. f
3. b
4. d
5. a
6. e

PREPARING CHILDREN FOR PROCEDURES

7. child's age, developmental level, personality, present level of knowledge and understanding, past experiences, coping skills, and family situation
8. T
9. T
10. T
11. F
12. F
13. T
14. F

TRANSPORTING INFANTS AND CHILDREN

15. age and development of the child, physical condition, destination, and safety

USING RESTRAINTS

16. T
17. T
18. T
19. F

INFECTION CONTROL

20. blood; all body fluids, secretions, and excretions except sweat; nonintact skin; and mucous membranes

BATHING INFANTS AND CHILDREN

21. 100° F
22. testing the water temperature on the inside of the wrist or elbow
23. 3 inches
24. Inhalation of powder into the lungs can cause severe respiratory consequences.

ORAL HYGIENE

25. T
26. F
27. F

FEEDING

28. There is a risk of aspiration when an infant drinks from a propped bottle.
29. Allow them to sit at a table; allow them to feed themselves; have their parents bring their own utensils from home; use colorful plates and utensils.

VITAL SIGNS

30. Take an axillary temperature if the child is less than 4 to 6 years of age or if the child has had oral surgery or is uncooperative, immunosuppressed, or neurologically impaired.
31. The measurement may be inaccurate if liquids were consumed within 30 minutes of measurement, if the child is crying, or if the child is undergoing oxygen therapy or nebulization treatments.
32. F
33. T
34. The child is under 2 years of age, has an irregular heartbeat, or has a congenital heart defect.
35. 1 minute
36. 60 seconds
37. 88/P

FEVER-REDUCING MEASURES

38. There is an association between Reye syndrome and aspirin use in children with viral illnesses such as influenza or varicella.
39. acetaminophen, ibuprofen
40. liver

SPECIMEN COLLECTION

41. standard
42. epiglottitis
43. clean
44. posterior iliac crest

GAVAGE AND GASTROSTOMY

45. Tube placement is verified when the tube is inserted, any time the feeding is interrupted, before each bolus feeding, and every 4 to 8 hours during continuous feedings.
46. auscultation of air entering stomach, aspiration of enteral fluid, and pH measurement of the aspirate
47. F
48. F
49. T
50. F

ENEMAS

51. 360–480 cc; 3 inches

CARE OF OSTOMIES

52. T
53. T

OXYGEN THERAPY

54. It differs very little except for the size of the equipment and the teaching and support of children and families. An oxygen hood can be used for infants, and toddlers and preschoolers can use a nasal cannula, blow-by, or face mask.

ASSESSING OXYGENATION

55. adequate oxygen saturation
56. Report it to the physician because the child may require oxygen therapy. (For some children with cardiac or respiratory diseases, a pulse oximetry reading of 89% may be normal.)

CHEST PHYSIOTHERAPY

57. Percussion is rhythmic clapping with a cupped hand over the affected part of the lung or the simulation of this movement with a percussion cup or mechanical percussor.
58. Postural drainage is positioning of the patient to promote gravity-assisted drainage of the lungs.
59. before meals or 1½ hours after meals. Stop a continuous enteral feeding one hour before chest PT.

TRACHEOSTOMY CARE

60. assessing the stoma area for signs of infection and skin breakdown, changing tracheostomy ties, cleaning the tracheostomy site and inner cannula, changing the tracheostomy tube, and suctioning
61. at least every 8 hours
62. 5 seconds
63. off

SURGICAL PROCEDURES

64. 2 hours before the time of arrival at the hospital
65. Auscultate lungs to identify any abnormal breath sounds or areas of diminished or absent sounds. Encourage early ambulation, deep breathing, and coughing. Incentive spirometers can increase respiratory movement. To facilitate air exchange, the nurse can engage the child in games such as blowing cotton, a windmill, or bubbles.
66. separation from significant others; care by strangers; unfamiliar procedures; pain, fear of mutilation; disruption in routine; lack of privacy; temporary disability

REVIEW QUESTIONS

1. b
2. a
3. b
4. b
5. c

6. b
7. a
8. d
9. c
10. a
11. d

CHAPTER 38: MEDICATING INFANTS AND CHILDREN

MATCHING KEY TERMS

1. c
2. b
3. d
4. f
5. e
6. a

PHARMACOKINETICS IN CHILDREN

7. gastric acidity, gastric emptying, gastrointestinal motility, and enzyme activity
8. T
9. F
10. F
11. The renal system is immature at birth. The newborn's glomerular filtration rate is about 30%–50% that of an adult, and the renal tubules function less efficiently. Infants and young children cannot concentrate urine as well as older children or adults. Because of renal immaturity, medications may not be excreted.
12. to monitor that the serum concentrations of certain drugs are at safe and therapeutic levels.
13. trough

PSYCHOLOGIC AND DEVELOPMENTAL DIFFERENCES

14. Nurses should ask parents about medication allergies, child's ability to take medications (e.g., liquid versus solid), and special techniques they use to give medicines. Allow parents to administer certain medications (e.g., oral, otic, ophthalmic) if the child will cooperate. Ask parents to report if a medication does not seem to be effective.
15. Toddler: Give explanations through play; allow the child to see and handle the equipment first; allow him to help place liquid preparations into his mouth. Allow the parent to give the medication if the child prefers. Use as little restraint as possible because the child will resist restraint. Offer praise when the child takes the medication. Rewards, such as stickers, are useful. Preschooler: Offer a choice about what to drink after taking oral medication. Offer a Band-Aid (preferably, a colorful one) after an injection. School-age child: Offer choices as much as possible. The child may need a source of distraction to cooperate with painful procedures such as venipuncture or injection. Praise for cooperation and use rewards such as stickers.

CALCULATING DOSAGES

16. F
17. F
18. F

ADMINISTRATION PROCEDURES

19. Use the six rights of medication administration. Double-check medication calculations before administering; double-check pharmacy calculations of unit dose medications before administering. Have two nurses check the following medications: insulin, narcotics, chemotherapy, digoxin, anticoagulants, potassium and calcium salts.
20. Absorption of oral medications is affected by the presence or absence of food in the stomach, gastric emptying time, GI motility, and stomach acidity. It is also less predictable because of medication loss due to spillage, leaking, or spitting out.
21. The nurse can check to see whether the medication is available as a liquid or can be crushed and mix it with a nonessential food.
22. Because medications can alter the flavor of the food, the child may associate that food with the undesirable flavor and refuse it in the future, even without the medication added. Thus, only foods not essential to the child's diet should be used for mixing with medications.

MEDICATION ADMINISTRATION

23. F
24. F
25. T
26. T
27. Place the child on nurse's lap with child's right arm behind the nurse's back and with the nurse's left hand holding the child's left hand. Support the child's head with the nurse's left arm and secure it between the arm and body. Secure the child's legs between the nurse's legs. (Reverse sides if the nurse is left-handed.)
28. Notify the physician and report what medication was vomited and how much time has elapsed since administration.
29. Verify tube is properly positioned before administering medication. Flush tube with water after medication is administered.

ADMINISTERING INJECTIONS

30. Explanations should be tailored to the child's cognitive level. Explain the reason for the injection and describe the sensations that the child can expect to feel. The child may need to be assured that the injection is not a punishment for any misbehavior.
31. Ice can be applied to the injection site for several minutes prior to the injection to numb the area. Children can be taught how to use guided imagery, deep breathing, or distraction to cope with the discomfort. Topical anesthetics such as EMLA cream are effective in reducing injection pain.

ADMINISTERING INTRAMUSCULAR INJECTIONS

32. b
33. c
34. d
35. a

36. T
37. F
38. T
39. F

ADMINISTERING SUBCUTANEOUS INJECTIONS

40. circulation
41. fat pads above the iliac crests, hips, lateral upper arms, and anterior thighs
42. T
43. F
44. F

INTRADERMAL INJECTIONS

45. testing (such as allergy testing or PPD)
46. inner aspect of the forearm or upper back
47. Insert needle bevel up at a 15-degree angle. The needle will barely penetrate the skin and when the medication is injected, it will form a wheal.

RECTAL ADMINISTRATION

48. F
49. F
50. T

OPHTHALMIC AND OTIC ADMINISTRATION

51. F
52. T
53. F

INHALATION THERAPY

54. spacer
55. whistle
56. 10 seconds

INTRAVENOUS THERAPY

57. Consider the rate and type of fluid to be administered, the projected length of time the IV line will be needed, availability of veins, and the child's developmental level. The child's dominant hand should be avoided as a site for injection.
58. Use guided imagery—for example, putting on a "magic" glove. Try distraction with music, toys, seek-and-find books.
59. Clean the area well and place a liberal amount of EMLA cream on the site. Cover with a bioclusive dressing and leave in place for 1–2 hours to anesthetize the area.
60. to prevent inadvertent fluid overload
61. at least every hour
62. Assess for signs of infiltration (edema, erythema, pain, blanching, and coolness) and phlebitis (streaking on the skin above the vein). Discontinue IV line if any of these signs is present and notify physician.
63. 0–10 kg: 100 ml/kg/day >10–20 kg: 1000 ml plus 50 ml/kg/day for each kg between 10 and 20 kg >20 kg: 1500 ml plus 20 ml/kg/day for each kg >20 kg

64. 1800 ml; 1300 ml
65. These medications are not diluted and are injected (pushed) directly into the IV catheter using the port closest to the patient.
66. The needle is placed into the injection port nearest the child, and the medication is injected away from the child into the tubing above the port.
67. to complete the delivery of the medication from the IV tubing into the patient
68. every 6–12 hours (to maintain patency)
69. to administer medications, blood products, IV fluids, and parenteral nutrition over the long term to chronically ill children
70. An implanted venous access device consists of a catheter that is connected to a port or reservoir. The catheter tip rests at the junction of the superior vena cava and right atrium. The port is located under the skin.
71. phlebitis, infection, and thrombosis

ADMINISTRATION OF BLOOD OR BLOOD PRODUCTS

72. F
73. T
74. T
75. T
76. T

CHILD AND FAMILY EDUCATION

77. name of the medication, reason it is to be given, action of the medication, expected side effects and what to do if they should occur, when to notify the health care provider, any dietary restrictions, how to take the medication, how to measure the dosage correctly, and how to use droppers or syringes

REVIEW QUESTIONS

1. a
2. c
3. a
4. d
5. c
6. b
7. c
8. d

CHAPTER 39: PAIN MANAGEMENT FOR CHILDREN

MATCHING KEY TERMS

1. c
2. h
3. f
4. b
5. e
6. g
7. a
8. d

DEFINITIONS AND THEORIES OF PAIN

9. whatever the experiencing person says it is, existing whenever the person says it does
10. an unpleasant sensational and emotional experience associated with actual or potential damage
11. T
12. F
13. F
14. T
15. T

RESEARCH ON PAIN IN CHILDREN

16. the World Health Organization (WHO)
17. the American Pain Society
18. JCAHO

MYTHS ABOUT PAIN AND PAIN MANAGEMENT IN CHILDREN

19. T
20. T
21. F
22. F

ASSESSMENT OF PAIN IN CHILDREN

23. behavioral; physiologic
24. more purposeful
25. agitation
26. restlessness
27. punishment
28. They fear bodily harm and have an awareness of death.
29. They may not report pain, believing that the nurse must already be aware of it.
30. These tools provide a more objective measure of the pain experience
31. 3–4
32. the Oucher and the FACES Pain Rating Scales

NONPHARMACOLOGIC AND PHARMACOLOGIC PAIN INTERVENTIONS

33. They provide a focus for distraction, and they produce relaxation.
34. Children who are distracted may be able to focus on something other than pain, but the pain still exists.
35. relaxation; focused concentration
36. a technique that allows a person to notice body states not usually noticed and to bring them under control
37. relaxation, decreased anxiety, decreased pain
38. a form of focused or narrowed attention, an altered state of consciousness accompanied by relaxation
39. transmission of pain signals
40. oxygen, a bag and mask, and naloxone (Narcan)
41. It is associated with Reye syndrome.
42. F
43. T
44. T

45. T
46. F
47. T
48. T

REVIEW QUESTIONS

1. d
2. b
3. d
4. a
5. c
6. c
7. b
8. d

CHAPTER 40: THE CHILD WITH AN INFECTIOUS DISEASE

MATCHING KEY TERMS

1. c
2. h
3. g
4. a
5. b
6. e
7. f
8. d

REVIEW OF DISEASE TRANSMISSION

9. d
10. e
11. b
12. c
13. a

INFECTION AND HOST DEFENSES

14. skin; intact mucous membranes

IMMUNITY

15. c
16. e
17. a
18. d
19. b

NURSING CARE: THE CHILD WITH AN INFECTION IN THE COMMUNITY SETTING

20. Ask the caregiver when and how the child was exposed to the infectious disease; obtain a history of symptoms. Inspect the type, configuration, and distribution of lesions. Measure vital signs, particularly temperature. Determine general wellness and whether any other disease manifestations are present.
21. Instruct families to use acetaminophen or ibuprofen for fever control. Do not use any products containing aspirin because of the possibility of the child developing Reye syndrome. Provide written information that explains the various preparations available, as well as the appropriate dosage and administration intervals for the child.
22. Report visual disturbances, headache, nausea, vomiting, muscle flaccidity, absence of sweating, delirium, and coma.

VIRAL INFECTIONS

23. f
24. c
25. i
26. h
27. a
28. e
29. b
30. j
31. g
32. d
33. k
34. AAP recommends the use of a four-dose schedule using the inactivated poliomyelitis vaccine in order to prevent vaccine-acquired polio.

BACTERIAL, RICKETTSIAL, BORRELIA, HELMINTH, AND FUNGAL INFECTIONS

35. T
36. T
37. T
38. T
39. T
40. F
41. F
42. F

SEXUALLY TRANSMITTED DISEASES (STDS)

43. c
44. e
45. b
46. a
47. f
48. d

REVIEW QUESTIONS

1. b
2. b
3. b

4. d
5. c
6. c
7. d
8. b

CHAPTER 41: THE CHILD WITH AN IMMUNOLOGIC ALTERATION

MATCHING KEY TERMS

1. d
2. f
3. j
4. i
5. b
6. k
7. h
8. e
9. a
10. g
11. m
12. c
13. l

REVIEW OF THE IMMUNE SYSTEM

14. c
15. f
16. i
17. d
18. g
19. b
20. h
21. e
22. a

THE CHILD WITH AN IMMUNODEFICIENCY

23. They can be inherited or acquired through infection, or they can result from using certain medications.
24. repeated or persistent infections, severe bacterial infections, opportunistic infections, poor response to appropriate therapy

HUMAN IMMUNODEFICIENCY VIRUS (HIV) INFECTION

25. via the placenta, during delivery, through breast-feeding
26. zidovudine (ZDV)
27. to suppress viral replication in order to preserve immune function and delay disease progression
28. Tanner staging of sexual maturity
29. trimethoprim-sulfamethoxale
30. a. acetaminophen and NSAIDs, b. codeine, c. morphine or methadone

CORTICOSTEROID THERAPY

31. They decrease monocytes and macrophage differentiation and lymphokine production leading to T cell inhibition.
32. The child may develop acute adrenal insufficiency.
33. ACTH
34. every other day
35. To minimize risk for GI bleeding, give corticosteroids with food or milk. To deal with increased appetite, offer low-calorie, low-salt snacks.

IMMUNE COMPLEX AND AUTOIMMUNE DISORDERS

36. Kawasaki disease and poststreptococcal glomerulonephritis
37. antibodies that act against the body's own cells

SYSTEMIC LUPUS ERYTHEMATOSUS (SLE)

38. T
39. F
40. T
41. T
42. T
43. T

ALLERGIC REACTIONS AND ANAPHYLAXIS

44. an immune response to an antigen (allergen) that causes a hypersensitivity reaction in various body systems
45. b
46. a
47. d
48. c
49. laryngospasm, edema, cyanosis, shock, vascular collapse, cardiac arrest
50. epinephrine
51. RASTs are more expensive but provide more precise information without the risk of hypersensitivity reactions.

REVIEW QUESTIONS

1. b
2. c
3. a
4. d
5. b
6. c
7. b
8. b

CHAPTER 42: THE CHILD WITH A FLUID AND ELECTROLYTE ALTERATION

MATCHING KEY TERMS

1. a
2. c
3. e
4. g
5. b
6. f
7. d
8. h
9. i
10. k
11. j

REVIEW OF FLUID AND ELECTROLYTE IMBALANCES IN CHILDREN

12. F
13. T
14. F
15. F
16. T
17. extracellular
18. water; solutes
19. sodium; potassium; magnesium
20. 7.35; 7.45
21. chemical buffers, respiratory system, and the kidneys
22. bicarbonate; proteins
23. increase
24. hydrogen ions; bicarbonate
25. b
26. f
27. a
28. e
29. c
30. d
31. a
32. d
33. c
34. b

DEHYDRATION

35. T
36. F
37. T
38. T
39. F
40. F
41. F

DIARRHEA

42. an increase in the frequency, fluidity, and volume of stools
43. gastroenteritis
44. food intolerance, medications, malabsorption, colon disease, obstruction, stress, other infectious diseases elsewhere in the body
45. The high carbohydrate content of these drinks may worsen diarrhea. In addition, they do not replace electrolytes lost through diarrhea.
46. to prevent dehydration, to reduce stool frequency and volume, and to reduce duration of diarrhea
47. complex carbohydrates, yogurt, cooked vegetables, lean meats
48. Change diaper immediately after bowel movement, wash skin with mild soap and pat dry, apply "barrier" ointment (e.g., A and D), and avoid using commercial baby wipes.

VOMITING

49. T
50. T
51. F
52. F

REVIEW QUESTIONS

1. d
2. b
3. b
4. d
5. a
6. a
7. b
8. c
9. b
10. a

CHAPTER 43: THE CHILD WITH A GASTROINTESTINAL ALTERATION

MATCHING KEY TERMS

1. f
2. j
3. a
4. l
5. g
6. d
7. h
8. k
9. c
10. m
11. e
12. i
13. b
14. n

REVIEW OF THE GASTROINTESTINAL SYSTEM

15. to ingest food and fluids, begin digestion, and propel food to intestines
16. to digest and absorb nutrients, detoxify and eliminate waste, and maintain fluid and electrolyte balance
17. phagocytosis, bile production, detoxification, glycogen storage and breakdown, vitamin storage
18. via the placenta

DISORDERS OF PRENATAL DEVELOPMENT

19. T
20. T
21. F
22. T
23. T
24. polyhydramnios
25. aspiration
26. coughing, cyanosis, choking with feedings
27. parenterally
28. Cover stoma with gauze, change gauze often, cleanse with half-strength hydrogen peroxide, assess for skin breakdown and inflammation.
29. c
30. e
31. b
32. a
33. d
34. f

MOTILITY DISORDERS

35. small, frequent feedings with frequent burping
36. a. cimetidine and ranitidine; b. metoclopramide; c. sucralfate
37. Over time, the rectum enlarges, resulting in failure to control external sphincter, leading to encopresis.
38. stress, psychological factors
39. diffuse abdominal pain, alternating constipation and diarrhea, undigested food and mucus in stool, normal growth

INFLAMMATORY AND INFECTIOUS DISEASES

40. F
41. F
42. T
43. T
44. T
45. T
46. F
47. T
48. F
49. Crohn's affects the entire GI tract and all layers. It has periods of remission. Ulcerative colitis affects only the colon and the mucosa and submucosa. It can be cured by a colectomy.
50. anti-inflammatory, antibacterial, antibiotics, and immunosuppressive drugs

OBSTRUCTIVE DISORDERS

51. progressive, projectile, nonbilious
52. stools with bloody mucus, sausage-shaped abdominal mass
53. with a barium or air enema or with an ultrasound-guided isotonic saline enema
54. volvulus
55. delayed passage or absence of meconium stool
56. enterocolitis

MALABSORPTION DISORDERS

57. T
58. F
59. F
60. T

HEPATIC DISORDERS

61. fecal-oral route; contaminated food and water
62. blood, secretions, sexual contact, breast milk, and prenatally and perinatally
63. blood and blood products, and perinatally
64. blood
65. fecal-oral route
66. bleeding, encephalopathy, ascites, acute hepatic failure
67. jaundice
68. A; B
69. F
70. F
71. T
72. T
73. biliary obstruction; hepatitis B infection
74. ascites, varices, encephalopathy
75. liver transplantation

REVIEW QUESTIONS

1. d
2. b
3. b
4. d
5. b
6. c
7. d
8. a
9. b
10. a
11. b
12. b
13. d

CHAPTER 44: THE CHILD WITH A GENITOURINARY ALTERATION

MATCHING KEY TERMS

1. f
2. d
3. i
4. e
5. j
6. b
7. h
8. g
9. c
10. a

REVIEW OF THE GENITOURINARY SYSTEM

11. abdominal
12. urinary tract infections
13. nephron
14. 10
15. 4.6–8.0

ENURESIS

16. F
17. T
18. T
19. T
20. T

URINARY TRACT INFECTIONS (UTIS)

21. b
22. c
23. d
24. a
25. urine culture
26. suprapubic aspiration
27. structural abnormalities
28. intravenous
29. pyelonephritis
30. Keep foreskin in males clean; cleanse perineal area in girls from front to back; encourage child to urinate at least 4 times/day; offer fluids throughout day; avoid bubble baths; avoid tight, synthetic clothing and tight diapers.

CRYPTORCHIDISM

31. T
32. F
33. T
34. T

HYPOSPADIAS AND EPISPADIAS

35. circumcised
36. epispadias; hypospadias
37. chordae
38. urethral stents

MISCELLANEOUS DISORDERS AND ANOMALIES OF THE GENITOURINARY TRACT

39. c
40. a
41. e
42. d
43. b

ACUTE POSTSTREPTOCOCCAL GLOMERULONEPHRITIS

44. hematuria, proteinuria (0 to 2+), edema, renal insufficiency, hypertension
45. They travel through the circulation and get trapped in glomeruli, creating an inflammatory response and damaging the glomeruli. This decreases the glomerular filtration rate, which leads to renal insufficiency.
46. increase
47. diuresis

NEPHROTIC SYNDROME

48. proteinuria (3+ to 4+), hypoalbuminemia, edema, anorexia, fatigue, respiratory infection, weight gain, hyperlipidemia, hypovolemia, decreased IgG
49. prednisone
50. when urine protein level is zero to trace for 5–7 consecutive days

ACUTE RENAL FAILURE

51. b
52. b
53. a
54. b
55. a
56. c
57. c
58. T
59. F
60. T
61. F

CHRONIC RENAL FAILURE AND END-STAGE RENAL DISEASE (ESRD)

62. waste products; excess body fluids; electrolytes; minerals
63. arteriovenous fistula or shunt
64. peritoneal
65. fluid and electrolyte imbalances, acid-base imbalances, osteodysthrophy; anemia, poor growth, hypertension, fatigue, decreased appetite, nausea and vomiting, neurologic changes

66. renal transplantation
67. rejection
68. the use of immunosuppressive drugs to prevent rejection

REVIEW QUESTIONS

1. b
2. d
3. b
4. a
5. d
6. b
7. d
8. a
9. b
10. d

CHAPTER 45: THE CHILD WITH A RESPIRATORY ALTERATION

MATCHING KEY TERMS

1. h
2. m
3. p
4. k
5. b
6. f
7. l
8. o
9. n
10. e
11. q
12. g
13. a
14. j
15. c
16. d
17. i

REVIEW OF THE RESPIRATORY SYSTEM

18. T
19. F
20. T
21. T
22. F
23. T

ALLERGIC RHINITIS

24. 2 years
25. rhinorrhea; itching eyes, nose, ears, and palate; paroxysmal sneezing; dark circles under eyes; rubbing nose upward with palm of hand
26. immunotherapy

SINUSITIS

27. upper respiratory infection
28. acute otitis media with effusion
29. acetaminophen; warm, moist compresses

OTITIS MEDIA

30. T
31. F
32. T

PHARYNGITIS AND TONSILLITIS

33. c
34. a
35. b

LARYNGOMALACIA

36. inspiratory; increases

CROUP

37. a
38. c
39. b
40. d
41. T
42. F
43. T
44. F

EPIGLOTTITIS

45. sudden onset, high fever, sitting in tripod position, nasal flaring, retracting, tachycardia, drooling, dysphagia, dysphonia
46. tongue blade

BRONCHITIS

47. virus
48. rest; humidification; increased fluid intake

BRONCHIOLITIS

49. 50
50. It can live on the skin for up to 1 hour and on nonporous surfaces for up to 6 hours.

51. It can cause burning of eyes and nasal passages. It can crystallize on contact lenses. It is teratogenic in some animals.
52. RSV immune globulin (RSV-16; RespiGam) or RSV monoclonal antibody (Synagis)

PNEUMONIA

53. Chest physiotherapy before meals and before bed; change position every 2 hours; elevate head of bed. Assist older children to cough and deep breathe.
54. 95

FOREIGN BODY ASPIRATION

55. nuts, grapes, hard candy, popcorn, hot dogs, raw carrots, large chunks of food
56. aphonia; apnea

PULMONARY NONINFECTIOUS IRRITATION

57. aspiration, trauma, drug ingestion, shock, massive transfusions
58. passive smoking
59. carbon monoxide

RESPIRATORY DISTRESS SYNDROME (RDS)

60. T
61. F
62. F
63. F

APNEA

64. b
65. a
66. c
67. time and duration of episode, skin color, heart rate, O_2 saturation, precipitating trigger, any actions taken to stimulate breathing
68. monitor use, CPR

SUDDEN INFANT DEATH SYNDROME (SIDS)

69. T
70. F
71. T
72. F

ASTHMA

73. increased
74. expiration
75. lowers
76. dilate airway and/or relieve bronchospasm
77. status asthmaticus
78. swimming
79. decrease inflammation
80. peak flowmeters

81. exposure to triggers
82. belly breathing; pursed lip breathing

BRONCHOPULMONARY DYSPLASIA (BPD)

83. T
84. T
85. F
86. F

CYSTIC FIBROSIS (CF)

87. F
88. T
89. F
90. T
91. T
92. T
93. F
94. T

TUBERCULOSIS (TB)

95. a
96. c
97. b
98. T
99. T
100. F
101. F

REVIEW QUESTIONS

1. b
2. a
3. b
4. b
5. c
6. c
7. b
8. c
9. c
10. a
11. b
12. c
13. a

CHAPTER 46: THE CHILD WITH A CARDIOVASCULAR ALTERATION

MATCHING KEY TERMS

1. f
2. h
3. c
4. k
5. g
6. j
7. i
8. l
9. e
10. b
11. a
12. d

MORE DEFINITIONS

13. T
14. F
15. T
16. T
17. T
18. F
19. F
20. T

REVIEW OF THE CARDIOVASCULAR SYSTEM

21. placenta
22. foramen ovale
23. ductus arteriosus
24. decreases; increases

CARDIOVASCULAR ASSESSMENT

25. T
26. F
27. T
28. T
29. T
30. F
31. F
32. T

PHYSIOLOGIC CONSEQUENCES OF CONGENITAL HEART DISEASE

33. resting tachycardia and difficulty feeding
34. e
35. b
36. a
37. d
38. c
39. weighing daily

40. the apical heart rate; the dose with another nurse; for signs of digoxin toxicity
41. chronic hypoxia
42. calming the child; placing the child in knee-chest position; administering oxygen and, if necessary, morphine; phenylephrine, a potent vasoconstrictor, may be necessary.

LEFT-TO-RIGHT SHUNTING LESIONS AND OBSTRUCTIVE LESIONS

43. patent ductus arteriosus
44. coarctation of the aorta
45. ventricular septal defect; atrial septal defect
46. atrioventricular septal defect
47. pulmonary stenosis
48. aortic stenosis

CYANOTIC LESIONS WITH ALTERED PULMONARY BLOOD FLOW

49. f
50. e
51. c
52. a
53. d
54. b

ACQUIRED HEART DISEASE

55. T
56. T
57. T
58. T
59. F
60. T
61. T
62. T
63. F
64. F

CARDIOMYOPATHIES

65. hypertrophic cardiomyopathy
66. dilated cardiomyopathy
67. beta blockers; calcium channel

DYSRHYTHMIAS

68. supraventricular tachycardia
69. hypoxia
70. asystole
71. vagal
72. epinephrine

HIGH CHOLESTEROL IN CHILDREN AND ADOLESCENTS

73. tobacco use; increased LDL and cholesterol; hypertension; decreased physical activity; obesity
74. 110–129; 130

REVIEW QUESTIONS

1. a
2. b
3. a
4. c
5. d
6. d
7. c
8. d
9. b
10. d
11. a
12. a

CHAPTER 47: THE CHILD WITH A HEMATOLOGIC ALTERATION

MATCHING KEY TERMS

1. i
2. k
3. f
4. a
5. j
6. h
7. d
8. e
9. c
10. g
11. b

REVIEW OF THE HEMATOLOGIC SYSTEM

12. a. to transport O_2 to the tissues; b. to destroy foreign cells; c. to prevent blood loss
13. a. decrease in number of RBCs or their hemoglobin content; b. increase in number of RBCs; c. decrease in production of WBCs; d. source of platelets

IRON DEFICIENCY ANEMIA (IDA)

14. Cow's milk, which is not iron-fortified, replaces formula, which is. It may also irritate the immature bowel, which can lead slowly to GI blood loss.
15. They have compromised tissue oxygenation resulting from decreased hemoglobin.
16. adolescent growth spurt, poor dietary intake; menstruation in females
17. cow's milk, formula, cereal

SICKLE CELL DISEASE (SCD)

18. low O_2 concentrations, acidosis, dehydration
19. pain, tissue ischemia, infarcts, organ damage
20. g
21. f
22. d

23. a
24. e
25. c
26. b

BETA-THALASSEMIA

27. autosomal recessive
28. hemosiderosis
29. iron
30. deferoxamine (Desferal)

HEMOPHILIA

31. Her father has hemophilia; her mother is a carrier.
32. factor VIII; factor IX
33. swelling, pain, and stiffness
34. X

VON WILLEBRAND'S DISEASE (VWD)

35. F
36. T
37. F
38. T

IMMUNE THROMBOCYTOPENIC PURPURA (ITP)

39. T
40. T
41. T
42. F
43. T

DISSEMINATED INTRAVASCULAR COAGULATION (DIC)

44. T
45. T
46. F

APLASTIC ANEMIA

47. granulocytes, erythrocytes, and megakaryocytes
48. petechiae, ecchymosis, pallor, epistaxis, fatigue, tachycardia, anorexia, infection
49. colony-stimulating factor

REVIEW QUESTIONS

1. c
2. b
3. c
4. c
5. c
6. d
7. d
8. b

CHAPTER 48: THE CHILD WITH CANCER

MATCHING KEY TERMS

1. f
2. a
3. h
4. g
5. j
6. c
7. i
8. d
9. b
10. e

REVIEW OF CANCER

11. neoplasm
12. invasion; metastasis
13. Tumor staging describes the extent of the disease locally, regionally, and systemically; it guides therapy for most solid tumors.
14. T
15. F
16. F
17. T
18. mass, purpura, pallor, weight loss, whitish reflex in the eye, vomiting in early morning, and recurrent or persistent fever
19. bone pain; headache; persistent lymphadenopathy; change in balance, gait, or personality; fatigue; and malaise.
20. The child is positioned prone with a small pillow under the hips to facilitate access to the posterior iliac crest.

THE CHILD WITH CANCER

21. chemotherapy, surgery, and radiation therapy
22. antineoplastic drugs
23. hematopoietic, gastrointestinal, and integumentary
24. The time of greatest bone marrow suppression, generally occurring 7–10 days following chemotherapy administration, depending on the specific agent used
25. neutropenia
26. R
27. B
28. C
29. B
30. C
31. B
32. 5-HT_3 serotonin antagonists
33. to obtain a small piece of the tumor for microscopic examination for the purpose of confirming tumor type and guiding therapy decisions
34. Provides easy access to venous system. Child does not have to undergo frequent, painful venipunctures.
35. dose; treatment site
36. 7–10
37. erythema at the irradiated site
38. any type of hematologic cell

39. transplant using child's own bone marrow that was collected prior to high-dose chemotherapy
40. transplant from a donor whose tissue type matches the child's tissue type
41. first-remission Philadelphia chromosome-positive ALL, AML, and stage IV neuroblastoma
42. preparation for a bone marrow transplant involving a regimen of chemotherapy, with or without radiation
43. graft-versus-host disease (GVHD)
44. naturally occurring substances found in small quantities in the body that influence immune system functions

LEUKEMIA

45. immature WBCs
46. fever, pallor, excessive bruising, bone or joint pain (usually leg pain), lymphadenopathy, malaise, hepatosplenomegaly, abnormal WBC counts (either lower or higher than normal for age), and mild to profound anemia and thrombocytopenia
47. biopsy of bone marrow aspirate
48. blast cells
49. combination chemotherapy
50. Remission is defined as the reduction of immature blast cells in the bone marrow to less than 5%.
51. to decrease serum uric acid levels and alkalinize the urine
52. central nervous system and the testes
53. Risk for infection related to immunosuppressed state; Risk for injury related to thrombocytopenia; Imbalanced nutrition: less than body requirements related to nausea and vomiting, mucositis, or taste changes; Deficient knowledge related to unfamiliarity with the disease process and treatment plan; Disturbed body image related to hair loss; Ineffective individual/family coping related to chronic illness; Acute and chronic pain related to the disease process and procedures
54. A rectal thermometer can damage delicate rectal tissues, resulting in abscesses.
55. 500 cells/mm^3
56. Use a soft-bristled toothbrush, perform oral hygiene 4 times a day, and at the first sign of mouth ulcers, notify physician to begin using an antifungal medication. Do not use alcohol-containing mouthwashes. If the child's platelet count is low, use a washcloth wrapped around a finger instead of a toothbrush.
57. Giving a live virus vaccine to an immunosuppressed child could produce infection.
58. Give the child varicella-zoster immune globulin (VZIG) within 96 hours of exposure.
59. Limit activities to prevent injury, particularly to the head. No contact sports. Use a soft-bristled toothbrush or gauze swab to clean teeth. Stool softeners but no suppositories. Check urine and stools for blood. Teach child how to control nosebleeds and to blow the nose gently. For adolescent girls, monitor menstrual flow. Avoid sharp foods like potato chips.
60. cool, clear liquids and soft, bland foods at room temperature
61. F
62. F
63. T
64. F
65. T

BRAIN TUMORS

66. tumor location; age and development of the child
67. headache and morning vomiting related to getting out of bed

68. magnetic resonance imaging (MRI)
69. surgery and chemotherapy
70. This position increases intracranial pressure and the risk of bleeding.

OTHER CHILDHOOD CANCERS

71. F
72. T
73. F
74. T
75. T
76. F
77. T
78. T

REVIEW QUESTIONS

1. a
2. d
3. c
4. b
5. c
6. a
7. c
8. b
9. c
10. b
11. a
12. a
13. a
14. b

CHAPTER 49: THE CHILD WITH AN INTEGUMENTARY ALTERATION

MATCHING KEY TERMS

1. k
2. d
3. i
4. h
5. e
6. b
7. j
8. f
9. a
10. c
11. g

REVIEW OF THE INTEGUMENTARY SYSTEM

12. protects deeper tissues from injury, drying, and foreign matter invasion; regulates temperature; aids in excretion of water; aids in production of vitamin D; and initiates the sensations of touch, pain, heat, and cold

13. T
14. F
15. T
16. F

INFECTIONS OF THE SKIN

Impetigo

17. impetigo
18. *Staphylococcus aureus*; group A beta hemolytic streptococci
19. It can spread if the child touches the affected area and then touches another part of the body. It can spread to others if the child's linens or utensils, which have been in contact with the infected area, are used by others.
20. The primary lesions of impetigo occur in two forms. Bullous impetigo presents as small vesicles, which can progress to bullae. The lesions are initially filled with serous fluid, and later become pustular. The bullae rupture, leaving a shiny, lacquered-appearing lesion surrounded by a scaly rim. Crusted impetigo appears initially as a vesicle or pustule, which ruptures to become an erosion with an overlay of honey-colored crust. When crusts are removed, the erosion bleeds easily.
21. Impetigo is treated with topical and oral antibiotics. Wash lesions 3 times a day with a warm, soapy washcloth. Then apply topical antibiotics. Severe cases are treated with oral antibiotics.
22. acute glomerulonephritis
23. Wash hands often and well, keep the child's nails short, do not share linens and eating utensils used by the child, have the child sleep alone, and complete the full course of antibiotics.

Cellulitis

24. Cellulitis is a bacterial infection of the subcutaneous tissues and dermis.
25. lower extremities, buccal and periorbital regions
26. Affected areas will appear red, hot, swollen, and painful; lymphangitis will occur with red streaking of the surrounding area; edema and purple discoloration of eyelids appear with decreased eye movement if the periorbital area is affected; and lymph node enlargement, fever, malaise, and headache occur.
27. Administer an initial intramuscular or intravenous dose of an antibiotic, then complete a 10-day course of antibiotics and warm compresses. Hospitalization and intravenous antibiotics are required if cellulitis affects a joint or face. Incision and drainage of the affected area may be necessary.
28. Have the child rest in bed with the affected leg elevated. Warm moist soaks should be applied every 4 hours. Administer antibiotics as ordered. Acetaminophen can be given for fever or pain. Assess for signs of sepsis or spread of infection. And, of course, practice frequent handwashing!

Candidiasis

29. *Candida albicans*
30. white, curd-like plaques on the tongue, gums, or buccal membranes that are difficult to remove
31. Does she have vaginal itching or discharge? Does she have any tenderness or redness of the nipples? Ask about her methods of cleaning bottles, nipples, and pacifiers and about the infant's prior feeding patterns.
32. Nystatin oral suspension
33. Swab 1 ml of oral nystatin suspension onto the infant's gums and tongue every 6 hours until 3 to 4 days after symptoms have disappeared.

Tinea Infections

34. a. scalp; b. trunk, face, and extremities; c. feet
35. a. griseofulvin orally for 6–8 weeks; b. antifungal preparations such as clotrimazole (Lotrimin) or miconazole (Monistat) topically 3 times a day to affected area until lesions are gone for 1 week; c. topical antifungal preparation applied twice daily to lesions and at least 1 inch beyond lesion borders; d. topical antifungal agent such as clotrimazole (Lotrimin), miconazole (Monistat), or oxiconazole (Oxistat) applied twice daily until lesions have been cleared for 1 week.
36. T
37. F
38. F

Herpes Simplex Virus (HSV) Infection

39. painful HSV-1 infection of the fingers that may be transmitted to caregiver during oral or tracheal care of a child with herpes infection
40. oral or topical acyclovir (Zovirax)
41. Try to feed the child frozen ice pops, noncitrus juices, milk, or flat soda. Small, frequent meals of soft, bland foods may be tolerated.

Lice Infestations

42. F
43. F
44. Nits are visible silvery, grayish white specks resembling dandruff that are firmly attached to the hair shafts near the scalp. Nits resemble dandruff but are more difficult to remove from the hair. They are commonly found ¼ to ½ inch from the scalp surface behind the ears and at the nape of the neck. An adult louse is a small gray speck that crawls quickly and is difficult to see.
45. Treatment involves an over-the-counter antilice product such as permethrin 1% (Nix) cream rinse, which kills both lice and eggs with one application.
46. After the hair is treated with a pediculocide, all nits must be removed from the hair. The child should be rechecked in 7–10 days for infestation. Parents should be advised to wash clothing, bedding, and linens in hot water and to dry at a hot dryer setting. Items that cannot be washed can be dry cleaned or sealed in plastic bags for 3 weeks. Combs and brushes must be cleaned through boiling or soaking in antilice shampoo or hot water for 15 minutes.

Mite Infestation (Scabies)

47. by close personal contact with infected individuals
48. intense itching, especially at night; papules, vesicles, and nodules on the wrists, finger webs, elbows, umbilicus, axillae, groin, and buttocks; presence of burrows (fine, grayish, threadlike lines) that are difficult to see because of inflammation and excoriation from scratching
49. A topical application is applied to the body and head, avoiding the eyes and mouth. Lotion is kept on the body for the recommended period of time (usually 8–14 hours), and then the child is bathed.

Atopic Dermatitis

50. High levels of histamine trigger an inflammatory response resulting in erythema, edema, and intense pruritis. Scratching increases itching, leading to an "itch-scratch-itch" cycle.

51. It is scaly on the flexor surfaces of the wrists, ankles, knees and elbows, neck creases, eyelids, and dorsum of hands and feet. Chronic lichenification results from persistent scratching. Areas may be weeping and possibly infected.
52. Avoid trigger factors such as overheating, soaps, wool clothing, or any skin irritant. Apply moisturizer while the skin is damp to hydrate the skin. Use corticosteroid creams for inflamed or lichenified areas. Oral antihistamines can be used to break the itch-scratch-itch cycle, particularly at night.

Seborrheic Dermatitis

53. cradle cap
54. nonpruritic oily yellow scales on the scalp, forehead, eyebrows, and behind the ears; confluent erythema in the diaper area and intertriginous areas and around the umbilicus
55. Remove scales daily by shampooing with a mild baby shampoo or an over-the-counter antiseborrheic shampoo containing sulfur and salicylic acid, selenium, or tar. Massage the scalp with warm mineral oil before shampooing to loosen the scales. Use a fine-toothed comb or clean soft-bristled toothbrush to loosen the scales.

Contact Dermatitis

56. an inflammatory reaction to irritants resulting from prolonged contact with irritants or from a delayed hypersensitivity response to an allergen
57. cool compresses, antipruritic lotions, Aveeno baths, topical steroid creams, and oral antihistamines; avoid overheating
58. Rinse the child's skin with cool water immediately and wash clothing in hot, soapy water.
59. T
60. T
61. T

Acne Vulgaris

62. sebaceous hair follicles on the face, neck, back, shoulders, and upper chest
63. When the sebaceous or sweat glands become blocked, a blackhead or a pimple is formed. If these rupture under the skin, inflammation occurs.
64. a. Use sunscreen to reduce photosensitivity; b. Avoid exposure to sunlight; c. If sexually active, use contraception because of drug's teratogenic effect on the fetus.
65. Wash the face twice a day with an antibacterial soap and shampoo hair daily. Avoid vigorous scrubbing and picking or squeezing pimples. Use only water-based cosmetics. Get adequate rest and exercise, and eat a balanced diet.

Insect Bites or Stings

66. Wear identification describing the allergy and stating the treatment. Keep an emergency kit containing antihistamine, epinephrine, and a syringe available.
67. If the stinger is in the skin, it can be removed by carefully scraping it out horizontally. Do not squeeze the area, because more venom will be released. Wash with soap and water. A meat tenderizer paste applied to the area may be soothing.
68. because of the risk for toxic encephalopathy

Miscellaneous Skin Disorders

69. Cover affected areas immediately with warm hands and clothing. Do not massage the area. Rewarm by immersion in a warm water bath (90°–106° F) until all parts are thawed and skin appears flushed.

70. Child should wear warm, layered clothing, hat, gloves, and two pairs of socks (one wool, one cotton). Teach children to warm their hands and feet when they begin to sting. Do not allow young children to play in extremely cold temperatures.
71. Remove with tweezers as close to the skin as possible, taking care to remove the head. If mouth parts remain, remove with sterile needle. Wash area with soap and water.
72. d
73. a
74. b
75. c

BURN INJURIES

76. b
77. a
78. b
79. c
80. c
81. a
82. b
83. c
84. Avoid sun exposure, especially between 10 A.M. and 3 P.M. during the summer. Apply ultraviolet A and ultraviolet B protective sunscreens with SPF >15 to the child's skin. Apply frequently. Use a waterproof sunscreen if children are in and out of water. Wear a hat and a shirt. Sunscreen is contraindicated for infants under age 6 months. Infants should be kept in the shade away from reflecting sun rays.
85. silver nitrate solution, mafenide acetate cream, and silver sulfadiazine cream
86. a hypovolemic condition that develops after burn injury affecting more than 15%–20% of total body surface area.
87. cardiac arrest or arrhythmia, tissue damage, myoglobinuria, and metabolic acidosis

REVIEW QUESTIONS

1. b
2. a
3. c
4. c
5. d
6. b
7. d
8. b
9. b
10. c
11. d
12. a

CHAPTER 50: THE CHILD WITH A MUSCULOSKELETAL ALTERATION

MATCHING KEY TERMS

1. e
2. c
3. h
4. o
5. l
6. n
7. f
8. m
9. d
10. a
11. k
12. g
13. j
14. b
15. i
16. a. adduction, b. inversion, c. external rotation, d. internal fixation
17. T
18. F
19. F
20. T
21. F
22. T
23. T
24. F

REVIEW OF THE MUSCULOSKELETAL SYSTEM

25. a. immovable joints, b. slightly movable joints, c. freely movable joints
26. a. in internal organs, b. along the skeleton, c. in the heart

Casts and Traction

27. pain, paresthesia, pallor, pulselessness, paralysis
28. osteomyelitis
29. muscle and nerve irritation of the shoulder and upper arm
30. skeletal
31. humerus
32. skin
33. Russell
34. cervical; thoracic

Limb Defects and Clubfoot

35. T
36. T
37. F
38. T
39. F
40. T
41. T
42. F
43. F

Developmental Dysplasia of the Hip

44. a. femoral head that can be displaced with manipulation, b. asymmetric gluteal skin folds, limited abduction, and shorter-appearing femur on affected side, c. gait variation with lurching toward affected side
45. abduction, flexion, external rotation
46. avascular necrosis
47. mobility, transportation, skin integrity, toileting, constipation, clothing, comfort, safety, keeping cast clean and dry, inactivity, isolation

Legg-Calvé-Perthes Disease (LCP)

48. T
49. T
50. F
51. F

Slipped Capital Femoral Epiphysis (SCFE)

52. above
53. knee, groin, or thigh
54. Buck extension
55. growth plate

Fractures

56. a fracture in which skin, tissue, or muscle has been damaged
57. Compartment syndrome is a serious complication occurring when swelling causes pressure to rise within the closed space of an extremity. The increased pressure compromises circulation to muscles and nerves, causing paralysis and necrosis.
58. blood loss
59. retention
60. internal fixation
61. nonaccidental
62. ulna, clavicle, tibia, femur
63. epiphyseal plate
64. crush; long

Soft Tissue Injuries

65. d
66. c
67. b
68. a

Osgood-Schlatter Disease

69. repetitive stress from sports, overuse of immature muscles and tendons, imbalance in strength of quadriceps muscle
70. insidious onset of knee pain, swelling of the tibial tubercle, difficulty with weight bearing

Osteogenesis Imperfecta

71. an inherited disorder characterized by connective tissue and bone defects
72. osteoporosis, bone fragility and fractures, blue sclerae, discolored teeth, deafness by age 20–30 years, shorter than average adult height

Osteomyelitis

73. T
74. T
75. F
76. T
77. F

Juvenile Arthritis

78. an autoimmune inflammatory disease that affects the body's connective tissue
79. inflammation of the eye structure in the uveal tract
80. when children with severe juvenile arthritis do not respond well to NSAIDs
81. blindness and disability

Muscular Dystrophies

82. a group of degenerative, inherited disorders that affect the muscle cells of specific muscle groups, causing weakness and atrophy
83. Duchenne
84. cardiopulmonary complications

Scoliosis, Kyphosis, and Lordosis

85. F
86. T
87. F
88. T
89. F
90. F
91. F
92. T

REVIEW QUESTIONS

1. c
2. d
3. a
4. b
5. a
6. c
7. a
8. b
9. c
10. a
11. d
12. d
13. a
14. d

CHAPTER 51: THE CHILD WITH AN ENDOCRINE OR METABOLIC ALTERATION

MATCHING KEY TERMS

1. b
2. e
3. a
4. f
5. h
6. g
7. c
8. d

REVIEW OF THE ENDOCRINE SYSTEM

9. P
10. A
11. A
12. A
13. P
14. A
15. A

DIAGNOSTIC TESTS AND PROCEDURES

16. laboratory testing
17. height; weight

NEONATAL HYPOGLYCEMIA

18. 40 mg/dl
19. premature; small for gestational age
20. jitteriness, poor feeding, lethargy, seizures, hypotonia, high-pitched cry, bradycardia, cyanosis, temperature instability, and respiratory alterations, including apnea
21. feed formula or D_5W
22. blood glucose level by 2 hours of age; ongoing monitoring for signs of hypoglycemia
23. infiltration of IV line can cause severe extravasation

HYPOCALCEMIA

24. 7.0 mg/dl
25. Maternal diabetes causes immature parathyroid function in the neonate.
26. Oral supplements are given with feedings because they can cause gastric irritation.

PHENYLKETONURIA AND INBORN ERRORS OF METABOLISM

27. autosomal recessive
28. central nervous system
29. Testing should be done after the infant is 48 hours old
30. special diet that restricts phenylalanine and protein
31. F
32. T
33. F

CONGENITAL ADRENAL HYPERPLASIA

34. glucocorticoid; androgens
35. ambiguous genitalia
36. glucocorticoid therapy

CONGENITAL AND ACQUIRED HYPOTHYROIDISM

37. F
38. T
39. T
40. T
41. F
42. a
43. b
44. b
45. a
46. a
47. a
48. Give one daily oral dose. Dissolve in a small amount of water and give by syringe or place into the nipple of a baby bottle with a small amount of formula. Do not put in a full bottle because the infant must drink all of the formula to receive a full dose. If the infant vomits within 1 hour, give it again. Parents must observe infant for both hypothyroidism and hyperthyroidism, so teach parents about signs and symptoms.

HYPERTHYROIDISM (GRAVES DISEASE)

49. antithyroid therapy with propylthiouracil or methimazole, radioactive iodine, or surgery
50. neutropenia and hepatotoxicity
51. to determine if the child has gone into remission

DIABETES INSIPIDUS

52. vasopressin or antidiuretic hormone (ADH)
53. increased urination (polyuria) and excessive thirst (polydipsia)
54. In diabetes insipidus, when fluid is restricted, the child continues to produce large amounts of dilute urine and the serum sodium may increase.
55. synthetic vasopressin (DDAVP)
56. intranasally, or by subcutaneous injection, or orally

SYNDROME OF INAPPROPRIATE ANTIDIURETIC HORMONE (SIADH)

57. The kidneys reabsorb too much free water.
58. a. decreased, b. increased, c. decreased, d. increased
59. seizures

PRECOCIOUS PUBERTY

60. premature appearance of secondary sexual characteristics, accelerated growth rate, and advanced bone maturation
61. rapid bone growth, which causes early fusion and ultimately results in short adult stature
62. administration of a GnRH agonist or blocker
63. It inhibits binding of GnRH to the pituitary gland, causing a decrease in hormone production. This slows or reverses sexual development

GROWTH HORMONE (GH) DEFICIENCY

64. F
65. T
66. T
67. T

DIABETES MELLITUS

68. glucose
69. glycogen
70. regulate blood glucose by controlling the rate of glucose uptake by cells
71. an autoimmune process that results in destruction of the insulin-secreting cells of the pancreas
72. When glucose is unable to move into the intracellular space, hyperglycemia occurs.
73. Glucose spills into the urine via osmotic diuresis, causing increased urination.
74. Excess fluid is lost through polyuria, causing thirst.
75. Cellular starvation from lack of glucose causes hunger.
76. Cellular starvation from lack of glucose causes weight loss.
77. 120 mg/dl; 160 mg/dl
78. F
79. F
80. T
81. T
82. T
83. F
84. F
85. T
86. 4 ounces of fruit juice; 6 ounces of regular cola, 6 Lifesavers, or a commercial glucose product.
87. Hypoglycemia could result from a missed or delayed meal, too much insulin, or an unusual amount of exercise without increasing carbohydrate intake.
88. Rub a small amount of glucose gel on the inner cheek and gums, or inject glucagon subcutaneously or intramuscularly. Position an unconscious child on his/her side. Once the child is conscious, replace lost glycogen stores with a large snack.

DIABETIC KETOACIDOSIS (DKA)

89. It is necessary to replace fluids lost from diuresis as a result of hyperglycemia. Fluids are essential in flushing ketones.
90. regular insulin administered intravenously

REVIEW QUESTIONS

1. c
2. c
3. d
4. b
5. d
6. a
7. d
8. c
9. c
10. d

11. c
12. b
13. a
14. a

CHAPTER 52: THE CHILD WITH A NEUROLOGIC ALTERATION

MATCHING KEY TERMS

1. c
2. d
3. g
4. e
5. a
6. f
7. b

REVIEW OF THE CENTRAL NERVOUS SYSTEM

8. a. 4 weeks, b. 15–20 weeks, c. 30 weeks, d. 16 weeks
9. cerebrum, cerebellum, brain stem
10. The CSF acts as a watery cushion, surrounding and absorbing any shock to the brain, spinal cord, and meninges.
11. b
12. d
13. e
14. f
15. a
16. c

INCREASED INTRACRANIAL PRESSURE

17. decreased CSF production, increased CSF absorption, and reduction in cerebral mass as a result of fluid displacement
18. Infants: bulging fontanel, high-pitched cry, poor feeding, vomiting, irritability, restlessness, distended scalp veins, eyes deviated downward, increased head circumference, separation of cranial sutures; Children: headache, diplopia, mood swings, slurred speech, nausea and vomiting (especially in the morning), altered level of consciousness, papilledema
19. a. decorticate, b. decerebrate
20. eye opening, verbal response, and motor response
21. b
22. d
23. c
24. f
25. a
26. e
27. T
28. F
29. F
30. F

SPINA BIFIDA

31. failure of the neural tube to close, resulting in incomplete closure of vertebrae
32. a. sac-like protrusion filled with spinal fluid and meninges, b. sac filled with spinal fluid, meninges, nerve roots, and spinal cord, c. failure of the vertebrae to fuse
33. T
34. T
35. F
36. F
37. T
38. T

HYDROCEPHALUS

39. surgical placement of a ventriculoperitoneal shunt
40. Position the child off the shunt site so that no weight is on the valve for the first 2 days.
41. poor feeding, nausea or vomiting, elevated temperature, redness or tenderness along the shunt tract
42. a
43. c
44. b
45. b
46. a
47. c
48. d

CEREBRAL PALSY

49. F
50. T
51. T

HEAD INJURY

52. evaluation of airway, breathing, and circulation (ABCs); baseline vital signs; Glasgow Coma Scale; complete history; neurologic examination
53. Notify the physician if bleeding does not stop after 10 minutes of holding pressure, if the wound requires sutures, if the child is <1 year of age, if the child has a seizure after head injury, if the child is unconscious or confused, or if the child has any of the following: severe headache, vomiting, slurred speech, blurred vision, difficulty walking or crawling, blood or watery drainage from nose or ear, unequal pupils or crossed eyes.
54. c
55. a
56. e
57. b
58. d
59. A condition following a concussion that may last for months. Common problems experienced include irritability, learning and memory difficulties, diplopia, dizziness, headache, fatigue, photosensitivity.

SPINAL CORD INJURY

60. T
61. F
62. T
63. T

SEIZURE DISORDERS

64. a
65. f
66. c
67. e
68. d
69. b
70. A seizure occurs when there is an excessive disorderly discharge of neuronal activity in the brain. Epilepsy refers to recurrent seizure activity that does not occur in association with an acute illness.
71. height; rapidity
72. precipitating events, behavior prior to and immediately after the seizure, detailed description of how the seizure progressed, and the duration of the seizure
73. Remove sharp objects or furniture from the area; do not put anything in the child's mouth; place child on the side; do not restrain the child; and loosen clothing around the neck.
74. Gums may become swollen and tender; brush and floss teeth after every meal using a soft toothbrush; have a dental examination every 3–6 months; and have blood levels monitored regularly.
75. pediatric emergency characterized by prolonged seizure activity that may be a single seizure lasting 10 minutes or recurrent seizures lasting longer than 30 minutes with no return to consciousness between seizures

MENINGITIS

76. lumbar puncture
77. pain with extension of leg and knee
78. Flexion of head causes flexion of hips and knees.
79. prompt initiation and uninterrupted administration of intravenous antibiotics
80. T
81. F
82. T

GUILLAIN-BARRÉ SYNDROME

83. upper respiratory infection
84. respiratory failure

HEADACHES

85. vascular, tension, increased intracranial pressure

REVIEW QUESTIONS

1. b
2. d
3. a

4. c
5. d
6. c
7. a
8. a
9. d
10. a
11. b
12. c
13. d
14. c
15. c

CHAPTER 53: THE CHILD WITH A PSYCHOSOCIAL DISORDER

DEFINITIONS

1. (across) addiction
2. (down) comorbidity
3. (across) bulimia
4. (down) abuse
5. (down) violence
6. (across) suicide
7. (across) threat

OVERVIEW OF CHILDHOOD PSYCHOPATHOLOGY

8. F
9. T
10. T

ANXIETY AND DEPRESSION

11. c
12. b
13. a
14. e
15. d
16. F
17. T
18. T
19. selective serotonin reuptake inhibitors (SSRIs)

SUICIDE

20. using cryptic verbal messages; giving away personal items; changes in expected patterns of behaviors; specific statements about suicide or self-harm; preoccupation with death; frequent risk-taking or self-abusive behaviors; use of drugs or alcohol to cope; overwhelming sense of guilt or shame; obsessional self-doubt; open signs of mental illness; history of physical or sexual abuse; homosexuality; and significant change or life event that is internally disruptive
21. Have you ever thought of trying to hurt yourself? How might you do this? Have you ever thought of trying to kill yourself? How might you do this? Have you ever told

anyone about wanting to kill yourself? How do you feel right now? Do you have access to firearms? Knives? (For more, see Box 53-1, "Questions to Assess Suicide Potential.")
22. Communicate with the adolescent in an empathetic and nonjudgmental way to decrease her sense of isolation and rejection. Use clear, direct, and supportive tone of voice and demeanor. Be physically and emotionally present, and offer opportunities for her to discuss feelings and thoughts. Remove any potentially harmful objects.
23. T
24. F
25. F
26. T

EATING DISORDERS: ANOREXIA NERVOSA AND BULIMIA NERVOSA

27. deliberate refusal to maintain adequate body weight, distorted body image, and amenorrhea
28. recurrent episodes of binge eating; a sense of lack of control over eating binges; self-induced vomiting or excessive use of laxatives, diuretics, and/or emetics to prevent weight gain; excessive exercise to prevent weight gain; and a persistent overconcern with body image
29. T
30. T
31. F
32. F

ATTENTION-DEFICIT/HYPERACTIVITY DISORDER (ADHD)

33. attention and concentration, impulse control, and overactivity
34. on the basis of reports by the child, parent(s), and teacher(s)
35. teach the family about the disorder
36. F
37. T
38. F

SUBSTANCE ABUSE

39. Phase 1: Drug is taken to see what it does or to appease peers. Phase 2: Drug is used somewhat regularly for pleasurable effects or to reduce anxiety. Phase 3: Drug is used regularly, physical dependence begins, and social functioning has drug as focus. Phase 4: Physical condition deteriorates, and all activities are related to obtaining and using drug.
40. increase in antisocial behavior, poor school performance, irregular school attendance, aggressive or rebellious behavior, excessive influence by peers, deterioration of relationships with family or former friends, history of lack of parental support and supervision, rapid or extreme changes in mood, loss of interest in hobbies, and changes in eating or sleeping patterns as manipulative behaviors increase
41. T
42. T
43. F
44. T

INFANTS OF ADDICTED MOTHERS AND INFANTS WITH FETAL ALCOHOL SYNDROME (FAS)

45. W: wakefulness, I: irritability, T: tremulousness, temperature variation, tachypnea, H: hyperactivity, high-pitched persistent cry, hypersensitivity to sound, hyperreflexia,

hypertonus, D: diarrhea, diaphoresis, dehydration, disorganized suck, R: respiratory distress, rub marks, rhinorrhea, A: apnea, autonomic dysfunction, W: weight loss or failure to gain weight, A: alkalosis (respiratory), L: lacrimation

46. Organize care to limit the number of times the infant is disturbed, keep noise and light levels to a minimum, provide comfort measures immediately when the infant becomes irritable.
47. microcephaly, microphthalmia, poorly developed philtrum, thin upper lip, and flattening or absence of the maxilla

CHILDHOOD PHYSICAL AND EMOTIONAL ABUSE AND NEGLECT

48. Isolation from community and social groups; intense competition for emotional resources within family; low levels of differentiation among family members; distrust of outsiders and family members; unpredictable and unstable family environment. (For more, see Box 53-3, "Characteristics of Abusive Family.")
49. It is a form of physical abuse that is caused by vigorous shaking while the infant is being held by the extremities or shoulders, causing whiplash-induced intracranial or retinal bleeding.
50. It is a form of physical abuse in which the child's primary caretaker falsifies or produces illness in the child and then takes the child in for medical care, claiming no knowledge of how the child became ill.
51. Have a nonjudgmental and supportive attitude, answer questions directly and specifically, and act as an advocate for the child and the family.
52. T
53. F
54. F
55. T

FAILURE TO THRIVE (FTT)

56. a maladaptive parent-infant relationship, in which the parent displays impaired skills in reading or responding to the infant's cues
57. weight below the 5th percentile, a sudden or rapid deceleration on the growth curve, delay in reaching developmental milestones, and decreased muscle mass
58. avoidance of eye contact and physical touch, intense watchfulness, sleep disturbances, lack of age-appropriate stranger anxiety or preference for own parents, and disturbed affect
59. T
60. T

REVIEW QUESTIONS

1. d
2. a
3. c
4. a
5. b
6. d
7. c
8. b
9. c
10. d

CHAPTER 54: THE CHILD WITH A COGNITIVE IMPAIRMENT

MATCHING KEY TERMS

1. c
2. b
3. d
4. a
5. intellectual; functional
6. manifests before 18 years; includes significant subaverage general intellectual functioning; has concurrent deficits in two or more adaptive areas, such as communication, home living, community use, health and safety, leisure, self-care, social skills, self-direction, functional academics, and work.
7. severe and chronic disability that is attributable to mental or physical impairment, or a combination of both; impairment present before age 22 years; impairment likely to continue, resulting in the need for lifelong individual services or supports; substantial functional limitations in three or more areas
8. This law required states to provide an education for all disabled children aged 3–21 years that is free and appropriate and in the least restrictive environment.
9. Each child with a disability must have a written IEP that outlines specialized instruction and services the school system must provide. It is designed by the child's parents and school personnel after an educational assessment.

COGNITIVE IMPAIRMENT

10. This may be related to intense stress experienced by families of disabled children, parental isolation, or unrealistic expectations for the child's performance due to a lack of knowledge about normal growth and development.
11. delayed achievement of developmental milestones
12. Down syndrome, fragile X syndrome
13. F
14. T
15. T
16. F
17. T

DOWN SYNDROME

18. trisomy 21
19. at home until early adulthood, after which group home placement is an option
20. characteristic physical features
21. the child's typical coping patterns, daily routines, understanding of language, learning abilities, social and motor skills
22. T
23. F
24. F
25. T

FRAGILE X SYNDROME

26. T
27. F
28. F

AUTISM

29. pervasive developmental disorder (PDD)
30. language; social
31. disturbance in the rate and appearance of physical, social, and language skills; abnormal responses to body sensations; presence of thinking capacity, but with absent or delayed speech and language; abnormal ways of relating to people, objects, and events
32. lack of social interaction and awareness
33. F
34. F
35. F
36. F
37. D
38. A
39. D
40. A
41. X
42. D
43. X
44. X

REVIEW QUESTIONS

1. d
2. c
3. d
4. a
5. c
6. b
7. b

CHAPTER 55: THE CHILD WITH A SENSORY ALTERATION

DEFINITIONS

1. (across) nystagmus
2. (down) astigmatism
3. (down) hyphema
4. (across) central
5. (down) amblyopia
6. (down) mixed
7. (across) mild
8. (across) exotropia
9. (across) ophthalmia

REVIEW OF THE EYE AND THE EAR

10. f
11. g
12. a
13. c
14. d
15. h

16. b
17. e
18. i
19. 22–50 days' gestation
20. 4–6 weeks' gestation
21. 6 months
22. 5 years

DISORDERS OF THE EYE

23. d
24. b
25. h
26. f
27. i
28. e
29. a
30. c
31. g
32. squinting, head tilting, holding a book close to the eyes, decreased attention span, and poor school performance
33. correction to 20/200 or less in the better eye or a visual field of 20° or less
34. amblyopia—decreased vision in the deviated eye
35. It strengthens the weak eye while the good eye is patched.
36. excessive tearing, light sensitivity, muscle spasm causing involuntary closing of the eyelid, corneal enlargement, and haziness
37. surgery
38. pain, nausea and vomiting, and increased inflammation
39. Elevate the head of the bed slightly and avoid any position in which the affected eye is dependent, because this would cause edema and pressure on the eye.
40. itching, burning, light sensitivity, scratchy eyelids, redness, edema, and discharge
41. chemical irritation from eye prophylaxis
42. Practice good handwashing habits, do not share the child's linens or eye medication with other family members, and do not allow child to return to school or daycare until he has received eyes drops for 24 hours.
43. excessive tearing and crusting of eyelids on awakening; a small mass just below the inner aspect of the eye
44. reduces the risk of rebleeding between 3 and 5 days following injury
45. wearing protective eyewear, such as goggles and face masks
46. rebleeding, change in the size of the area, presence of bright red blood, signs of increased intraocular pressure (pain, nausea and vomiting, increased inflammation), and side effects from medications
47. Irrigate immediately with water or saline solution. For a mild burn use at least 2 L of fluid for 30 minutes; for a severe burn, use at least 10 L for 2–4 hours.
48. F
49. T
50. F
51. F
52. F
53. T
54. T
55. T
56. T

HEARING LOSS IN CHILDREN

57. b
58. d
59. a
60. c
61. excessive cerumen, foreign bodies, perforated tympanic membrane, or otitis media
62. infection, heredity, exposure to loud noises, ototoxic medications, and prematurity
63. auditory brain stem response; evoked otoacoustic emissions test
64. audiometry
65. Have child use hearing aid if he has one, look at the child when speaking, speak clearly and slightly slower, eliminate background noise, and use visual aids.
66. T
67. F
68. T
69. F
70. T

LANGUAGE DISORDERS

71. a
72. b
73. c
74. pitch and intonation, articulation, and fluency
75. Describe any activities to the child; expand on what the child says; add new information; build the child's vocabulary; and repeat the child's words using adult pronunciations.
76. T
77. F
78. T
79. T

REVIEW QUESTIONS

1. b
2. a
3. c
4. b
5. c
6. a
7. b
8. c
9. d
10. d
11. d